Evaluating Outbreak Potential of Infections in Tropical Climates

Fingani Annie Mphande ·
Peter Suwirakwenda Nyasulu
Editors

Evaluating Outbreak Potential of Infections in Tropical Climates

Preventing the Pandemics of the Future

Springer

Editors
Fingani Annie Mphande
Faculty of Medicine
King Mongkut's Institute of Technology
Ladkrabang
Bangkok, Thailand

Peter Suwirakwenda Nyasulu
Division of Epidemiology and Biostatistics
Faculty of Medicine and Health Sciences
Stellenbosch University
Cape Town, South Africa

ISBN 978-981-95-0617-0 ISBN 978-981-95-0618-7 (eBook)
https://doi.org/10.1007/978-981-95-0618-7

This Springer imprint is published by the registered company Springer Nature Singapore Pte Ltd.
The registered company address is: 152 Beach Road, #21-01/04 Gateway East, Singapore 189721, Singapore

Contents

Contributors

Nebiyu Dereje Abebe Africa Centres for Disease Control and Prevention, Addis Ababa, Ethiopia;
School of Public Health, Wachemo University, Hosainna, Ethiopia

Furaha Akimanimpaye School of Nursing, University of the Western Cape, Cape Town, South Africa

Natalya Andreeva Institute of Fundamental Medicine and Biology, OpenLab "Gene and Cell Technologies", Kazan Federal University, Kazan, Russia

Paul Armah Aryee Department of Nutritional Sciences, School of Allied Health Sciences, University for Development Studies, Tamale, Ghana

Manoj Baranwal Department of Biotechnology, Thapar Institute of Engineering and Technology, Patiala, India

Mulekya Francis Bwambale School of Public Health, Makerere University, Kampala, Uganda;
International Organisation for Migration (IOM), Juba, South Sudan;
Department of Research and Innovations, Faculty of Public Health, Nursing and Midwifery, Uganda Christian University - Kagando University College, Kasese, Uganda

Sara Chandy Childs Trust Medical Research Foundation, Kanchi Kamakoti Childs Trust Hospital, Chennai, India

Christine Chawhanda School of Public Health, Faculty of Health Sciences, University of the Witwatersrand, Johannesburg, South Africa;
Department of Community and Social Development, Faculty of Social and Behavioural Sciences, University of Zimbabwe, Harare, Zimbabwe

Yuriy Davidyuk Institute of Fundamental Medicine and Biology, OpenLab "Gene and Cell Technologies", Kazan Federal University, Kazan, Russia

Julius T. Dongdem Department of Biochemistry and Molecular Medicine, School of Medicine, University for Development Studies, Tamale, Ghana

Calvin Bisong Ebai Division of Epidemiology and Biostatistics, Department of Global Health, University of Stellenbosch, Cape Town, South Africa; Department of Medical Laboratory Science, University of Bamenda, Bamenda, Cameroon

Mosoka Fallah Africa Centres for Disease Control and Prevention, Addis Ababa, Ethiopia

Gideon Kofi Gelegbe Department of Biochemistry and Molecular Medicine, School of Medicine, University for Development Studies, Tamale, Ghana

Emmanuel Kabwe Institute of Fundamental Medicine and Biology, OpenLab "Gene and Cell Technologies", Kazan Federal University, Kazan, Russia

Svetlana Khaiboullina Institute of Fundamental Medicine and Biology, OpenLab "Gene and Cell Technologies", Kazan Federal University, Kazan, Russia

Ekaterina Martynova Institute of Fundamental Medicine and Biology, OpenLab "Gene and Cell Technologies", Kazan Federal University, Kazan, Russia

Regis Rugira Marie Modeste Department of Nursing and Midwifery, Stellenbosch University, Cape Town, South Africa

Fingani Annie Mphande Faculty of Medicine, King Mongkut's Institute of Technology Ladkrabang, Bangkok, Thailand

Peter Suwirakwenda Nyasulu Division of Epidemiology and Biostatistics, Faculty of Medicine and Health Sciences, Stellenbosch University, Cape Town, South Africa

Olesia Ohlopkova Virology Research Institute of the Federal Research Center for Fundamental and Translational Medicine, Novosibirsk, Russia

Albert Rizvanov Institute of Fundamental Medicine and Biology, OpenLab "Gene and Cell Technologies", Kazan Federal University, Kazan, Russia; Division of Medical and Biological Sciences, Tatarstan Academy of Sciences, Kazan, Russia

Doris Yasinti Sakala Division of Epidemiology and Biostatistics, Department of Global Health, University of Stellenbosch, Cape Town, South Africa

Ilnur Salafutdinov Institute of Fundamental Medicine and Biology, OpenLab "Gene and Cell Technologies", Kazan Federal University, Kazan, Russia; Department of Medical Biology and Genetics, Kazan State Medical University, Kazan, Russia

Kristina Stolbunova Virology Research Institute of the Federal Research Center for Fundamental and Translational Medicine, Novosibirsk, Russia

Jacques Lukenze Tamuzi Division of Epidemiology and Biostatistics, Faculty of Health Sciences, School of Public Health, University of the Witwatersrand, Johannesburg, South Africa

Abbreviations

ACTs	Artemisinin based Combination Therapies
AKI	Acute Kidney Infection
ART	Antiretroviral Therapy
AWD	Acute Watery Diarrhoea
BVD	Bundibugyo Virus Disease
CAC	COVID-19 Associated Candidiasis
CAM	COVID-19 Associated Mucormycosis
CAPA	COVID-19 Associated Pulmonary Aspergillosis
CARICOM	Caribbean Community
CARPHA	Caribbean Public Health Agency
CATI	Case Area Targeted Interventions
CDC	Centre for Disease Control
CFR	Case Fatality Rate
CORT	Community Outbreak Response Teams
COVID-19	Corona Virus Disease -2019 (SARS-CoV-2)
COVID-19	Coronavirus Disease 2019
DALYs	Disability Adjusted Life Years
DOBV	*Orthohantavirus dobravaense*
DRC	Democratic Republic of Congo
EOC	Emergency Operations Centre
ESKD	End Stage Kidney Disease
ETU	Ebolavirus Disease Treatment Unit
EVD	Ebola Virus Disease
GHS	Ghana Health Service
GM-CSF	Granulocyte-Macrophage Colony-Stimulating Factor
GMIS	Ghana Malaria Indicator Survey
GPC	Gn and Gc, Glycoprotein Precursor
GPI	Glycosylphosphatidylinositol
HCPS	Hantavirus Cardiopulmonary Syndrome
HFRS	Hemorrhagic Fever with Renal Syndrome
HIV	Human Immunodeficiency Virus

HNTV	*Orthohantavirus hantaanense*
ICTV	International Committee on Taxonomy of Viruses
ICU	Intensive Care Unit
IDSR	Integrated Disease Surveillance Response
IPC	Infection Prevention and Control
ITN	Insecticide Treated Nets
KHAV	Orthohantavirus khaba-rovskense
L	Large
LGA	Local Government Area
LLINs	Long-Lasting Insecticidal Nets
LMIC	Low and Middle Income Countries
M	Medium
MPXV	Monkeypox Virus
MVA-BN	Modified Vaccinia Ankara-Bavarian Nordic
N	Protein, Nucleocapsid Protein
NCD	Non-Communicable Diseases
NFP	National Focal Point
NTCP	National Tuberculosis Control
NTD	Neglected Tropical Diseases
OCV	Oral Cholera Vaccine
PAHO	American Health Organization
PEP	Post Exposure Prophylaxis
PHEIC	Public Health Emergency of International Concern
PICT	Pacific Island Countries and Territories
PJP	*Pneumocystis jirovecci* pneumonia
PMTCT	Prevention of Mother-Child Transmission
PoC	Point of Contact
PoE	Point of Entrance
PoE	Point of Entry
PUUV	*Orthohantavirus puumalaense*
RAT	Rapid Assessment Tool
RCCE	Risk Communication and Community Engagement
RdRp	Viral RNA-dependent RNA polymerase
RDT	Rapid Detection Kit
RDTs	Rapid Diagnostic Tests
RRT	Rapid Response Team
S	Small
SARS-CoV-2	Severe Acute Respiratory Syndrome Coronavirus 2
SEOV	*Orthohantavirus seoulense*
SIDS	Small Island Developing States
SMC	Seasonal Malaria Chemoprevention
SVD	Sudan Ebolavirus Disease
TB	Tuberculosis
THAIV	Orthohantavirus Thailandense
TULV	Orthohantavirus Tulaense

VLP	Virus-Like Particle
WASH	Water Sanitation and Hygiene
WHO AFRO	World Health Organization African regional Office
WHO	World Health Organization

Part I
Zoonotic Diseases

Chapter 1
Rabies, a Neglected Tropical Disease

Peter Suwirakwenda Nyasulu, Jacques Lukenze Tamuzi, Gideon Kofi Helegbe, and Fingani Annie Mphande

Abstract Rabies is a zoonotic disease caused by a *Lyssavirus*, Family *Rhabdovirus.* The infection clinically manifests as fulminating encephalomyelitis. The disease remains a public health threat worldwide, with about 15.69 million people potentially exposed to the virus annually, requiring post-exposure prophylaxis (PEP), and an estimated 59,000 human deaths. Nearly all human rabies cases are reported from the developing countries of Africa and Asia. Data showing the burden of rabies in Tanzania remains scanty owing to the lack of a systematic reporting mechanism. Rabies disease kills an estimated 500 people annually in Malawi, with more deaths occurring in children. There is potential for underestimating rabies, as most cases remain undiagnosed, hence untreated, and unreported. This paradigm is driven by an absence of a national rabies control programme, inadequate laboratory infrastructure as well a lack of a surveillance system. Furthermore, the burden of human rabies due to dog bites is on the rise because of poor intersectoral collaboration between human and animal health. Diagnosis of rabies remains poor due to the non-existence of such services in many African countries, where access to such services in rural and remote areas in catchment areas for pastoralist communities is key. Associated with the lack of diagnostic services, surveillance activities are also poor, consequently

P. S. Nyasulu (✉) · J. L. Tamuzi
Division of Epidemiology and Biostatistics, Faculty of Medicine and Health Sciences, Stellenbosch University, Cape Town, South Africa
e-mail: pnyasulu@sun.ac.za

J. L. Tamuzi
e-mail: drjacques.tamuzi@gmail.com

P. S. Nyasulu
Division of Epidemiology and Biostatistics, School of Public Health, Faculty of Health Sciences, University of the Witwatersrand, Johannesburg, South Africa

G. K. Helegbe
Department of Biochemistry and Molecular Medicine, School of Medicine, University for Development Studies, Tamale, Ghana
e-mail: ghelegbe@uds.edu.gh

F. A. Mphande
Faculty of Medicine, King Mongkut's Institute of Technology, Ladkrabang, Bangkok, Thailand
e-mail: yadoster@gmail.com

F. Mphande and P. Nyasulu (eds.), *Evaluating Outbreak Potential of Infections in Tropical Climates*, https://doi.org/10.1007/978-981-95-0618-7_1

leading to a misappreciation of the impact of rabies on affected communities. The African continent still faces numerous challenges in achieving zero dog-mediated rabies deaths by 2030. The data produced by well-established surveillance systems support health policymakers to establish the burden of rabies morbidity, mortality, and other associated complications and lobby for sustained surveillance and control and prevention programs. For example, such data is crucial to guide strategies for effective interventions including among others access and availability of anti-rabies vaccines. In Malawi, some community sensitization and mobilization have been initiated to report animal bites mostly from dogs, and any sudden occurrence of deaths of domestic dogs or humans who might have experienced a dog bite. While some data exist for countries like Tanzania, Uganda, and Ghana, it is important to note that this information is made available only through routine surveillance, and most of these cases reported are not laboratory confirmed due to a lack of diagnostic facilities. Often, diagnosis is done mainly using a syndromic approach because of the lack of readily available diagnostic capability in the country. For this reason, developing accurate point-of-care diagnostics tests (POCTs) for rabies based on temporo-spatial data is user-friendly and would make a significant difference in early detection, reporting, and making clinical decisions among individuals presumed to have been exposed to rabies virus at the community level. Furthermore, an integrated rabies surveillance, One Health surveillance, and response system are thus essential.

Keywords Rabies · Burden of rabies in Africa · Research Gaps · Diagnostic Challenges · Surveillance · Rabies Control · Prevention of Rabies · Elimination of rabies · One Health

Abbreviations

NTD Neglected tropical diseases
PEP Post exposure prophylaxis
WHO World Health Organization

1.1 Introduction: Rabies and Endemicity

Rabies is a vaccine-preventable, zoonotic, viral disease affecting the central nervous system. In up to 99% of human rabies cases, dogs are responsible for virus transmission (World Health Organization, 2024b). The natural history of rabies disease in Africa is not well known, but it is well accepted that the disease must have been present in northern Africa for hundreds of years, particularly as an urban dog disease, and was also associated with cycles in the Middle East (Nel, 2013). European colonization influenced the spread of dog rabies in Western and Central Africa (Talbi et al.,

2009). In many African countries, rabies has become epizootic only in the nineteenth and twentieth centuries involving domestic dogs and free-ranging wildlife species (Nel, 2013; Nel & Rupprecht, 2007; Nyasulu et al., 2021; Talbi et al., 2009).

Over the past few years, many countries have acted to strengthen rabies control efforts—scaling up dog vaccination programmes, making human biologicals for post-exposure and pre-exposure prophylaxis more accessible, and engaging communities on rabies (Minghui et al., 2018). Dog-mediated rabies has been eliminated from Western Europe, Canada, the USA, and Japan (Minghui et al., 2018). Twenty-eight (28) of the 35 Latin American countries report no human deaths from dog-transmitted rabies (M. A. Vigilato et al., 2013). Great strides have been made in reducing rabies deaths in countries such as Bangladesh, the Philippines, Sri Lanka, Tanzania, Vietnam, and South Africa, to mention a few (Minghui et al., 2018). These experiences have generated important collective knowledge on what works, and have strengthened both the quality of rabies-related data and the arsenal of tools for the development of rabies-related control programmes, capacity building, education, and surveillance (Minghui et al., 2018). Rabies is a neglected tropical disease (NTD), predominantly affecting marginalized populations. Although effective human vaccines and immunoglobulins exist for rabies, these are often inaccessible or unaffordable to those in need (World Health Organization, 2024b).

To achieve the 2030 dog-mediated rabies elimination goal, it is important to place the global rabies response on a sustainable footing over the next 5 years (Minghui et al., 2018). This requires a phased, multi-pronged strategy in all affected countries, based on close coordination between the human and veterinary sectors and the extended community of practice (Minghui et al., 2018). It requires engaging communities and health workers to build awareness of the problem and prevent bite exposures; to prevent transmission by managing dog populations and ensure herd immunity through dog vaccination; and to provide post-exposure prophylaxis and care for exposed victims (Minghui et al., 2018).

1.2 Burden of Rabies, and Gaps

Rabies have devastating human, social, and economic burden especially on the poor, vulnerable, and marginalized populations. The disease has huge consequences on achieving the Sustainable Development Goals (SDGs) 1, 3, 10 and 17. It has been estimated that 50,000–60,000 human deaths occur every year globally, with 95% deaths in Asia and Africa, and 40% of children under 15 years of age affected (Akinsulie et al., 2024; World Health Organization, 2024b). In Africa, about 25,000 humans' deaths are associated with rabies every year, and approximately 40% of these rabies deaths occur in children under 15 years of age (CDC-Africa, 2023). In this review, we identified 66.67% African countries reporting poor rabies diagnostic capacity, 50% reported the lack of coordinated surveillance, 50% showed the lack of PEP course completion, 22.22% had insufficient rabies control and 77.78% had low dog vaccination coverage. Insufficient knowledge and practice on rabies prevention was also identified as a gap (Nyasulu et al., 2021). Comparing Africa and other continents in reporting deaths from rabies from 2010 to 2022 (WHO, 2025; World Health Organization, 2024a), our analysis showed rabies deaths were less reported during this period as well as no data on reporting rabies mortality was commonly found in Africa compared to other continents. Kenya, Tanzania, Uganda, Angola, Ghana, Zimbabwe, Lesotho, Algeria, Morocco, and Egypt had the highest number of human rabies deaths among the 76.6% of countries that reported it between 2010 and 2022 (WHO, 2025). This study should be viewed as limited because some countries did not report for all eleven years (Fig. 1.1). This report should be interpreted with caution because several countries did not report for the entire eleven-year period. Weak surveillance systems mean these numbers are probably underestimates, masking the true scale of the problem and perpetuating health inequities across the African continent (Amani et al., 2024). Besides, the majority of deaths in Africa occurred in rural areas and in populations living in healthcare underserved regions with mortality in young children being particularly high (Fooks et al., 2014; Hampson et al., 2015; Haselbeck et al., 2021; World Health Organization, 2018b).

There are numerous gaps in tropical countries' efforts to effectively manage rabies (Table 1.1). Nyasulu et al. summarized mapped human rabies research gaps and strengths in Africa (Nyasulu et al., 2021). The most important gaps included weak legislative protections for rabies control and poor animal protection regulations, management of Rabies in Africa, and a scarcity of data about dog populations or vaccination coverage. Furthermore, challenges of rabies control include a limited budget, limited human resources, a lack of public awareness and political support, limited surveillance data, weak coordination, difficulty controlling animal

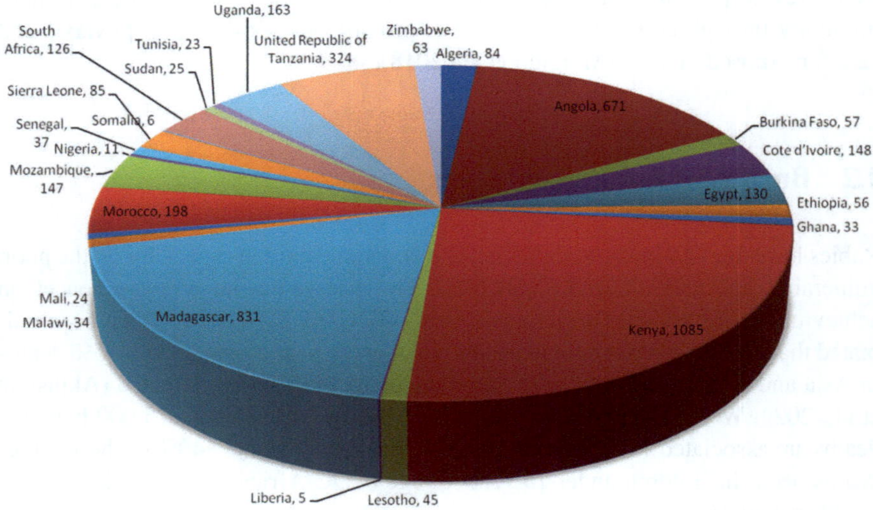

Fig. 1.1 Report of human rabies deaths in Africa from 2010–2022 (*Source* WHO, 2025 https://www.who.int/data/gho/data/indicators/indicator-details/GHO/reported-number-of-human-rabies-deaths)

movement, and low participation from local administration officials and dog owners (Yang et al., 2018). In this review, we identified 66.67% African countries reporting poor rabies diagnostic capacity, 50% reported the lack of coordinated surveillance, 50% showed the lack of rabies post-exposure prophylaxis (PEP) course completion, 22.22% had insufficient rabies control and 77.78% had low dog vaccination coverage. Insufficient knowledge and practice on rabies prevention was also identified as a gap (Nyasulu et al., 2021). Inadequate education for veterinarians and physicians, insufficient resources for proper confirmatory diagnosis and risk assessment, and the lack of effective communication channels between Ministries of Health and Agriculture frequently have led to failures of prophylactic intervention, even in regions where vaccines and immunoglobulins were available (Franka et al., 2013). A recent study conducted in Africa and Asia revealed that Rabies Immune Globulins (RIGs) were found to be less available than the vaccine, with access restricted in almost two-thirds of the countries surveyed (Sreenivasan et al., 2019). This review showed that eleven African countries had comprehensive access to RIG (Sreenivasan et al., 2019). Of the seven countries with broad access to vaccines, six of them had a national rabies prevention programme or policy (Sreenivasan et al., 2019). Two of the countries had only a monitoring programme/strategy in place (Sreenivasan et al., 2019). This is worrisome as it exposes a huge absence of surveillance and prevention policies in most African countries. The absence of a robust monitoring process is mostly attributed to the lack of rabies in national communicable disease plans and reporting systems at national level in Africa (Abela-Ridder et al., 2016). Therefore, widespread under-reporting is likely to occur in many affected countries due to lack of health information, civil registration and vital statistical systems, and inaccessibility of clinical care and diagnostic confirmation as symptoms of the disease may be non-specific and similar to other encephalitic infections (Abela-Ridder et al., 2016; Nyasulu et al., 2021). Even where data exist in Africa, the lack of communication and exchange of data between the animal and human health sectors also hinders the collection, storage, and reporting of coherent data to international databases (Abela-Ridder et al., 2016; Nyasulu et al., 2021). Given Africa's rabies epidemiology and gaps, the calls for urgent and effective efforts to prevent and control rabies with the goal of zero dog-mediated rabies deaths by 2030 cannot be overemphasized.

1.3 Diagnostic Tests for Rabies

Antemorterm and post-mortem diagnostic tests for rabies exist and are currently replaced by advanced methods that utilize rabies viral antigens, antibody detection assays and detection of viral nucleic acids as well as specific biomarkers (Mani & Madhusudana, 2013). Clinically, human rabies consists of two forms, the encephalitic (furious) form which makes up 80% of human rabies cases and the atypical/paralytic (dumb) form which constitutes 20% of the cases. The encephalitic form presents with symptoms distinctive of rabies while the atypical form presents with symptoms that can be confused with other diseases including Guillain Barre Syndrome, viral

Table 1.1 Mapping research gaps and strengths in Africa (*Source* Nyasulu et al., 2021 https://doi.org/10.1136/bmjopen-2020-048551)

African countries	Mapping research gaps and strengths in Africa					
	Diagnostic capacity	Coordinated surveillance	Lack of PEP course completion /PEP unavailable	Inefficient control	Insufficient knowledge and practice on rabies prevention	Low dog vaccination coverage (<70%
Algeria	N/A	N/A	N/A	√	N/A	X
Cameroon	√	√	X	√	N/A	X
Chad	X	X	X	X]	N/A	X
Democratic Republic of Congo	X	X	X	X	N/A	X
Ethiopia	X	N/A	X	X	X	X
Ghana	XA	X	X	X	N/A	X
Ivory Coast	√	√	X	X	N/A	X
Kenya	X	X	X	X	N/A	N/A
Madagascar	√	X	X	X	N/A	X
Malawi	X	√	√	√	N/A	N/A
Mozambique	X	X	X	X	N/A	X
Namibia	X	X	N/A	X	N/A	N/A
Nigeria	X	N/A	X	X	N/A	X
Senegal	X	√	X	X	√	X

(continued)

Table 1.1 (continued)

African countries	Mapping research gaps and strengths in Africa					
	Diagnostic capacity	Coordinated surveillance	Lack of PEP course completion /PEP unavailable	Inefficient control	Insufficient knowledge and practice on rabies prevention	Low dog vaccination coverage (<70%
Tanzania	X	√	X	X	X	N/A
Uganda	X	X [	X	X	N/A	X
South Africa	√	√	X	√	N/A	N/A
Zimbabwe	√	√	N/A	X	N/A	X

X: research gaps identified in different studies; √: research strengths identified in different studies; N/A: Not applicable encephalitis, cerebral malaria, tetanus, herpes simplex (Mani & Willoughby, 2017; Willoughby, 2015) Diagnosis of atypical rabies remains a challenge globally and more so in limited resource settings (Sheikh et al., 2005). Current laboratory diagnostic tests include detection of viral antigen (fluorescent antibody technique (FAT); direct rapid immunohistochemical test (dRIT); rapid immunochromatographic diagnostic test (RIDT); detection of viral antibodies (rapid fluorescent focus inhibition test (RFFIT); fluorescent antibody virus neutralization test; (FAVN), enzyme-linked immunosorbent assay (ELISA); nucleic acid detection techniques (reverse transcriptase–polymerase chain reaction (RTPCR); viral isolation techniques (rabies tissue culture infection test (RTCIT), mouse inoculation test (MIT); and histopathological techniques (H and E: Haematoxylin and Eosin) (Ashwini et al., 2024).

Furthermore, lack of monitoring data on rabies or low data quality is problematic, resulting in rabies being poorly addressed in most African countries (Amani et al., 2024). Laboratory-based surveillance is critical to rabies prevention, control, and management activities. Then, diagnostic tests for rabies should be addressed clearly and explored in African countries. Then, diagnostic testing for rabies should be properly addressed and researched in African countries. To improve rabies reporting and periodic assessment, appropriate diagnostic tests for rabies should be selected based on the country's environment in terms of rabies gaps and epidemiology. Table 1.2 summarized test methods available for the diagnosis of rabies and their purpose.

1.4 Rabies Diagnosis in Animals

A diagnosis of rabies can be made after detection of rabies virus from any part of the affected brain, but to rule out rabies, the test must include a full cross-section of tissue from both the brain stem and cerebellum (CDC, 2024). Rabies testing requires that the animal be euthanized. There are no approved methods for ante-mortem rabies testing of animals (CDC, 2024).

1.5 Rabies Diagnosis in Humans

Several tests are necessary to diagnose rabies antemortem (before death) in humans; no single test is sufficient. Tests are performed on samples of saliva, serum, spinal fluid, and skin biopsies of hair follicles at the nape of the neck (CDC, 2024). Post-mortem (after death) testing requires the collection of brainstem and cerebellum tissues (CDC, 2024). Due to the risk of rabies exposure to healthcare workers and close community contacts, deceased patients suspected of rabies should always undergo an autopsy and post-mortem rabies testing (CDC, 2024).

Table 1.2 Test methods available for the diagnosis of rabies and their purpose

Method	Purpose					
	Population freedom from infection	Individual animal freedom from infection prior to movement	Contribute to eradication policies	Confirmation of clinical cases	Prevalence of infection and surveillance	Immune status in individual animals or populations post-vaccination
Detection and identification of the agent						
DFA (antigen detection)	+++	–	+++	+++	+++	–
dRIT (antigen detection)	+++	–	+++	+++	+++	–
RTCIT (virus isolation)	–	–	+++	+++	+++	–
MIT (virus isolation)	–	–	+	+	+	–
Conventional RT-PCR (RNA detection)	+++	–	+++	+++	+++	–
Real-time RT-PCR (RNA detection)	+++	–	+++	+++	+++	–
Detection of immune response						
VN	–	+++	+++	–	–	+++
ELISA	–	–	+++	–	–	+++
Histologic Examination						
Biopsy or autopsy tissues	–	–	–	++	–	–
Diagnostic test kits						
Antigen detection	+++	–	+++	+++	+++	–
Antibody detection	+	–	+	+	+	–

Abbreviations: Key: +++ = recommended for this purpose; ++ recommended but has limitations; + = suitable in very limited circumstances; – = not appropriate for this purpose. DFA = direct fluorescent antibody test; dRIT = direct rapid immunohistochemistry test; RTCIT = rabies tissue culture infection test; RT-PCR = reverse-transcription polymerase chain reaction; MIT = mouse inoculation test; VN = virus neutralization; ELISA = enzyme-linked immunosorbent assay

1.6 Diagnostic Testing Methods

Detection of rabies virus antigen or RNA by any of the below methods can confirm a rabies infection, but gold standard tests should be used to rule out infection. Ruling out infection also requires that appropriate tissues are tested, which include a full cross-section of the brainstem and cerebellum for post-mortem human and animal testing (CDC, 2024). Ante-mortem human rabies testing that is negative is a strong indication that the patient does not have rabies, however, post-mortem confirmatory testing should be pursued if an alternative diagnosis is not identified (CDC, 2024). Current diagnostic tools are not suitable for detecting rabies infection before the onset of clinical disease, and unless the rabies-specific signs of hydrophobia or aerophobia are present, clinical diagnosis may be difficult. Human rabies can be confirmed intra-vitam and postmortem by various diagnostic techniques that detect whole viruses, viral antigens, or nucleic acids in infected tissues (brain, skin, urine, or saliva) (WHO/Africa, 2024). Lack of surveillance, related to limited diagnostic capabilities, contributes to the underestimation of the burden of this disease. Among the rabies diagnostic assays that are potentially advantageous for low-resource settings, the dRIT has, to date, shown promise in preliminary applications (Coetzer et al., 2014). Given the consequences of a false-negative rabies diagnosis, regular interlaboratory comparisons are essential, and a secondary or confirmatory method, such as immunohistochemistry (IHC), should be performed on all submitted specimens, especially negative cases with a history of human contact. Furthermore, quick rabies tests, such as the Antigen quick Rabies Ag Test Kit, which employs an immunochromatographic technique to identify rabies virus antigen, should be investigated in Africa.

1.6.1 Direct Fluorescent Antibody (DFA) Test

The DFA test is based on the fact that animals infected with the rabies virus contain rabies virus proteins (antigens) in their tissues. Because rabies is found in neural tissue (rather than blood, as many other viruses are), brain tissue is the best place to test for rabies Antigen. Other innervated tissues may include antigens; however, testing using these tissues were less accurate at diagnosing rabies when compared to brain tissues (CDC, 2024). The most crucial component of a DFA test is the fluorescently labelled anti-rabies antibody. When labelled antibody is treated with rabies-suspect brain tissue, it binds to the rabies antigen. The DFA test is one of the "gold standard" diagnostic tests for identifying rabies due to its excellent sensitivity and specificity. It has been carefully validated by international, national, and state health laboratories (CDC, 2024). The DFA test is an important diagnostic technique in rabies surveillance and control, particularly for post-mortem detection of rabies in animals. While the

DFA is the most often used test for routine rabies diagnosis (Patrick et al., 2019), the expense of obtaining and maintaining a fluorescence microscope might be prohibitive in African nations.

1.6.2 Direct Rapid Immunohistochemistry Test (DRIT)

The DRIT for rabies, like the DFA test, detects the presence of rabies virus antigen in animal tissues. DRIT, like DFA, is based on the discovery that rabies virus proteins are prevalent in affected tissues, particularly the neurological system. Brain tissue is the chosen tissue for DRIT testing due to its high rabies antigen content. DRIT, like DFA, has great sensitivity and specificity, making it a reliable diagnostic test for rabies. It has been rigorously tested by international, national, and state health laboratories, confirming its status as a "gold standard" approach for rabies diagnosis (CDC, 2024). The DRIT is a flexible tool for field-based surveillance to detect the presence of the rabies virus that may be utilized in decentralized laboratory locations (Patrick et al., 2019), making it helpful in African countries. The DRIT has several advantages over the DFA, including lower costs, the ability to perform the test outside of a centralized laboratory, the need for only light microscopy rather than a fluorescent microscope, and the relatively straightforward training process for people administering and reading the test (Dürr et al., 2008; Patrick et al., 2019). A study reported that DRIT shows excellent performance qualities both in regard to user friendliness and reliability compared to standard fluorescent antibody test (FAT) and real-time reverse transcriptase polymerase chain reaction (RT-PCR) in developing countries (Léchenne et al., 2016).

1.6.3 Real-Time Reverse Transcriptase Polymerase Chain Reaction (RT-PCR)

The LN34 PCR test for rabies is a modern diagnostic test that uses RT-PCR to identify the presence of rabies virus genetic material (CDC, 2024). The brain is the best tissue for rabies testing by any test, and the LN34 test requires a full cross-section of the brainstem and representative samples from the cerebellum to rule out rabies (CDC, 2024). The World Health Organization (WHO) and the World Organization for Animal Health (WOAH) regard the LN34 test as a "gold standard" test, and it is increasingly recognized and implemented globally for rabies diagnosis and surveillance (CDC, 2024). RT-PCR is an important method for rabies detection and control. It detects rabies virus genetic material quickly and sensitively, allowing for earlier diagnosis and control measures. A study conducted in Namibia found that RT-PCR led to much higher reliability and flexibility in laboratory-based rabies diagnosis in Namibia and sustainably strengthened the diagnostic pillar of the Namibian dog rabies elimination strategy (Freuling et al., 2023). RT-PCR is an excellent and adaptable method for rabies diagnosis, providing a good balance of speed, sensitivity, and cost-effectiveness (Marston et al., 2019).

1.6.4 Immunohistochemistry (IHC)

Immunohistochemistry (IHC) methods are sensitive and specific for detecting the rabies virus antigen in formalin-fixed tissues. Rabies virus antigen is identified with anti-rabies monoclonal or polyclonal antibodies (CDC, 2024). IHC testing is more sensitive and specific than histologic staining procedures such as hematoxylin and eosin and Seller's stains (CDC, 2024). IHC plays an important role in rabies diagnosis, control, and surveillance in low and middle-income countries. It is a sensitive and specific approach for detecting the rabies virus antigen in tissues, particularly brain tissue, and can be employed in both field and laboratory settings (Lembo et al., 2006; Patrick et al., 2019). IHC, notably the dRIT, provides a cost-effective and timely alternative to traditional diagnostic procedures such as DFA testing, which can be difficult to implement in resource-constrained environments (Dürr et al., 2008).

1.6.5 Histologic Examination

Histologic examination of biopsy or autopsy tissues is occasionally useful in diagnosing unsuspected cases of rabies that have not been tested by routine methods (CDC, 2024). This method is nonspecific and not considered diagnostic for rabies (CDC, 2024). Prior to the availability of contemporary diagnostic technologies, this procedure was used in conjunction with the clinical case history to diagnose rabies.

1.6.6 Detection of the Replication of Rabies Virus After Inoculation

These tests determine the infectiousness of a tissue suspension in cell cultures or laboratory animals. They should be employed if the FAT provides an ambiguous result or if the FAT is negative in the case of confirmed human exposure (Mani & Madhusudana, 2013). The inoculation in cell culture tests and mouse inoculation can be used to investigate the detection of rabies virus replication. This in-vivo test should be avoided wherever possible due to concerns about animal suffering. It is also more expensive, especially if specific pathogen-free (SPF) mice are used, and the findings are not as fast (compared to in-vitro inoculation testing), but when the test is positive, a considerable amount of virus can be isolated from a single mouse brain for strain identification. Another benefit of this low-tech test is that it can be readily and practically employed in settings where skills and facilities for other tests (for example, cell culture) are not available (Mani & Madhusudana, 2013).

1.6.7 Rabies Serology and Point-of-Care Rabies Tests (POCTs)

Serological tests are ineffective for diagnosing rabies infections in humans and animals because virus-specific antibodies in serum develop late, if at all, following the onset of clinical symptoms. Rabies virus neutralizing antibody tests, such as the quick fluorescent focus inhibition test, are typically used to monitor antibody levels in those who may have an occupational risk of rabies virus exposure (e.g. veterinarians, rabies virus laboratory workers, etc.) (CDC, 2024). In rare situations, such serological testing is utilized to assess the immune response of a person taking rabies post-exposure prophylaxis when there are significant deviations from the vaccination schedule or there are concerns about a patient's immunity. The CDC's National Rabies Reference Laboratory provides serological testing for humans and animals on a case-by-case basis. Approval is required before submitting the serum (CDC, 2024). Recently, point-of-care diagnostic tests have been more widely available to the public. Promising research conducted in Africa, Asia, and the United States discovered that certain point-of-care rabies tests (POCTs) can display high sensitivity and specificity (CDC, 2024). However, no POCT has been systematically validated, and none are approved for use by the United States Department of Agriculture (USDA), CDC's National Rabies Reference Laboratory, WHO, or WOAH (CDC, 2024). However, POCTs will provide rapid, on-site rabies diagnosis, potentially increasing treatment outcomes, particularly in African countries. POCTs may be beneficial in African countries for animal illness surveillance and diagnosis, which is sometimes difficult in remote locations, with turnaround times ranging from days to weeks (Hobbs et al., 2021). However, accurate and rapid field diagnosis of infectious and zoonotic animal diseases in Africa has many benefits in controlling rabies in Africa (Hobbs et al., 2021). Rabies POCTs may be beneficial for animal rabies diagnosis and surveillance. Unfortunately, accurate, independent test validation data for commercial rabies POCTs are often incomplete or absent.

1.7 Integrated Surveillance and One Health

The new rabies-focused partnership known as United Against Rabies gives a platform to mobilize resources and leverage existing tools and expertise in a coordinated way. It is fully aligned with the priorities of the Tripartite Memorandum of Understanding signed in May 2018, between WHO, the FAO and the WOAH (Minghui et al., 2018; World Health Organization, 2018a). Through that agreement, the three organizations are intensifying their collaboration to combat critical health risks at the human-animal-environment interface—i.e. challenges that require a genuine One Health approach (Minghui et al., 2018). FAO supports member countries in their efforts to prevent and control rabies, including disease surveillance and outbreak responses, laboratory capacity building, public awareness promotion, dog vaccinations, cross-sectoral collaboration, and rabies national control plan development and implementation through a One Health (https://www.fao.org/one-health/overview/one-health-overview/en) approach (FAO, 2024). The WHO advocates for nations to enhance the capabilities of their One Health workforce by leveraging rabies elimination initiatives as a foundation for multi-sectoral collaboration; and promotes the utilization of the United Against Rabies (UAR) multi-stakeholder forum, established in partnership with WHO, the FAO, and the WOAH, to champion action and investment in rabies management (World Health Organization, 2024b). The 'One Health' approach urges implementation of a national rabies control programme that includes mass dog vaccination, laboratory-based surveillance, stable budget allocation, a rapid reporting system, management of dog populations, international cooperation, prevention of animal introductions from other countries, and risk assessment to analyze the programme's weaknesses. As several developed countries have shown, an effective rabies control strategy leads to rabies-free status (Yang et al., 2018). A widespread educational activity on rabies prevention and control in schools, community committees, instructional pamphlets, and network media is a requirement for the achievement of the goal (Shafaati et al., 2023). To achieve the goal of "Zero by 30", the global strategy to tackle the rabies should also emphasize on the intersectoral collaboration including the medical doctors, veterinarians, ecologists, environmentalists, and law-enforcement agents (Kardjadj & Ben-Mahdi, 2019; Shafaati et al., 2023). Furthermore, emphasis should also be made on the cross-border spread of rabies between African bordering nations, which has an impact on disease control and elimination efforts throughout the area. Canine rabies can be eliminated, and this should be the ultimate goal of rabies control efforts. To do this, regional and continental plans based on and encouraging strong national programmes are required. Rabies will continue to spread into rabies-free or disease-free areas unless neighbouring countries cooperate.

According to the theory of change announced by WHO, three global strategic objectives for the elimination of rabies have been prioritized: (1) Effective use of vaccines, drugs, tools, and technologies to reduce human rabies risk through dog vaccination and increased public awareness; (2) The development, innovation, and coordination of policies and guidelines coordinated with international and national strategies, encouraging technology and health innovations, and strengthening health and treatment systems; (3) The impact of international partnerships against rabies at national, regional, and global levels. A strong rabies programme also needs to have access to qualified people in the fields of education, human health, and animal health (Minghui et al., 2018; Shafaati et al., 2023). The three three-phase strategies used by One Health to implement its global Zero by 30 goals include phase 1: Startup (countries where rabies is a priority, countries that are currently engaged in rabies control or countries with projects that might learn to implement projects more effectively in the future), phase 2: Scale up (maintaining support for Phase 1 participating countries while involving more countries), and phase 3: Mop up (engaging the remaining countries and completing the prospective program) (Shafaati et al., 2023). One of the most significant examples is the One Health India action plan, which is a model of leadership in India and can serve as an example for other rabies-endemic African countries by 2030 (Shafaati et al., 2023). As India bears almost one-third of the worldwide rabies burden, it can play an important role in accomplishing this global goal. India has made it a priority to end this preventable disease (Shafaati et al., 2023). Mass vaccination of dogs as a key component of national rabies elimination programmes has been successful in eliminating dog-transmitted rabies in Europe, North, and Latin America, and Japan (Athingo et al., 2020; Müller et al., 2012; Nyasulu et al., 2021; Velasco-Villa et al., 2017). By far, the most significant public health threat comes from rabies virus variant, and over 99% of all globally reported human cases are caused by exposure to unvaccinated dogs infected with canine rabies virus variant, mostly in Asia and Africa (Nyasulu et al., 2021; "WHO Expert Consultation on Rabies. Second Report," 2013). The higher engagement of the community in reporting dog bite cases during the one health intervention led to a higher calculation of the rabies burden in the animal and human health sectors in Indonesia compared to the period before the one health intervention (Aptriana et al., 2024).

Rabies cases have declined in Bangladesh, the Philippines, Sri Lanka, Tanzania, Vietnam, and South Africa (Shafaati et al., 2023). Mexico was the first country to get WHO permission to end dog-borne rabies as a public health issue. To combat frequent killer diseases among humans and animals, including rabies, One-Health approaches are crucial to the sustainable prevention of neglected tropical diseases and eliminating health inequalities in underdeveloped communities (Shafaati et al., 2023). In Mozambique, the human component, the system presents regular data quality, timely, with limitations in terms of acceptability and simplicity. It was not possible to evaluate the animal component (da Costa et al., 2023). It is recommended that a multi-sectoral platform be created to share and visualize rabies surveillance data in Mozambique (da Costa et al., 2023). In Chad, Côte d'Ivoire, and Mali, major challenges arose from the lack of data collection and documentation experience of human health and veterinary workers and weak infrastructural capacities of the veterinary and human health systems of the project countries (Léchenne et al., 2021). In Tunisia, rabies remains a worrying health problem with a high percentage reported among youth and males. Targeting children and adolescents with education and information campaigns about preventive measures and mass dog vaccination are the keys to ending this scourge (Ben Nasrallah et al., 2024). Gaps and strengths should be explored as shown in Table 1.1 to eliminating dog-transmitted rabies in African countries. In African countries where rabies is endemic, the following backbone policy is substantial: (1) Assessment of local rabies epidemiology, (2) preparation of a short-term rabies action plan, (3) development of national rabies preventive and control strategy, (4) full-scale implementation of the national rabies control strategy, and (5) preservation of human rabies freedom, and elimination of dog rabies (Fig. 1.2).

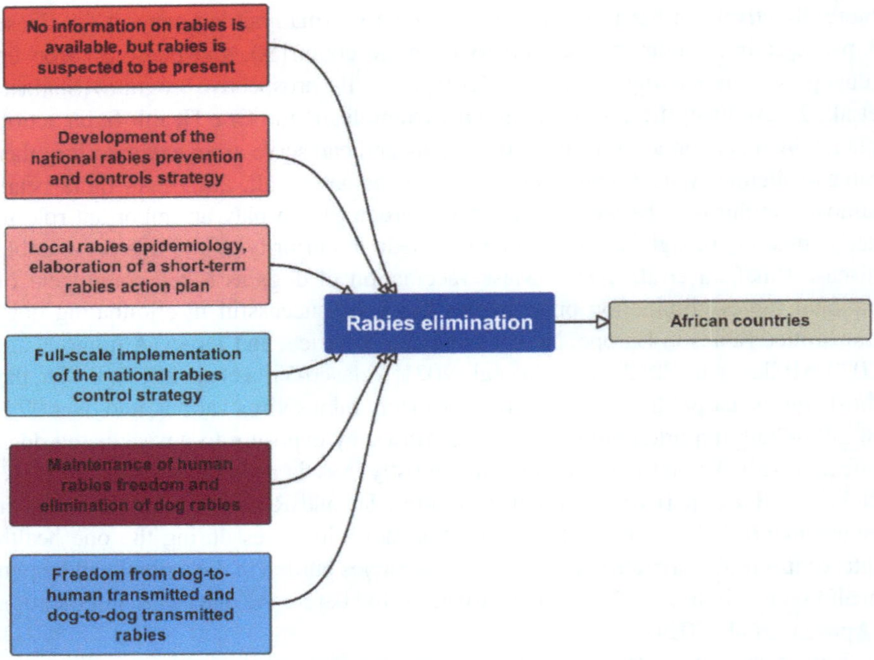

Fig. 1.2 Mind map showing the approach towards rabies elimination in African endemic countries

1.8 Way Forward

Rabies is included in WHO's 2021–2030 Roadmap for the global control of NTDs (https://www.who.int/publications/i/item/9789240010352), which sets regional, progressive targets for the global strategic plan to end human deaths from dog-mediated rabies by 2030 which entails (World Health Organization, 2024b): (1) improving access to human rabies vaccines through the efforts of the WHO and its partners, and (2) providing technical guidance to African countries in developing and implementing their national rabies elimination plans, focusing on strengthening surveillance and reporting. One health approach as described above is needed all over the African continent, including the approach towards rabies elimination in African endemic countries.

The relatively little attention given to coordinated control and prevention of rabies makes the global target of achieving elimination by 2030 challenging in African countries. Now is the time to act as the rabies' neglected disease master plans or national plans in African countries. Recognizing the complexity of the disease and transmission mode would better inform prevention and control methods (Haselbeck et al., 2021). The design of effective rabies elimination strategies and implementation should span healthcare sectors including veterinarians, public health workers, physicians, ecologists, and vaccine producers in African countries. Synchronization of activities through a multi-disciplinary approach will increase the chances of overcoming technical and infrastructural barriers towards regional forces that drive disease control under the One Health approach (Haselbeck et al., 2021). However, strategies to eliminate human rabies in Africa should adapt the rabies programme directors in the Americas (REDIPRA) model in African context, which emphasizes that people exposed to rabies have timely access to quality immunobiologicals, that appropriate levels of vaccination coverage in dogs in highly enzootic areas are maintained, that national rabies plans are strengthened and that systematic implementation is ensured, that the surveillance system for human rabies transmitted by dogs is strengthened and that systematic implementation is ensured, and that training and the development of a laboratory quality control system, particularly in highly enzootic areas, strengthen education, communication and advocacy in enzootic areas, to ensure the continuous political support that is necessary, develop and adopt a guide that delineates the requirements for declaring countries or areas free of human rabies transmitted by dogs (Nyasulu et al., 2021; Vigilato et al., 2018). Rabies requires a comprehensive, strategic, and targeted control and prevention approach with collaboration from human, animal, and environmental health disciplines at local, national, and global levels to achieve more effective control (Acharya et al., 2020; Nyasulu et al., 2021). Infact most of African countries lack a One Health approach to prevent human rabies deaths (Nyasulu et al., 2021; Otu et al., 2021). Targeting domestic dogs through mass dog vaccination campaigns is the method of choice despite its costs. However, the turn-over in African dog populations remains a great challenge in order to reach the expected 70% coverage recommended by WHO Therefore, in some cases, vaccination needs to be associated with dog population management programmes, also expensive (e.g. sterilization) [6]. Outstanding examples from African countries include South Africa and Malawi, where vaccine coverage of dog populations is at ≥70%. Several years, of pilot programmes have shown that the global elimination of dog-mediated human rabies by 2030 is an achievable goal.

1.9 Conclusion

This chapter shows that African countries are still facing multiple challenges and gaps in rabies prevention, control, and even elimination through a combination of strategies, including data reporting, diagnostics, mass vaccination of dogs, and public awareness campaigns. The description of this chapter shows that strategic and/or operational plans for the national elimination of dog-mediated human rabies by 2030 should be strengthened with particular emphasis on "One Health Approach". Given that dog bites cause 99% of human rabies deaths, reducing canine rabies in Africa could significantly lower the number of human cases and potentially eradicate human rabies deaths by 2030. Furthermore, developing POCTs for rabies with accurate tests and based on temporo-spatial data will be user-friendly and will make a significant difference in early detection, reporting, and clinical decision-making among individuals suspected of having been exposed to the rabies virus at the community level. Furthermore, an integrated rabies surveillance, One Health monitoring, and response system are required.

References

Abela-Ridder, B., Knopf, L., Martin, S., Taylor, L., Torres, G., & De Balogh, K. (2016). 2016: The beginning of the end of rabies? *The Lancet. Global Health, 4*(11), e780–e781. https://doi.org/10.1016/S2214-109X(16)30245-5

Acharya, K. P., Acharya, N., Phuyal, S., Upadhyaya, M., & Lasee, S. (2020). One-health approach: A best possible way to control rabies. *One Health (Amsterdam, Netherlands), 10*, Article 100161. https://doi.org/10.1016/j.onehlt.2020.100161

Akinsulie, O. C., Adebowale, O. O., Adesola, R. O., Banwo, O. G., Idris, I., Ogunleye, S. C., Fasakin, O., Bakre, A., Oladapo, I. P., Aliyu, V. A., Waniwa, E. O., Fasiku, O., Joshi, M., & Olorunshola, M. (2024). Holistic application of the one health approach in the prevention and control of rabies: Plausible steps towards achieving the 2030 vision in Africa. *One Health Outlook, 6*(1), 22. https://doi.org/10.1186/s42522-024-00108-6

Amani, A., Abela, B., Biey, J., Traore, T., & Impouma, B. (2024). Accelerating rabies elimination in Africa by 2030. *Lancet.* https://doi.org/10.1016/S0140-6736(24)02141-X

Aptriana, C. D., Sudarnika, E., Basri, C., Indrawan, D., Daryono, J., & Suseno, P. P. (2024). Assessment of the burden of rabies in one health approach control program in Ketapang District Indonesia: Using zDALY. *Preventive Medicine Reports, 45*, Article 102838. https://doi.org/10.1016/j.pmedr.2024.102838

Ashwini, M. A., Pattanaik, A., & Mani, R. S. (2024). Recent updates on laboratory diagnosis of rabies. *The Indian Journal of Medical Research, 159*(1), 48–61. https://doi.org/10.4103/ijmr.ijmr_131_23

Athingo, R., Tenzin, T., Shilongo, A., Hikufe, E., Shoombe, K. K., Khaiseb, S., van der Westhuizen, J., Letshwenyo, M., Torres, G., & Mettenleiter, T. C. (2020). Fighting dog-mediated rabies in Namibia—Implementation of a rabies elimination program in the Northern communal areas. *Tropical Medicine and Infectious Disease, 5*(1), 12.

Ben Nasrallah, C., Abroug, H., Ghoul, M., Grira, S., Ben Fredj, M., Kacem, M., Dhouib, W., Zemni, I., Bouanene, I., & Belguith Sriha, A. (2024). Rabies epidemiology in the central of Tunisia: A call for a one-health approach. *European Journal of Public Health, 34*(Supplement_3), ckae144-1081.

CDC. (2024). *Information for diagnostic laboratories.* https://www.cdc.gov/rabies/php/laboratories/diagnostic.html

CDC-Africa. (2023). *World Rabies Day 2023 Campaign: "All for 1 One Health for All."* https://africacdc.org/news-item/world-rabies-day-2023-campaign-all-for-1-one-health-for-all/

Coetzer, A., Sabeta, C. T., Markotter, W., Rupprecht, C. E., & Nel, L. H. (2014). Comparison of biotinylated monoclonal and polyclonal antibodies in an evaluation of a direct rapid immunohistochemical test for the routine diagnosis of rabies in southern Africa. *PLoS Neglected Tropical Diseases, 8*(9), Article e3189. https://doi.org/10.1371/journal.pntd.0003189

da Costa, I. A., Gatambire, A. C., Tivane, A. R., Chicanequisso, M. V., Chilengue, I., Ali, S., Rossetto, É., Baltazar, C., Chongo, I., & Inlamea, O. F. (2023). Evaluation of rabies surveillance system using the one health approach-Mozambique, 2020–2021. *American Journal of Field Epidemiology, 1*(4 (Supplement)), S20.

Dürr, S., Naïssengar, S., Mindekem, R., Diguimbye, C., Niezgoda, M., Kuzmin, I., Rupprecht, C. E., & Zinsstag, J. (2008). Rabies diagnosis for developing countries. *PLoS Neglected Tropical Diseases, 2*(3), Article e206. https://doi.org/10.1371/journal.pntd.0000206

FAO. (2024). *One Health approach to rabies*. https://www.fao.org/one-health/areas-of-work/rabies/en

Fooks, A. R., Banyard, A. C., Horton, D. L., Johnson, N., McElhinney, L. M., & Jackson, A. C. (2014). Current status of rabies and prospects for elimination. *Lancet, 384*(9951), 1389–1399. https://doi.org/10.1016/S0140-6736(13)62707-5

Franka, R., Smith, T. G., Dyer, J. L., Wu, X., Niezgoda, M., & Rupprecht, C. E. (2013). Current and future tools for global canine rabies elimination. *Antiviral Research, 100*(1), 220–225. https://doi.org/10.1016/j.antiviral.2013.07.004

Freuling, C. M., van der Westhuizen, J., Khaiseb, S., Tenzin, T., & Müller, T. (2023). From field tests to molecular tools—Evaluating diagnostic tests to improve rabies surveillance in Namibia. *Viruses, 15*(2), 371.

Hampson, K., Coudeville, L., Lembo, T., Sambo, M., Kieffer, A., Attlan, M., Barrat, J., Blanton, J. D., Briggs, D. J., Cleaveland, S., Costa, P., Freuling, C. M., Hiby, E., Knopf, L., Leanes, F., Meslin, F.-X., Metlin, A., Miranda, M. E., Müller, T., & Dushoff, J. (2015). Correction: Estimating the global burden of endemic canine rabies. *PLoS Neglected Tropical Diseases, 9*(5), Article e0003786. https://doi.org/10.1371/journal.pntd.0003786

Haselbeck, A. H., Rietmann, S., Tadesse, B. T., Kling, K., Kaschubat-Dieudonné, M. E., Marks, F., Wetzker, W., & Thöne-Reineke, C. (2021). Challenges to the fight against rabies-the landscape of policy and prevention strategies in Africa. *International Journal of Environmental Research and Public Health, 18*(4). https://doi.org/10.3390/ijerph18041736

Hobbs, E. C., Colling, A., Gurung, R. B., & Allen, J. (2021). The potential of diagnostic point-of-care tests (POCTs) for infectious and zoonotic animal diseases in developing countries: Technical, regulatory and sociocultural considerations. *Transboundary and Emerging Diseases, 68*(4), 1835–1849. https://doi.org/10.1111/tbed.13880

Kardjadj, M., & Ben-Mahdi, M. H. (2019). Epidemiology of dog-mediated zoonotic diseases in Algeria: A One Health control approach. *New Microbes and New Infections, 28*, 17–20. https://doi.org/10.1016/j.nmni.2019.01.001

Léchenne, M., Naïssengar, K., Lepelletier, A., Alfaroukh, I. O., Bourhy, H., Zinsstag, J., & Dacheux, L. (2016). Validation of a rapid rabies diagnostic tool for field surveillance in developing countries. *PLoS Neglected Tropical Diseases, 10*(10), Article e0005010. https://doi.org/10.1371/journal.pntd.0005010

Léchenne, M., Traore, A., Hattendorf, J., Kallo, V., Oussiguere, A., Tetchi, M., Moyengar, R., Traore, A. K., Moto, D. D., & Ngandolo, R. (2021). Increasing rabies data availability: The example of a One Health research project in Chad, Côte D'ivoire and Mali. *Acta Tropica, 215*, Article 105808.

Lembo, T., Niezgoda, M., Velasco-Villa, A., Cleaveland, S., Ernest, E., & Rupprecht, C. E. (2006). Evaluation of a direct, rapid immunohistochemical test for rabies diagnosis. *Emerging Infectious Diseases, 12*(2), 310.

Mani, R. S., & Madhusudana, S. N. (2013). Laboratory diagnosis of human rabies: Recent advances. *The Scientific World Journal, 2013*(1), Article 569712.

Mani, R. S., & Willoughby, R. E. (2017). Human rabies in South Asia. In S. K. Singh (Ed.), *Neglected tropical diseases—South Asia* (pp. 349–371). Springer International Publishing. https://doi.org/10.1007/978-3-319-68493-2_11

Marston, D. A., Jennings, D. L., MacLaren, N. C., Dorey-Robinson, D., Fooks, A. R., Banyard, A. C., & McElhinney, L. M. (Directors). (2019, July 10). *Pan-lyssavirus real time RT-PCR for rabies diagnosis* (Issue 149) [Video recording]. https://doi.org/10.3791/59709

Minghui, R., Stone, M., Semedo, M. H., & Nel, L. (2018). New global strategic plan to eliminate dog-mediated rabies by 2030. *The Lancet. Global Health, 6*(8), e828–e829. https://doi.org/10.1016/S2214-109X(18)30302-4

Müller, T., Demetriou, P., Moynagh, J., Cliquet, F., Fooks, A. R., Conraths, F. J., Mettenleiter, T. C., & Freuling, C. M. (2012). Rabies elimination in Europe: A success story. In *Rabies control: Towards sustainable prevention at the source, Compendium of the OIE Global Conf. on Rabies Control, Incheon-Seoul, 7–9 September 2011, Republic of Korea* (pp. 31–44).

Nel, L. H. (2013). Discrepancies in data reporting for rabies, Africa. *Emerging Infectious Diseases, 19*(4), 529–533. https://doi.org/10.3201/eid1904.120185

Nel, L. H., & Rupprecht, C. E. (2007). Emergence of lyssaviruses in the old world: The case of Africa. *Current Topics in Microbiology and Immunology, 315*, 161–193. https://doi.org/10.1007/978-3-540-70962-6_8

Nyasulu, P. S., Weyer, J., Tschopp, R., Mihret, A., Aseffa, A., Nuvor, S. V., Tamuzi, J. L., Nyakarahuka, L., Helegbe, G. K., Ntinginya, N. E., Gebreyesus, M. T., Doumbia, S., Busse, R., & Drosten, C. (2021). Rabies mortality and morbidity associated with animal bites in Africa: A case for integrated rabies disease surveillance, prevention and control: A scoping review. *British Medical Journal Open, 11*(12), Article e048551. https://doi.org/10.1136/bmjopen-2020-048551

Otu, A., Effa, E., Meseko, C., Cadmus, S., Ochu, C., Athingo, R., Namisango, E., Ogoina, D., Okonofua, F., & Ebenso, B. (2021). Africa needs to prioritize One Health approaches that focus on the environment, animal health and human health. *Nature Medicine, 27*(6), 943–946. https://doi.org/10.1038/s41591-021-01375-w

Patrick, E. M., Bjorklund, B. M., Kirby, J. D., Nelson, K. M., Chipman, R. B., & Rupprecht, C. E. (2019). Enhanced rabies surveillance using a direct rapid immunohistochemical test. *JoVE, 146*, Article e59416. https://doi.org/10.3791/59416

Shafaati, M., Akbarpour, S., Priyanka, Saied, A. A., & Choudhary, O. P. (2023). Tackling rabies by one health approach: Pitfalls on the road to global eradication. *New Microbes and New Infections, 52*, 101098. https://doi.org/10.1016/j.nmni.2023.101098

Sheikh, K. A., Ramos-Alvarez, M., Jackson, A. C., Li, C. Y., Asbury, A. K., & Griffin, J. W. (2005). Overlap of pathology in paralytic rabies and axonal Guillain-Barré syndrome. *Annals of Neurology, 57*(5), 768–772. https://doi.org/10.1002/ana.20482

Sreenivasan, N., Li, A., Shiferaw, M., Tran, C. H., Wallace, R., Blanton, J., Knopf, L., Abela-Ridder, B., & Hyde, T. (2019). Overview of rabies post-exposure prophylaxis access, procurement and distribution in selected countries in Asia and Africa, 2017–2018. *Vaccine, 37*(Suppl 1), A6–A13. https://doi.org/10.1016/j.vaccine.2019.04.024

Talbi, C., Holmes, E. C., de Benedictis, P., Faye, O., Nakouné, E., Gamatié, D., Diarra, A., Elmamy, B. O., Sow, A., Adjogoua, E. V., Sangare, O., Dundon, W. G., Capua, I., Sall, A. A., & Bourhy, H. (2009). Evolutionary history and dynamics of dog rabies virus in western and central Africa. *The Journal of General Virology, 90*(Pt 4), 783–791. https://doi.org/10.1099/vir.0.007765-0

Velasco-Villa, A., Escobar, L. E., Sanchez, A., Shi, M., Streicker, D. G., Gallardo-Romero, N. F., Vargas-Pino, F., Gutierrez-Cedillo, V., Damon, I., & Emerson, G. (2017). Successful strategies implemented towards the elimination of canine rabies in the Western Hemisphere. *Antiviral Research, 143*, 1–12.

Vigilato, M. A., Cosivi, O., Knöbl, T., Clavijo, A., & Silva, H. M. (2013). Rabies update for Latin America and the Caribbean. *Emerging Infectious Diseases, 19*(4), 678.

Vigilato, M. A. N., Molina-Flores, B., Del Rio Vilas, V. J., Pompei, J. C., & Cosivi, O. (2018). Canine rabies elimination: Governance principles. *Revue Scientifique et Technique (International Office of Epizootics), 37*(2), 703–709. https://doi.org/10.20506/rst.37.2.2859

WHO. (2025). *The Global Health Observatory*. https://www.who.int/data/gho/data/themes/topics/rabies

WHO Expert Consultation on Rabies. Second report. (2013). *World Health Organization Technical Report Series, 982*, 1–139, back cover.

WHO/Africa. (2024). *Rabies*. https://www.afro.who.int/health-topics/rabies

Willoughby, R. E. (2015). Rabies: Rare human infection–common questions. *Infectious Disease Clinics, 29*(4), 637–650.

World Health Organization. (2018a). *International partnership to address human-animal-environment health risks gets a boost*. https://www.who.int/news/item/30-05-2018-international-partnership-to-address-human-animal-environment-health-risks-gets-a-boost

World Health Organization. (2018b). *WHO expert consultation on rabies: Third report* (Vol. 1012). World Health Organization.

World Health Organization. (2024a). *Global Health Observatory (2024)—Processed by Our World in Data. "Reported deaths from rabies"*. World Health Organization, "Global Health Observatory." https://ourworldindata.org/grapher/reported-rabies-deaths

World Health Organization. (2024b). *Rabies*. https://www.who.int/news-room/fact-sheets/detail/rabies/

Yang, D.-K., Cho, I. S., & Kim, H. H. (2018). Strategies for controlling dog-mediated human rabies in Asia: Using "One Health" principles to assess control programmes for rabies. *Revue Scientifique et Technique (International Office of Epizootics)*, *37*(2), 473–481. https://doi.org/10.20506/rst.37.2.2816

Chapter 2
Orthohantaviruses: A Zoonotic Public Health Threat in the Old World

Natalya Andreeva, Yuriy Davidyuk, Ekaterina Martynova, Kristina Stolbunova, Olesia Ohlopkova, Ilnur Salafutdinov, Albert Rizvanov, Sara Chandy, Manoj Baranwal, Emmanuel Kabwe, and Svetlana Khaiboullina

Abstract Orthohantaviruses cause emerging infections such as hemorrhagic fever with renal syndrome (HFRS) and hantavirus pulmonary syndrome in Eurasia and the Americas, respectively. Humans become infected by inhaling the virus-contaminated aerosols or dust and, in isolated cases, via bites/direct contact with infected rodents. Pathogenic orthohantaviruses such as Hantaan, Dobrava, Seoul, and Puumala are found in countries of the Old World, with the mortality rate ranging from 0.4 to 15%. These viruses continue to cause many infections in Asian and European countries. In recent years, orthohantaviruses have been diagnosed in countries where they were not considered endemic, such as India, Vietnam, Thailand, and some African countries. This chapter will provide a synopsis of orthohantaviruses distribution and genetic diversity in endemic areas in the Old World. We will also describe the data on clinical presentation, treatment and current vaccines for orthohantavirus infections.

N. Andreeva · Y. Davidyuk · E. Martynova · I. Salafutdinov · A. Rizvanov · E. Kabwe (✉) · S. Khaiboullina (✉)
Institute of Fundamental Medicine and Biology, OpenLab "Gene and Cell Technologies", Kazan Federal University, Kazan, Russia
e-mail: emmanuelkabwe@ymail.com; EmKabve@kpfu.ru

M. Baranwal
Department of Biotechnology, Thapar Institute of Engineering and Technology, Patiala, India

K. Stolbunova · O. Ohlopkova
Virology Research Institute of the Federal Research Center for Fundamental and Translational Medicine, Novosibirsk, Russia

S. Chandy
Childs Trust Medical Research Foundation, Kanchi Kamakoti Childs Trust Hospital, Chennai, India

A. Rizvanov
Division of Medical and Biological Sciences, Tatarstan Academy of Sciences, Kazan, Russia

I. Salafutdinov
Department of Medical Biology and Genetics, Kazan State Medical University, Kazan, Russia

F. Mphande and P. Nyasulu (eds.), *Evaluating Outbreak Potential of Infections in Tropical Climates*, https://doi.org/10.1007/978-981-95-0618-7_2

Additionally, the impact of interventions on the HFRS outbreak during the COVID-19 pandemic is discussed. The information provided in this chapter will help optimize and develop strategies for preventing HFRS, a serious human health threat.

Keywords Emerging viruses · Orthohantaviruses · Therapeutics · Vaccines · Immunology · Hemorrhagic fever with renal syndrome · COVID-19

List of Abbreviations

HNTV	*Orthohantavirus hantaanense*
SEOV	*Orthohantavirus seoulense,*
PUUV	*Orthohantavirus puumalaense*
DOBV	*Orthohantavirus dobravaense*
HFRS	Hemorrhagic Fever with Renal Syndrome
HCPS	Hantavirus Cardiopulmonary Syndrome
S	Small
M	Medium
L	Large
N	Protein, nucleocapsid protein
GPC	Gn and Gc, glycoprotein precursor
RdRp	Viral RNA-dependent RNA polymerase
COVID-19	Coronavirus disease 2019
KHAV	Orthohantavirus khaba-rovskense
ICTV	International committee on taxonomy of viruses
THAIV	Orthohantavirus thailandense
TULV	Orthohantavirus tulaense
AKI	Acute kidney infection
VLP	Virus-like particle
GPI	Glycosylphosphatidylinositol
GM-CSF	Granulocyte–macrophage colony-stimulating factor
SARS-CoV-2	Severe acute respiratory syndrome coronavirus 2

2.1 Introduction

Orthohantaviruses are zoonotic pathogens belonging to the genus *Orthohantavirus* family *Hantavirdae* (*ICTV Current ICTV Taxonomy Release. Available online:* https://ictv.global/taxonomy *(ac-cessed on 8 August 2022).*; Laenen et al., 2019). Multiple members of the genus *Orthohantavirus* are human pathogens: *Orthohantavirus hantaanense* (HNTV), *Orthohantavirus seoulense* (SEOV), *Orthohantavirus puumalaense* (PUUV), and *Orthohantavirus dobravaense* (DOBV). Presently, 38 orthohantavirus species have been identified (*ICTV Current ICTV Taxonomy Release. Available online:* https://ictv.global/taxonomy *(ac-cessed on 8 August 2022).*), out of which at least 12 are capable of causing infectious diseases in humans (Kuhn & Schmaljohn, 2023; Noack et al., 2020). Orthohantaviruses can cause two acute febrile diseases: Hemorrhagic Fever with Renal Syndrome (HFRS) and Hantavirus Cardiopulmonary Syndrome (HCPS) in the Old and New World, respectively (Chandy et al., 2008; Kariwa et al., 2007a, 2007b). The group of orthohantaviruses which cause HFRS circulate primarily in small rodents inhabiting the Asian and European regions (Brummer-Korvenkontio et al., 1986; Lee et al., 1982; Taller et al., 1993).

Orthohantaviruses have a negative sense single-stranded RNA genome, which is organized into three segments: small (S), medium (M), and large (L) (Fig. 2.1). Orthohantavirus S, M, and L segments are approximately 1828, 3650, and 6550 nucleotides (nt) long, respectively (Kukkonen et al., 2005; Schmaljohn et al., 1983). The length of the coding sequences is 1299, 3444, and 6468 nt for S, M, and L segments, respectively. These RNAs encode nucleocapsid (N) protein (433 amino acid sequences (aa), glycoprotein precursor (GPC), which is processed into two glycoproteins (Gn and Gc) (1138 aa), and the viral RNA-dependent RNA polymerase (RdRp) protein (2155 aa), respectively (Jiang et al., 2017).

(A) The structure is spherical, having a diameter of 8–120 nm, enveloped with a lipid bilayer containing spikes of glycoproteins (Gn and Gc). Inside the virion are three segments of single-stranded RNA: small (S), medium (M) and large (L). (B) The S, M, and L genomic segments encode for the nucleocapsid protein (433 aa), glycoprotein precursor (1138 aa) and the RNA-dependent RNA polymerase (2155 aa), respectively.

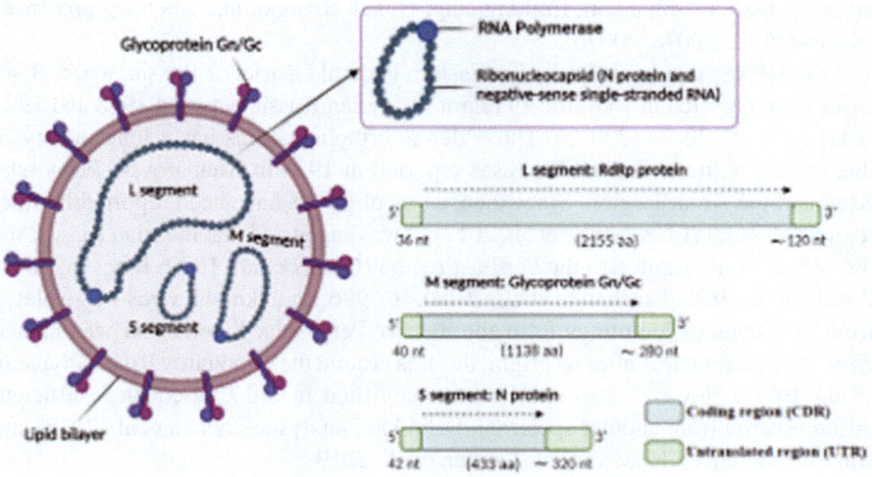

Fig. 2.1 Schematic representation of an orthohantavirus virion

Orthohantaviruses are endemic in many Eurasian countries, with the largest number of cases reported in China, South Korea, and the Volga Federal District of Russia (VFD) (Jiang et al., 2017). During the COVID-19 pandemic, the infection of orthohantaviruses dropped to the lowest level seen in decades (Jiang et al., 2017). This chapter provides a history of the orthohantaviruses and the disease they cause in Eurasian countries, particularly emphasizing the geographical distribution and genetic diversity of pathogenic orthohantaviruses, clinical manifestation and pathogenesis. We will also define clinical manifestation and address challenges in preventing, treating, and diagnosing orthohantaviruses, particularly in Eurasia. Finally, the impact of interventions on the HFRS outbreak during the COVID-19 pandemic will be discussed.

2.2 History of Orthohantaviruses and the Disease They Cause

In China, febrile disease with renal dysfunction was documented as early as 1931 (Kariwa et al., 2007a, 2007b). Since then, HFRS has been acknowledged as an endemic disease in this country, where 40–50% of worldwide HFRS cases are diagnosed (Jiang et al., 2017). China remains the most active HFRS endemic region, where cases increased from 10,378 reported in 1931–1949 (Chen & Qiu, 1993) to 1,557,622 diagnosed between 1950 and 2007 (Zhang et al., 2010). In recent decades, the incidence of HFRS in China has decreased. During 2004–2019, 209,209 cases of the disease were registered, of which 1855 were fatal (Zou & Sun, 2020). Epidemiological analysis indicated several "hot spots" in China with a high risk of orthohantavirus infections: Shandon, Heilongjiang, Hunan, Jiangxi, and Zhejiang provinces (Kariwa et al., 2007a, 2007b).

Still, HFRS is endemic in the Far Eastern Federal District of Russia, where 3145 cases were reported in 15 of the 29 regions of Asian Russia between 1978 and 1995 (Kariwa et al., 2007a, 2007b). The endemic orthohantavirus has a long history in this region, with the first HFRS cases reported in 1934 in Khabarovsk, Primorsky Krai, and the Amur Region. Since then, cases of HFRS have been reported in other regions of Russia (Tkachenko et al., 2019). It was suggested that in Asian Russia, the disease was only limited to the Far East region (Casals et al., 1970; Johnson, 2001; Povalishina, 1965; Tkachenko et al., 2014). In 1996, an unknown virus was isolated from the lungs of lemmings from the Taimyr Peninsula, Siberia and was named *Topografov* hantavirus after its origin, the area around the Topogafov River (Plyusnin et al., 1996). However, this species was abolished in 2017 based on insufficient differentiation from another species in DEmARC analysis (Laenen et al., 2018) and was considered a KHAV variant (Laenen et al., 2019).

Symptoms like HFRS were also described in approximately 1700 US soldiers during the Korean War (1950–1953), with less than 5% resulting in deaths (Smadel, 1953). Later, symptoms similar to HFRS from the Far East region were noticed in patients from Scandinavia (Casals et al., 1970). At that time, knowledge of the infectious agent causing HFRS remained limited (Myhrman, 1951; Smorodintsev et al., 1959). Human infection was usually associated with exposure to excreta from small rodents (Lokugamage et al., 2002).

Following a retrospective study of clinical cases, the identity of an infectious agent was revealed several years later. In 1978, Dr. Lee isolated the etiologic agent of hemorrhagic fever from the *Apodemus agrarius* lung tissue, which reacted with convalescent serum from HFRS patients (Lee et al., 1978). The morphology of a new virus, the *Hantaan virus*, was identified as a member of the family *Bunyaviridae (*McCormick et al., 1982*)*.

In 1980, antibodies to the causative agent of epidemic nephropathy (NE) were detected in the bank vole (Brummer-Korvenkontio et al., 1980). Later, a causative agent was identified as Hantavirus and named *Puumala* (PUUV) after the Puumala municipality in Finland. Two years later, Lee et al. discovered a variant of the *Hantaan* virus, now known as SEOV, which caused severe HFRS in Seoul city residents (Lee et al., 1982). Since patients had no history of travelling outside the city, urban rats were suggested as the natural reservoir of this virus in South Korea. The retrospective research showed that 15% of the rats in Seoul and 28% in Tokyo carried the newly identified virus (Pljusnin & Elliott, 2011). In southeastern Slovenia, hemorrhagic fever was observed in patients, and subsequently, DOBV was isolated from a yellow-necked mouse (*Apodemus flavicollis*) found in the village forest (Avsic-Zupanc et al., 1992).

The first cases of suspected orthohantavirus infection in India were reported in 1964 in Vellore (Song, Baek, et al., 2007a, 2007b). Investigation of these outbreaks led to the identification of a novel member of the genus *Orthohantavirus* (Song, Baek, et al., 2007a, 2007b) named *Thottapalayam virus* (TPMV) (Carey et al., 1971; Song, Baek, et al., 2007a, 2007b). Initially, this virus was isolated from a non-rodent host, the house musk shrew (*Suncus murinus*) (Song, Baek, et al., 2007a, 2007b). Although TPMV had morphological and genetic similarities with members of the genus *Orthohantavirus* of the family *Hantaviridae,* later, TPMV was shown to form a phylogenetically distinct genus (*ICTV Current ICTV Taxonomy Release. Available online:* https://ictv.global/taxonomy *(ac-cessed on 8 August 2022).*). Therefore, a new name was assigned, a *Thottapalayam thottimvirus*, a proto-type shrew-borne orthohantavirus belonging to the genus *Thottimvirus*. In addition to Vellore, a high rate of orthohantavirus seropositivity was reported in healthy individuals from the Cochin and Chennai regions of India (Clement et al., 2006). Analysis of serum samples revealed the cross-reactivity with SEOV in 12% and PUUV in 5% of individuals, respectively (Clement et al., 2006). In another study of 152 serum samples, 23 reacted with HTNV, PUUV, or SEOV (Chandy et al., 2005). These results suggest that orthohantaviruses could be endemic in India.

Hantavirus-reactive antibodies were found in serum samples from 5461 small mammals belonging to 16 species in Taiwan (Chin et al., 2000). It was demonstrated that *Rattus norvegicus* was the most common rodent species captured in that region, and these rodents were major contributors to orthohantavirus circulation in small mammals in the region. Using reverse transcriptase polymerase chain reaction (RT-PCR), SEOV was detected in *Rattus norvegicus* in lung tissues. As a result of further analyses, it was discovered that almost all orthohantavirus infections in Taiwan were caused by SEOV (Chin et al., 2000).

Also, 3.8% of rodents captured in the Nakhon Pathom region were seropositive for orthohantavirus antigens (Elwell et al., 1985). All the sera-positive rodents were *Bandicoot indica* species. These rodents were shown to carry the Hantaan-like virus (Elwell et al., 1985). Antibodies to the Hantaan-like virus were found in humans living near locations of infected rodents. The positive titer of antibodies to Hantavirus varied from 5–7% to 31–33 (Elwell et al., 1985). Later this virus was named *Thailand orthohantavirus* (THAIV).

For the first time after the detection of hantaviruses, the prevailing opinion was that rodents were their carriers; however, later studies have identified hantavirus antigen (virus) or/and specific antibodies in domestic animals, such as cats, rabbits, and dogs (Song, 1999). A case of human infection with Hantavirus from a domestic rat has also been reported (Jameson et al., 2013).

2.3 The Evolution of Viruses Belonging to Hantaviridae Family: Bats as One of the Important Hosts for These Viruses

Between 1964 and 2006, higher percentage of viruses of Hantaviridae family were detected in rodents, with the exception of Thottapalayam virus (TPMV) isolated from shrew specimens in India (Zeller et al., 1989). Consequently, rodents were considered the only natural reservoir for viruses belonging to Hantaviridae family during this period. In the shift of hypothesis, since 2007, most newly discovered Hantaviridae family virus genotypes have been isolated from either shrews or moles. This discovery highlighted the new order Eulipotyphla as a potential small mammal for these virus hosts and the role they could play in the evolution. Additionally, since 2012, bats have been found to carry different viruses circulating worldwide (Fig. 2.2). Currently, 18 viruses have been detected in bats and 10 are already classified by the International Committee on Taxonomy (Fig. 2.2).

Information about the first bat hantavirus was published in 2012. In this year, Magboi virus (MGBV) was found in the lungs of hairy bat (*Nycteris hispida*) collected in 2009 in Sierra Lona, West Africa. It is also worth noting that in 1994, Kim and colleagues found that bats such as the greater horseshoe bat (*Rhinolophus ferrumequinum*) and the lesser bat (*Eptesicus serotinus*) collected in South Korea were serologically positive for a virus closely related to HTNV (Kim et al., 1994). The genetic analysis of the isolated virus revealed that it is HTNV, though the authors suspected the bias results (Jung & Kim, 1995), indicating that bats could be carries of hantaviruses (Weiss et al., 2012). Complete list of bat viruses belonging to Hantaviridae family are presented in Table 2.1. Recently, the authors of this book

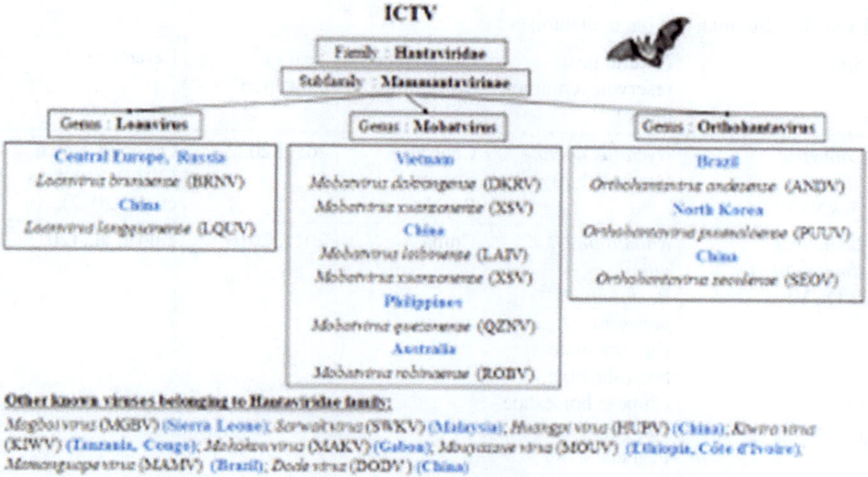

Fig. 2.2 Classification of known bats Hantaviridae family viruses

chapter detected Brno virus (BRNV) in the red noctule (*Nyctalus noctula*) in the Rostov region of Russia, marking the first time of detecting viruses of Hantaviridae family from bats in Russia (Ohlopkova et al., 2024).

Taken together, these data indicate that viruses of Hantaviridae family have a wide range of natural hosts. Phylogenetic analysis of viral sequences suggests that these viruses may have first evolved in chiropterans (bats) or soricomorphs (moles and shrews) before circulating in rodents (Fig. 2.3). The phylogenetic history of viruses does not always coincide with that of their hosts, indicating that interspecies transmission events have occurred at all taxonomic levels. Overall, both interspecies transmission and co-divergence have resulted in the high genetic diversity of viruses of Hantaviridae family described to date (Zhang, 2014). The discovery of these viruses in bats highlights the importance of interspecies transmission in viral evolution. This transmission may have occurred between bats, insectivores, and rodents at different stages of evolution, which also explains the diversity of modern hantaviruses.

This data demonstrate that bats are important natural reservoir hosts for viruses of Hantaviridae family. The global distribution of bats, high abundance, ability to migrate long distances, and density of breeding colonies potentially facilitate efficient maintenance, evolution, and dissemination of viruses. Efforts are needed to elucidate the potential importance of bats viruses, the possibility of spillover of bat-borne viruses to animals, including humans, and the study of their pathogenicity in humans (Guo et al., 2013). Bat viruses of Hantaviridae family are not associated with pathogenicity in humans. However, comparisons of pathogenic and nonpathogenic strains may help to understand the genetic changes that make viruses dangerous to humans.

Table 2.1 Summary of bat hantaviruses

Species	Natural host reservoir (common name)	Geographic distribution	Year of collection	Reference
Loanvirus brunaense (BRNV)	*Nyctalus noctule* (Noctule bat)	Central Europe, Russia	2012; 2022	Ohlopkova et al., (2024), Strakova et al., (2017)
Loanvirus longquanense (LQUV)	*Rhinolophus affinis, R. sinicus, P. pearsoni* (Intermediate horseshoe bat, Chinese horseshoe bat, Pearson's horseshoe bat)	China	2011, 2016	Guo et al., (2013)
Mobatvirus ribinaense (ROBV)	*Pteropus alecto* (Black flying fox)	Australia	2017	GenBank
Mobatvirus dakrongense (DKRV)	*Aselliscus stoliczkanus* (Stoliczka's Asian trident bat)	Viet Nam	2013	Arai et al., (2019)
Mobatvirus xuansonense (XSV)	*Hipposideros pomona, H. cineraceus* (Pomona leaf-nosed bat, Ashy roundleaf bat)	Viet Nam; China	1997; 1999; 2012; 2015	Arai et al., (2013, 2019), Gu et al., (2014)
Mobatvirus quezonense (QZNV)	*Rousettus amplexicaudatus* (Geoffroy's rousette)	Philippines	2009	Arai et al., (2016)
Mobatvirus laibinense (LAIV)	*Taphozous melanopogon* (black-bearded tomb bat)	China	2012	Xu et al., (2015)
Orthohantavirus andesense (ANDV)	*Carollia perspicillata* (Seba's short-tailed bat)	Brazil	2013	GenBank MF094269.1
Orthohantavirus puumalaense (PUUV)	*Rhinolophus ferrumequinum* (Greater horseshoe bat)	South Korea	ND	GenBank AF352567.1

(continued)

Table 2.1 (continued)

Species	Natural host reservoir (common name)	Geographic distribution	Year of collection	Reference
Orthohantavirus seoulense (SEOV)	*Hipposideros armiger, H. pomona, H.larvatus, Rhinolophus pusillus* *(Great roundleaf bat,* Pomona leaf-nosed bat, Horsfield's leaf-nosed bat, Least horseshoe bat)	China	2009	GenBank KF699336.1
Magboi virus (MGBV)	*Nycteris hispida* (Hairy slit-faced bat)	Sierra Leone	2009	Weiss et al., (2012)
Huangpi virus (HUPV)	*Pipistrellus abramus* (Japanese pipistrelle)	China	2012; 2023	Guo et al., (2013)
Dode virus (DODV)	*Hipposideros Pomona* (Pomona leaf-nosed bat)	China	2016	GenBank
Sarawak mobatvirus (SWKV)	*Murina aenea* (Bronze tube-nosed bat)	Malaysia	2015	Zana et al., (2019)
Kiwira virus (KIWS)	*Mops condylurus* (Angolan free-tailed bat)	Tanzania	2017	Weiss et al., (2022)
Makokou virus (MAKV)	*Hipposideros ruber* (Noack's roundleaf bat)	Gabon	2009	Witkowski et al., (2016)
Mouyassue virus (MOUV)	*Neoromicia nanus* (Banana but)	Cote d'Ivoire	2011	Sumibcay et al., (2012)
Mamanguape virus (MAMV)	*Carollia perspicillata* (Seba's short-tailed bat)	Brazil	2015	GenBank PP258966.1

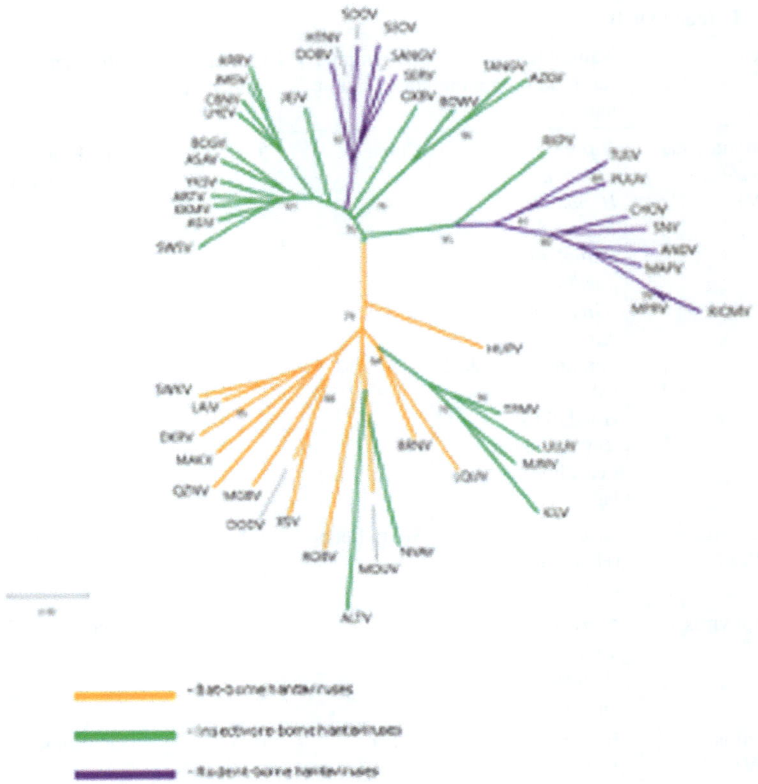

Fig. 2.3 Phylogenetic tree constructed based on L-segment regions of small mammal hantaviruses, constructed by the maximum likelihood method with a bootstrap support of 1000. General Time Reversible model. Abbreviations: ALTV—Altai virus; ANDV—Andes virus; ARRV—Ash River virus; ARTV—Artybash virus; ASAV—Asama virus; ASIV—Asikkala virus; AZGV—Azagny virus; BOGV—Boginia virus; BOWV—Bowe virus; BRNV—Brno virus; CBNV—Cao Bang virus; CHOV—Choclo virus; DKRV—Dakrong virus; DOBV—Dobrava-Belgrade virus; DODV—Dode virus; HTNV—Hantaan virus; HUPV—Huanqpi virus; JEJV—Jeju virus; JMSV—Jemez Springs virus; KILV—Kilimanjaro virus; KKMV—Kenkeme virus; LAIV—Laibin virus; LHEV—Lianghe virus; LQUV—Longquan virus; MAKV—Makokou virus; MAPV—Maporal virus; MGBV—Magboi virus; MJNV—Imjin virus; MOUV—Mouyassue virus; MPRV—Maripa virus; NVAV—Nova virus; OXBV—Oxbow virus; PUUV—Puumala virus; QZNV—Quezon virus; RIOMV—Rio Mamore virus; RKPV—Rockport virus; ROBV—Robina virus; SANGV—Sangassou virus; SEOV—Seoul virus; SERV—Serang virus; SNV—Sin Nombre virus; SOOV—Soochong virus; SWKV—Sarawak virus SWSV—Seewis virus; TANGV—Tanganya virus; TPMV—Thottapalayam virus; TULV—Tula virus; ULUV—Uluguru virus; XSV—Xuan Son virus; YKSV—Yakeshi virus

2.4 Geographical Distribution

The location of the natural host reservoir determines the geographic distribution of orthohantavirus, as these viruses establish chronic infection in specific rodents (considered natural host reservoirs) (de Oliveira et al., 2014; Jonsson et al., 2010; Watson et al., 2014). Rodent species associated with orthohantaviruses are divided into two families: *Muridae* ("Guénet, Jean Louis, Annie Orth and François Bonhomme. "Origins and Phylogenetic Relationships of the Laboratory Mouse." (2012)."') and *Cricetidae* ("Poor, A. Cricetidae World Rats and Mice, Voles, Hamsters, and Relatives Available online: https://animaldiversity.org/accounts/Cricetidae/."), which are found in Eurasia and the Americas. *Muridae* is divided into multiple subfamilies, where the subfamily *Murinae* includes rats and mice (Mir, 2010; Vaheri et al., 2008). Rodents in this subfamily were shown to carry orthohantaviruses such as HTNV, SEOV, THAIV and DOBV (de Oliveira et al., 2014; "Guénet, Jean Louis, Annie Orth and François Bonhomme. "Origins and Phylogenetic Relationships of the Laboratory Mouse." (2012). "; "Hussein, I.; Haseeb, A.; Haque, A.; MA Mir Recent Advances in Hantavirus Molecular Biology and Disease. Advances in applied 2011,"). The second family, Cricetidae, is divided into several subfamilies, whereas the Arvicolinae subfamily includes voles and lemmings (Mir, 2010; Vaheri et al., 2008). These small rodents are natural carriers of PUUV and TULV (de Oliveira et al., 2014; "Hussein, I.; Haseeb, A.; Haque, A.; MA Mir Recent Advances in Hantavirus Molecular Biology and Disease. Advances in applied 2011,"). A notable exception is the TPMV, which is carried by Suncus murinus (Asian house shrew), an insectivore of the Soricidae family. This shrew is mainly found in India (Song, Baek, et al., 2007a, 2007b).

Around 1,500,000 to 2,000,000 cases of orthohantavirus infection are reported annually worldwide. Therefore, orthohantavirus infection remains a serious threat to public health (Bi et al., 2008; Singh et al., 2022; Watson et al., 2014). Orthohantavirus infection has historically been prevalent in Asia, with most orthohantavirus cases clinically presenting as HFRS and endemic in China, Korea, and the Far East of Russia. Over 90% of HFRS cases worldwide originate in China (de Oliveira et al., 2014; Kruger et al., 2015). Approximately 300–500 HFRS cases are reported annually in Korea (Kruger et al., 2015). The SEOV is demonstrated in multiple countries due to the widespread distribution of domestic rats, a reservoir host. Still, SEOV infection is more common in Asia. The finding supports this assumption that 14–34% of rats were positive for anti-SEOV antibodies in Vietnam and Singapore (Kruger et al., 2015; Zhang et al., 2010). Orthohantavirus infection cases were also reported in Middle Eastern countries, where TULV-like orthohantavirus was isolated in the North West Iran outbreak ("Aude Lalis The First Identification of Tula Hantavirus in Iran. Malaria Control & Elimination, 2020, 9"). Another study identified a new orthohantavirus strain, Serang virus (SERV), circulating in an Asian house rat in Indonesia (Plyusnina et al., 2009). This virus was shown to be related to TPMV from Thailand. The geographical distributions of viruses in the Old World according to the classification of their host reservoirs are summarized in the Table 2.2.

Table 2.2 The geographic distribution of orthohantaviruses endemic to Asia and their small mammal hosts

Orthohantavirus species	Natural host reservoir (common name)	Geographic distribution	Associated disease	References
Orthohantavirus hantanense (HTNV) *	*Apodemus agrarius* (Striped field mouse)	China, Korea, Russia	HFRS	Fang et al., (2015), Plyusnina et al., (2009)
Orthohantavirus dabieshanense (DBSV)	*Niviventer confucianus* (Chinese white-bellied rat)	China	Unknown	Wang et al., (2000a, 2000b)
Orthohantavirus fugongense (FUGV)	*Eothenomys eleusis* (Small oriental vole)	China	Unknown	Ge et al., (2016)
Orthohantavirus fusongense (FUSV)	*Microtus fortis* (Reed vole)	China	Unknown	Zou et al., (2008)
Soochong orthohantavirus (SOOV) *	*Apodemus peninsulae* (Korean field mouse)	Korea	Unknown	Jiang et al., (2007)
Amur orthohantavirus (AMRV) *	*Apodemus peninsulae* (Korean field mouse)	Asia	HFRS	Jiang et al., (2007)
Orthohantavirus seoulense (SEOV)	*Rattus norvegicus Rattus* (Rats)	Worldwide	HFRS	Fang et al., (2015)
Orthohantavirus thailandense (THAIV)	*Bandicoot indica* (Bandicoot rat)	Southeast Asia (Thailand)	HFRS	Kutanan et al., (2018)
Orthohantavirus puumalaense (PUUV) **	*Myodes glareolus* (Bank vole)	Eurasian continent	Mild HFRS/NE	Garanina et al., (2009)
Orthohantavirus khabarovskense (KHAV)	*Microtus maximowiczii* (Maximowicz's vole)	Mongolia, northeast China	Unknown	Zou et al., (2008)
Hokkaido virus (HOKV) **	*Myodes rufocanus* (Grey red-backed vole)	Japan	HFRS	Daud et al., (2007)
Muju virus (MUJI) **	*Myodes regulus* (Royal vole)	South Korea	Unknown	Arai et al., (2012)

(continued)

Table 2.2 (continued)

Orthohantavirus species	Natural host reservoir (common name)	Geographic distribution	Associated disease	References
Orthohantavirus luxiense (LUXV)	*Eothenomys miletus* (Yunnan red-backed vole)	Asia (China)	Unknown	Zhang et al., (2011)
Orthohantavirus jejuense (JJUV)	*Crocidura shantungensis* (Asian lesser white-toothed shrew)	Asia (South Korea)	Unknown	Arai et al., (2012)
Orthohantavirus caobangense (CBNV)	*Anourosorex squamipes* (Chinese mole shrew)	China and Vietnam	Unknown	Song, Kang and et al., (2007a, 2007b)
Orthohantavirus yakeshiense (YKSV)	*Sorex isodon* (Taiga shrew)	Asia (China)	Unknown	Guo et al., (2013)
Orthohantavirus kenkemeense (KKMV)	*Ulotrichous talpoides* (Japanese shrew mole)	Asia (Japan)	unknown	Arai et al., (2008)
Orthohantavirus kenkemeense (KKMV)	*Sorex roboratus* (Flat-skulled shrew)	Altai (Russia), northeast China	Unknown	Wang et al., (2014)
Orthohantavirus asikkalaense (ASIV)	*Sorex minutus, S. araneus* (Common shrew)	Central Europe	Unknown	Ling et al., (2014), Radosa et al., (2013)
Orthohantavirus boweense (BOWV)	*Crocidura douceti* (Doucet's musk shrew)	Guinea	Unknown	Gu et al., (2013)
Orthohantavirus brugesense (BRGV)	*Talpa europaea* (European mole)	Central Europe	Unknown	Laenen et al., (2018)
Orthohantavirus dobravaense (DOBV)	*Apodemus agrarius* (Striped field mouse)	Eurasian continent	HFRS	Leopardi et al., (2022)
Orthohantavirus sangassouense (SANGV)	*Hylomyscus simus* (African wood mouse)	Guinea, Kenya	Unknown	Klempa et al., (2012)
Orthohantavirus seewisense (SWSV)	*Sorex araneus* (Common shrew)	Eurasian continent	Unknown	Kikuchi et al., (2023), Yashina et al. (2021)

(continued)

Table 2.2 (continued)

Orthohantavirus species	Natural host reservoir (common name)	Geographic distribution	Associated disease	References
Orthohantavirus tatenalense (TATV)	*Microtus agrestis* (Short-tailed field vole)	Central Europe	Unknown	Chappell et al., (2020)
Orthohantavirus tigrayense (TIGV)	*Stenocephalomys albipes* (Ethiopian white-footed mouse)	Ethiopia	Unknown	Meheretu et al., (2019)
Orthohantavirus tulaense (TULV)	*Microtus arvalis* (Common vole)	Eurasian continent	HFRS	Schlegel et al., (2012)
Orthohantavirus robinaense (ROBV)	*Pteropus alecto* (Black fruit bat)	Australia	Unknown	(GenBank)

* According to ICTV taxonomy, SOOV and AMRV are genetic variants of HNTV. ** According to ICTV taxonomy, HOKV and MUJV are genetic variants of PUUV

2.5 Genetic Diversity of Pathogenic Orthohantaviruses

Phylogenetic analysis of orthohantaviruses demonstrated two distinct clades formed by viruses in Europe and Asia. PUUV and TULV orthohantaviruses, circulating in rodents in Europe, appear genetically related. In contrast, DOBV from Europe and HTNV and SEOV from Asia form a separate clade (Plyusnin & Sironen, 2014). Also, these viruses are closely related to THAIV from Asia (Kariwa, 2007). Interestingly, orthohantaviruses circulating in Europe could also be endemic in Asia, as PUUV was found in *Myodes rufous*, *Apodemus speciosus*, and *Apodemus argenteus* from Japan (Kikuchi et al., 2021). Several other endemic orthohantaviruses were also identified in Asia (Milholland et al., 2018; Wang et al., 2014; Yanagihara et al., 2014; Yashina et al., 2022).

Analysis of the complete S, M, and L segment sequences indicated that orthohantavirus species could have consisted of several genetic lineages. Nine, six, four and eight lineages could be identified for HNTV, SEOV, DOBV and PUUV species, respectively (Cao et al., 2016; Klempa et al., 2013; Razzauti et al., 2012). Nucleotide sequence analysis of the M segment showed higher genetic variability in the HNTV compared to SEOV strains (Wang et al., 2000). The genetic diversity among HNTV lineages differs between 12 to 15%, while the sequence variation between DOBV lineages could reach up to 14% (Avsic-Zupanc et al., 2000). The highest level of the genome (S, M, and L segments) diversity is found among the PUUV strains, reaching 11 to 19% (de Vries et al., 2016). It is also demonstrated that the PUUV M segment is the most variable, while changes in the L segment are rare compared to the S segment (Kabwe et al., 2020).

The S segment coding region of PUUV is divided into N and NSs (non-structural) proteins of 433 aa and 90 aa long, respectively (Binder et al., 2020). The identity of N protein is 94–100%, while the NSs go up to 70% between PUUV lineages (Binder et al., 2020). Among the glycoprotein (Gn and Gc) aa sequences coded by the M segment, the identity ranges from 89–100% and 99–100% between inter-lineage and intra-lineage sequences, respectively (Lober et al., 2001; Pljusnin & Elliott, 2011). Among some PUUV strains, aa sequence differences in Gn and Gc proteins reach 7%. This percentage is higher than the agreed value for the classification of PUUV strains by the international taxonomy between different orthohantaviruses (de Oliveira et al., 2014). However, this observation indicates the circulation of two distinct genes of PUUV at the same location. As a result, individual rodents could be found with a mixture of closely related variants of strains.

The aa sequence identity for the RdRp, coded by the L segment, among PUUV strains of the same lineage, is 93.4% to 96.1% (Ali et al., 2015; Pljusnin & Elliott, 2011). When the RdRp aa sequences are compared between PUUV lineages, the identities go up to 94% (Ali et al., 2015; Pljusnin & Elliott, 2011). The RdRp plays an important role in virus replication, essential for preserving the aa sequence accuracy. This could be explained by the high sequence identities observed.

In Asia and Europe, orthohantaviruses circulate in specific small rodent hosts such as *Apodemus agrarius*, *Rattus norvegicus*, *A. flavicollis*, *Myodes glareolus*, *Microtus arvalis*, and *Bandicota indica* (Kabwe et al., 2020; Milholland et al., 2018). Orthohantavirses are also isolated from insectivores and bats (Guo et al., 2013). Studies have demonstrated the congruency in the phylogenetic tree for orthohantaviruses and their corresponding hosts (Holmes & Zhang, 2015; Yanagihara et al., 2014).

Orthohantaviruses' phylogeny and host relationships analysis demonstrated a host-virus phylogenetic congruence, which supports the hypothesis of their co-evolution and co-divergence from a common ancestor (Plyusnin & Morzunov, 2001). However, hypotheses are challenging this assumption (Holmes & Zhang, 2015). Souza et al. data suggest that the co-speciation of orthohantaviruses resulted from the host switch from Murinae to Arvicorinae and happened about 500–700 years ago (Souza et al., 2014). It was proposed that orthohantavirus' common ancestor had originated from China approximately 2000 years ago. After that, new species of orthohantaviruses evolved and spread out due to natural hosts' migration. This migration could make them geographically isolated, where orthohantavirus strains continue evolving independently (Souza et al., 2014).

Within the co-evolution theory, calculating the evolution rate of PUUV, HNTV, TULV, and Japanese PUUV-like viruses demonstrated values in interval 0.7 × 10–7–2.2 × 10–6 synonymous nucleotide substitutions/site/year (Sironen et al., 2001). In another study by Ramsden et al., a lower rate, ~ 3 × 10–4 and ~ 5.5 × 10–4 substitutions/site/year was calculated for DOBV and PUUV, respectively (Souza et al., 2014). The use of different methods for substitution/site/year calculations calculation could explain these variations. Other authors noted that genetic drift due to the accumulation of deletions and point mutations contributes more to orthohantavirus genome variations (Razzauti et al., 2013). The leading cause of genetic drift is the limited proofreading activity of viral RdRp, which leads to the incorporation of many mismatched nucleotides during genome replication (Choi, 2012).

Studies have shown that the reassortment and recombination could contribute to orthohantaviruses' genome variability (Klempa, 2018). Reassortment is characterized by an exchange of the genome segments among virus species coinfecting the same host cell. This exchange is mainly found between different strains of the same orthohantavirus species or between strains circulating in closely related host species (Kim et al., 2016; Razzauti et al., 2008). Among the orthohantaviruses circulating in Asia and Europe, reassortment was studied more in PUUV strains. For example, some PUUV strains isolated from bank voles in Finland were found to be reassortants (Razzauti et al., 2008). Most of these reassortants had the S-L/M or M-L/S genome variants, while the S-M/L variants were rare (Razzauti et al., 2013). Additionally, reassortment was reported in HNTV isolated in the Republic of Korea, where HTNV strains had S and M segments from one genetic group while the L segment was from another (Kim et al., 2016). In contrast, Lee et al. later showed that HNTV reassortants could include M and L segments from one ancestor and an S segment from another (Kim et al., 2016).

Indications of reassortment events were found within DOBV species but are still regarded as inter-lineage events (Meheretu et al., 2019). Compared with other orthohantaviruses associated with a single host, DOBV lineages are identified in distinct species of *Apodemus* sp. mice and are designed as genotypes (Meheretu et al., 2012). Assortments were observed among the DOBV lineages identified in striped field mice (*A. agrarius*) on Saaremaa island and Estonia; the M segment clustered within another *A. agrarius*-associated genotype designated Kurkino virus, while the S segment was closely related to the *A. flavicollis*- and *A. ponticus*-associated Dobrava and Sochi genotypes, respectively (Ali et al., 2015). The reassortment pattern $S_AM_BL_A$ was identified in MJNV from the Republic of Korea (Lee et al., 2017). Conflict in the L and S segments tree topologies was found among the Seewis viruses, suggesting multiple reassortment events (Ling et al., 2018).

It should be noted that the resulting reassortants are genetically distinct from both parental viruses and could have altered replication in the host cell (Rodriguez et al., 1998). Some data suggested that the inter-reassortants retain L and S segments from one parental species. This could be explained by the co-operating role of encoded proteins, RdRp and N protein, in viral RNA transcription and protein synthesis, respectively (Rizvanov et al., 2004). M segment codes for G proteins, which bind to the host cell receptors and initiate membrane fusion (Rey, 2021). It was suggested that M-segment reassortants could have altered the ability to infect cells, leading to a higher replication rate (Muyangwa et al., 2015; Rizvanov et al., 2004). These studies suggest that the exchange with the M segment could change the ability of the virus to infect cells and potentially increase virulence.

Recombination also plays a role in the genetic diversity of orthohantaviruses. Unlike reassortment, recombination refers to the exchange of genome fragments within the segment. Recombination in orthohantavirus has been reported in nature (Asikainen et al., 2000) and in laboratories (Zhang et al., 2010). Phylogenetic analysis of 3′ noncoding region (3′-NCR) of TULV strains from eastern Slovakian, western

Slovakia and the Czech Republic revealed disparities in the tree topologies. Interestingly, the eastern Slovakian strains clustered with western Slovakia and the Czech Republic strains, suggesting a recombinant pattern of the S segment in the eastern Slovakian TULV lineage.

Further analysis of these strains by boots can search showed two recombination points in the S sequences of eastern Slovakian TULV strains (nt 400 to 415 and around 1200). This was confirmed by the pattern of amino acid substitutions in the N protein (Sibold et al., 1999). Asikainen et al. showed the possible recombinant origin of the PUUV S segment genome from the Danish genetic lineage (Asikainen et al., 2000). In addition, it was suggested that the M segment of the PUUV Mo47 strain, circulating in the territory of Belgium, originated as a result of recombination (Escutenaire & Pastoret, 2001; Escutenaire et al., 2001). A similar pattern has been seen later for the Baltic PUUV strains (Sironen et al., 2001).

Our understanding of the mechanisms of natural recombination and its effect on orthohantavirus pathogenicity still needs to be discovered.

It is also suggested that the genetic diversity and molecular evolution of orthohantaviruses are affected by host switches (Bennett et al., 2014). Guo et al. proposed the order of orthohataviruses host switches: from shrews to bats and subsequently to rodents (Guo et al., 2013). Such host switches lead to virus adaptation to the new host and the emergence of new orthohatavirus species (Bennett et al., 2014).

Thus, genetic drift, recombination and reassortment, host switches, virus and host co-evolution could affect the speed of orthohantavirus evolution.

2.6 Transmission

Virus transmission is the most crucial stage in establishing infection. The most common route of orthohantavirus transmission is inhaling aerosol contaminated with the virus released by rodents (Lokugamage et al., 2002). It was demonstrated that orthohantaviruses could be transmitted by intramuscular injection; however, the aerosol route appears to have about 100 times higher efficacy in establishing infection. This data supports the notion that the orthohantaviruses spread primarily by inhaling aerosol contaminated with the virus (Fig. 2.4). The virus-containing aerosol could be produced when fresh rodent urine, droppings, or nesting materials are stirred, and small droplets containing the virus are released into the air (Pljusnin & Elliott, 2011). In addition to aerosol, orthohantaviruses could be transmitted by: (a) rodent bites, which is rare, (b) contact with rodents' urine, faeces, or saliva, or (c) ingesting food contaminated with urine, faeces, or saliva from infected rats (Song, Baek, et al., 2007a, 2007b).

The objective to reduce the spillover of viruses from natural hosts to humans requires a better understanding of the ecology and epizootiology of zoonotic pathogens. Studies have shown that the prevalence and transmission rates of viruses within host populations depend on the ecosystem, affecting the incidence of orthohantavirus diseases (Dearing & Dizney, 2010; Khalil et al., 2014). Environmental

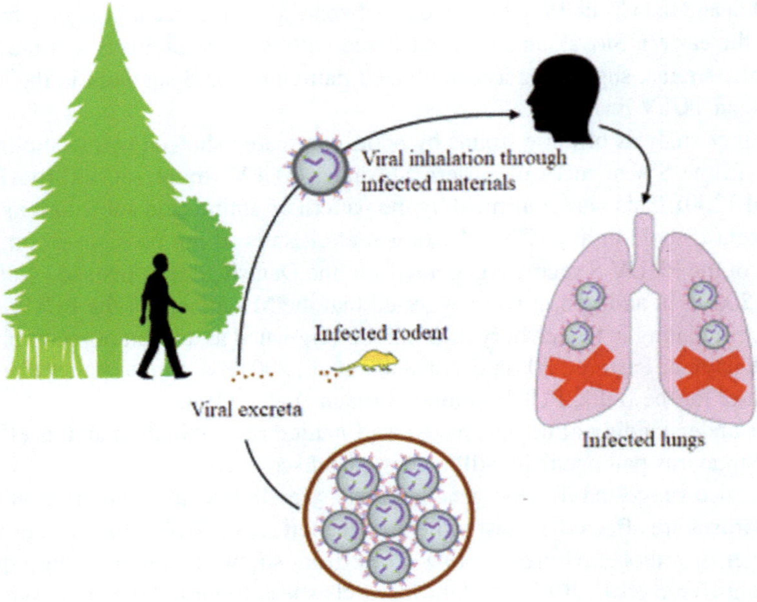

Fig. 2.4 Schematic presentation of orthohantavirus infection cycle. As the rodent population densities increase, the spread of orthohantaviruses among rodents increases proportionally. In rodent and or insectivore populations, orthohantaviruses are horizontally transmitted through aggressive behaviour and exposure to aerosolized contaminated droppings. Usually, humans are considered to be the dead-end hosts of orthohantaviruses and become infected by breathing aerosolized rodent excreta containing the virus. The Fig. was adapted from Kabwe et al. (2020)

changes, such as global warming, habitat reduction, and changes in the landscape, could affect the behaviour, host density, and diversity of small mammals carrying orthohantaviruses (Khalil et al., 2014). Supporting the role of the environment was the study by Dearing and Dizney demonstrating that natural climate cycles such as El Ni˜no and anthropogenic climate changes could enhance orthohantavirus prevalence (Dearing & Dizney, 2010). Territories highly affected by human activity are often associated with a high rate of zoonotic disease emergence (Jonsson et al., 2010; Mills, 2005). Five regulators of zoonotic virus prevalence and transmission have been suggested, such as (i) environmental regulators, (ii) anthropogenic factors, (iii) genetic factors, (iv) behavioural factors, and (v) physiological factors (Jonsson et al., 2010). Therefore, the disease incidence rate control could be improved by investigating how environmental changes affect the transmission of the viruses among the hosts (Lokugamage et al., 2002).

2.7 Clinical Presentation

More than 38 orthohantavirus species are identified worldwide; nevertheless, 12 are associated with the disease in humans (de Oliveira et al., 2014; Jiang et al., 2017; Jonsson et al., 2010; Kuhn & Schmaljohn, 2023; Noack et al., 2020; Reusken & Heyman, 2013). The spectrum ranges from acute febrile illness with or without renal impairment, fever with shock, and multi-organ failure to hemorrhagic illness such as HFRS. Hemorrhage and acute renal injury (AKI) are common clinical manifestations in severe HFRS cases (Krautkramer & Zeier, 2014).

The clinical presentation of HFRS may range from subclinical to mild to moderate to severe. HTNV, DOBV, and AMRV more often cause severe HFRS, while the moderate form is frequently diagnosed in SEOV causes. Also, Nephropathia epidemica (NE), a mild form of HFRS linked to PUUV infection, is diagnosed in Russia and European countries (Jonsson et al., 2010).

The incubation period of HFRS generally ranges between two and four weeks; however, in some cases, it could be as long as six weeks (Jonsson et al., 2010). Clinically, HFRS progresses through five phases: febrile, hypotensive, oliguric, polyuric, and convalescent. These phases are demarcated in severe HFRS but may overlap or be absent in mild and moderate forms of the disease (Jiang et al., 2016; Jonsson et al., 2010).

The febrile phase usually lasts three to seven days and is characterized by high fever, chills, headache, backache, abdominal pains, nausea, and vomiting. Symptoms are non-specific, making orthohantavirus infection diagnosis challenging during this phase. By day three to four post-onset, hemorrhagic manifestations appear in diffuse petechiae on the conjunctiva and the palate. AKI symptoms of hematuria and proteinuria become evident by day seven of the disease (Guang et al., 1989).

Shock is typical for the severe form of HFRS. Approximately 11–40% of febrile patients develop hypotension, and one-third have a shock (Jonsson et al., 2010). The hypotensive phase could last from several hours to a couple of days. Thrombocytopenia and leukocytosis are commonly documented during this phase. Also, symptoms of an AKI, such as acute tubulointerstitial nephritis, necrotizing glomerulonephritis, and IgA nephropathy, are characteristic of this phase (Sehgal et al., 2023).

The oliguric phase lasts three to seven days. Patients are at risk of hypotension, severe pulmonary oedema, and AKI, as symptoms of oliguria, anuria, proteinuria, hematuria, and azotemia are commonly described. The severe form of HFRS could require hemodialysis at this phase. This is the critical phase, as half of the total fatalities occur during this phase. Typical laboratory findings are elevated serum creatinine and urea (Jiang et al., 2017; Kruger et al., 2001). The polyuric phase, which could last for days or weeks, is characterized by increased urinary output. The renal function is restored, and symptoms of AKI dissolve.

Convalescence is usually extended and could last up to six months. Recovery is complete, though sequelae of chronic renal failure and hypertension have been reported (Vaheri et al., 2013; Wang et al., 2013). The fatality rate of 5–15% in

HTNV/DOBV-related HFRS is likely due to complications, such as renal insufficiency, oedema, haemorrhages, encephalopathy, and shock. SEOV infection causes a moderate form of HFRS with a clinical presentation similar to HFRS caused by HTNV (Linderholm & Elgh, 2001). The SEOV infection fatality rate is 1% (Shastri et al., 2019). Even lower than 1.0% is the mortality rate of PUUV infection (Bergstedt Oscarsson et al., 2016).

2.8 Treatment

There are no specific post-exposure therapeutics for HFRS. Therefore, treatment may differ between healthcare facilities adapting to patient management protocols based on the local regulatory authority's recommendations. Therapeutics for HFRS could be classified as targeting viruses, immune response, or supportive therapy.

Therapeutics targeting viruses could block virus entry and replication. Neutralizing antibodies can bind to surface glycoproteins, preventing binding to integrin receptors. Transfer of orthohantavirus convalescent serum containing neutralizing antibodies was shown to have a protective effect in the non-randomized multi-centre trial (Vial et al., 2015). Also, the protection efficacy of convalescent serum was confirmed in vivo experiments (Xu et al., 2002; Zhang et al., 1989). Several monoclonal antibodies with neutralizing activity were generated against HNTV (Hooper et al., 2001; Xu et al., 2002). Phase I and II clinical studies have demonstrated the therapeutic efficacy of these neutralizing antibodies in the early stage of HFRS(Xu et al., 2002, 2009).

Novel therapeutic approaches targeting orthohantavirus entry are still in the development stage. One is based on the peptides binding to αvβ3 integrin receptors (Hall et al., 2010). Orthohantaviruses bind to this integrin receptor for cell entry (Antoine et al., 2021). Therefore, the initial interaction between orthohantavirus and the integrin receptor is crucial in virus replication. Virus entry could be abrogated by preventing this interaction, protecting cells from infection. A study by Song et al. supported this hypothesis, where monoclonal antibodies to β3 integrin protected mice from HNTV infection (Song et al., 2005). This concept was further developed by Hall et al., where peptides binding to integrin receptors were shown to block orthohantavirus entry (Hall et al., 2008). A follow-up study demonstrated the efficacy of neutralizing SNV, ANDV, and HTNV by selected cyclic nonapeptides (Hall et al., 2010). In vivo, studies could evaluate the therapeutic efficacy of these peptides against orthohantaviruses.

Another approach targets virus replication. Ribavirin is one of the earliest drugs tested for its therapeutic efficacy against orthohantavirus infection. Ribavirin is a nucleotide analogue (1-beta-D-ribofuranosyl 1,2,4-triazole-3-carboxamide) used to treat HFRS (Huggins et al., 1991; Malinin & Platonov, 2017). The primary mechanism of antiviral activity of this drug is the induction of mutation into the viral RNA, leading to fatal errors (Severson et al., 2003). Clinical trials demonstrated reduced morbidity and mortality in HFRS when treatment was initiated early after HNTV

Jameson exposure (Huggins et al., 1991). However, later initiation of treatment was less effective. A lack of Ribavirin therapeutic efficacy was reported when treating PUUV-infected patients (Malinin & Platonov, 2017). Another drug used is Favipiravir, an antiviral drug that selectively inhibits the RdRp of negative strand segmented viruses (Furuta et al., 2017). The efficacy of Favipiravir was demonstrated against New World orthohantaviruses SNV and ANDV in vitro and in vivo (Mayor et al., 2021). Similar to Ribavirin, the protective effect of this drug was demonstrated only when used at the early stage of infection. Late administration failed to reduce virus load and protect hamsters from lethal ANDV infection.

Targeting the immune response: Activation of the kinin–kallikrein system and liberation of bradykinin were shown in endothelial cells infected by HNTV and ANDV (Taylor et al., 2013). This bradykinin was suggested to contribute to increased vascular permeability in ortho hantavirus-infected patients. Inhibition of bradykinin was introduced as a novel approach for treating orthohantavirus infection. Icatibant, a blocker of bradykinin binding to its receptor, was effective in some case reports. Antonen et al. have shown the efficacy of icatibant in PUUV infection cases, where a single dose stabilizes the patient's condition and complete recovery (Antonen et al., 2013). Similar to this case study, Laine et al. reported a successful outcome using icatibant (Laine et al., 2015) in another PUUV infection case.

Corticosteroids are most commonly used to treat orthohantavirus infection because of their anti-inflammatory effect (Rhen & Cidlowski, 2005). Also, decreased corticosteroids were demonstrated in orthohantavirus-infected rats (Easterbrook & Klein, 2008), suggesting the role of these hormones in the pathogenesis of this infection. Data from HNTV and PUUV-infected patients supported the hypothesis of corticosteroids' contribution to the pathogenesis of HFRS. Damage to hypophysis and the adrenal gland could lower cortisol levels and potentially contribute to inflammation (Hautala et al., 2002; Steer, 1955). This data supported the inclusion of corticosteroids in the HFRS treatment protocol. Rapid recovery was demonstrated in two severe PUUV cases after administering corticosteroids (Seitsonen et al., 2006). Also, thrombocyte counts were restored in NE patients after initiating prednisolone treatment (Dunst et al., 1998; Latus et al., 2015). However, the lack of corticosteroid therapeutic effect in ANDV-infected patients was reported by Vial et al. in a double-blind, randomized controlled clinical trial (Vial et al., 2013).

Supportive therapy: Supportive therapy is fundamental for HFRS management. Fluid and electrolyte replacement therapy maintains blood pressure ((HFRS)—). Thrombocyte transfusion is used in severe thrombocytopenia; however, caution should be exercised to prevent thrombosis (Connolly-Andersen et al., 2018). Additionally, continuous renal replacement therapy was effective in patients with multiple organ dysfunction syndromes (Ying et al., 2020).

2.9 Vaccines

Treatment of orthohantavirus infection is supportive and not specific (*Centers for Disease Control and Prevention Technical/Clinical Information: HPS Treatment—Hantavirus. Available online:* https://www.cdc.gov/hantavirus/technical/hps/treatment.html *(12.07.2022).*; Dheerasekara et al., 2020). Therefore, the main form of orthohantavirus control is to prevent infection. Prevention measures include minimizing exposure to rodents and utilizing vaccination.

Minimizing human exposure: Inhaling virus-contaminated aerosol or direct contact with rodent excreta are routes of orthohantavirus infection ("Centers for Disease Control and Prevention Facts about Hantaviruses. What You Need to Know to Prevent the Disease Pulmonary Syndrome (HPS). Available online: https://www.cdc.gov/hantavirus/pdf/hps_brochure.pdf (23.08.2022)."). In order to minimize exposure, measures should be taken to prevent small rodent entry into buildings ("PAHO/WHO Hantavirus. Available online: https://www3.paho.org/hq/index.php?option=com_content&view=article&id=14911:hantavirus&Itemid=40721&lang=en#:~:text=Hantavirus%20(HV)%20is%20an%20emerging,of%20respiratory%20distress%20and%20hypotension (13.10.2022)."; Zhang et al., 2004). Also, rodent control inside and around the home and workplaces will reduce contact with infected small mammals. Rodent urine and droppings should be removed regularly ("Centers for Disease Control and Prevention Cleaning Up after Rodents|Rodents|CDC. Availa-ble online: https://www.cdc.gov/rodents/prevent_infestations/clean_up.html#:~:text=Clean%20up%20rodent%20urine%20and,or%20droppings%20and%20cleaning%20product (15.09.2022)."). Clean-up starts with ventilation of the space for at least 30 min (Jonsson et al., 2010), followed by spraying and soaking urine and droppings with disinfectant before removal.

Monitoring the rodent population by local authorities is essential for predicting and preventing orthohantavirus outbreaks. Multiple small mammals identified in Asia could carry HNTV, SEOV, and THAIV (Tian & Stenseth, 2019). These carrier mammals include *A. agrarius*, the primary reservoir host for HTNV (Park et al., 2021), and *R. norvegicus*, the carrier for SEOV (Ling et al., 2019). Also, such species as *B. indica*, *R. rattus*, and Major's tufted-tailed rat should be included in the monitoring as they are shown to be reservoirs for THAIV (Raharinosy et al., 2018; Reynes et al., 2014). Studies have shown that the density of the population could affect the horizontal transmission of orthohantavirus, increasing the number of infected small rodents (Mills, 2005; Olsson et al., 2002). It was also demonstrated that the threshold density of the rodent population is required to maintain orthohantavirus (Khalil et al., 2014; Mills, 2005; Tian et al., 2017). A higher number of infected small mammals could increase the chance of human contact and exposure to orthohantavirus. Therefore, the efficacy of zoonotic carrier population control remains a necessary measure to prevent orthohantavirus infection.

Hantavirus vaccine: There is no World Health Organization (WHO) approved vaccine to prevent orthohantavirus infection. Likewise, local authorities do not approve the orthohantavirus vaccine in endemic areas such as Europe and North and

South America (Schmaljohn, 2012). However, inactivated orthohantavirus vaccines are licensed in China and Korea (Liu et al., 2019). Inactivated rodent brain or cell culture-derived HFRS vaccines are used in China (Dong et al., 2005). In 1993, the first inactivated orthohantavirus vaccine was approved in China [11]. Since then, four inactivated HTNV and SEOV-based vaccines have been used in China and demonstrated the safety and efficacy of protection ("Chen, H.X.; Luo, Z.Z.; Zhang, J.J. Hantavirus Vaccine Efficacy Evaluation Working Group. Large Scale Field Evaluation on Vaccines of Hemorrhagic Fever with Renal Syndrome in Chi-na. Chin. J. Epidemiol. 2002, 23, 145–147.,"). An inactivated HFRS vaccine was also used in Korea 1990 (Cho et al., 2002). Since the beginning of vaccination, the number of HFRS cases has reduced significantly (Cho et al., 2002). The vaccine's effectiveness was also reported by Park et al.; however, the authors state that using a large cohort and an extended monitoring period is required to make conclusions regarding vaccine efficacy (Park et al., 2004).

During the 30 years of the HFRS vaccine development, novel approaches were developed to improve the delivery, orthohantavirus antigens expression, the efficacy of the immune system activation, and reducing side effects.

Inactivated vaccines: These were the first type of vaccines containing inactivated orthohantavirus virion (Cho et al., 2002). HNTV was propagated in the brains of suckling mice, followed by chemical inactivation before being tested for immunogenicity (Yamanishi et al., 1988). In 1990, under the commercial name Hantavax, this vaccine was tested in a clinical trial where safety and seroconversion of over 90% were demonstrated (Cho & Howard, 1999; Song et al., 2016). Neutralizing antibodies were also demonstrated in 75% vaccinated one month after the booster (Cho & Howard, 1999). Several studies demonstrated less antibody prevalence, 23 and 41%, (Sohn et al., 2001; Song et al., 2016). Studies have demonstrated anti-orthohantavirus antibodies several months after immunization (Sohn et al., 2001; Song et al., 2020). Also, the immune response was detected one year after immunization (Song et al., 2016). The protective efficacy of the Hantavax vaccine was suggested to explain the decline in the number of HFRS cases in South Korea between 1991 and 1997 (Cho et al., 2002). Later studies aimed to analyse the Hantavax vaccine's effect on disease progression and demonstrated the reduction of stage 3 acute kidney injury and the requirement for dialysis in the vaccinated cohort (Yi et al., 2018). In another study, the efficacy of the anti-orthohantavirus vaccine was demonstrated in an immunized cohort from Yugoslavia ("Chu, Y.K.; Gligic, A.; Tomanovic, S.; Bozovjc, B.; Obradovic, M.; Woo, Y.D.; An, C.N.; Kim, H.; Jiang, Y.S.; Park, S.C.; et al. A Field Efficacy Trial of Inactivated Hantaan Virus Vaccine (Hantavax(TM)) Against Hemorrhagic Fever with Renal Syndrome (HFRS) in the Endemic Areas of Yugoslavia from 1996 to 1998. Journal of the Korean Society of Virology 1999, 29, 55–64.,"). Also, the developers of Hantavax, in collaboration with the Yugoslavia research team, demonstrated the vaccine's protective efficacy (Park et al., 2004).

Inactivated hantavirus vaccines in South Korea have been controversial regarding their effectiveness (Jung et al., 2018). In contrast, studies of vaccines in China showed that the absorbance value of HFRS-IgG was four times higher in vaccinated persons than those nonimmunized in the epidemic areas (Wang et al., 2012).

Later, the protective effectiveness of the three-dose regimen of the inactivated HFRS vaccine compared to the two-dose regimen was demonstrated (Wang et al., 2012).

Bivalent, HNTV, and SEOV inactivated orthohantavirus vaccines were manufactured in China (Maes et al., 2009). The persistence of anti-orthohantavirus antibodies was demonstrated after a three-dose series in China (Zheng et al., 2018). In another study, the bivalent inactivated vaccine induced anti-orthohantavirus antibodies one month after immunization (Li et al., 2017). Antibodies were detectable 33 months after vaccination. Recently, pre-clinical studies of inactivated polyvalent HFRS vaccine demonstrated the activation of a balanced immune response to PUUV, HNTV, and DOBV (Dzagurova et al., 2020).

Virus-like particle (VLP) vaccine: Inactivated vaccines effectively activate the humoral immune response. However, these vaccines had substantial limitations, such as failure to induce long-term antibody response, multiple immunizations, and potential side effects. Therefore, there was still an interest in developing vaccines to address these obstacles. VLP vaccine could provide a solution to some of these limitations. Several VLP are nano-sized self-assembly competent structures made by viral proteins (*Wagenknecht, H.-A. Book Review. Protein Science, 2009, 13, 3331–3332.* https://doi.org/https://doi.org/10.1110/ps.041082704.). The VLP have spike proteins, which could bind to the host receptor (Acuna et al., 2014; Fougeroux et al., 2021). Therefore, VLP host cell entry resembles a natural infection. However, VLPs lack nucleic acid, rendering them incapable of replication (*Wagenknecht, H.-A. Book Review. Protein Science, 2009, 13, 3331–3332.* https://doi.org/https://doi.org/10.1110/ps.041082704.). As a result, VLPs could deliver the viral antigens to the host cells without virus replication and, subsequently, disease symptoms. This feature of VLP made them an attractive tool for developing second-generation vaccines.

The efficacy of the VLP containing HNTV N and Gn/Gc proteins was tested in a mouse model (Cheng et al., 2016). To enhance the immunogenicity, HNTV chimeric VLPs containing glycosylphosphatidylinositol (GPI)-anchored granulocyte–macrophage colony-stimulating factor (GM-CSF) or CD40 ligand (CD40L) were generated. These chimeric VLPs induce humoral and cellular immune responses, which are more potent than HNTV VLP or commercially available inactivated vaccines. It should be noted that chimeric VLPs also protected mice from the HTNV challenge. Cheng et al. obtained similar results using GM-CSF-CD40L chimeric VLP (Cheng et al., 2016). Additionally, authors have demonstrated that incorporating GM-CSF-CD40L stimulated macrophages and dendritic cells. In another study by Dong et al., chimeric VLPs were shown to induce long-term immune responses with neutralizing antibodies circulating six months after immunization (Dong et al., 2019).

Production of anti-orthohantavirus antibodies was evidenced after immunization with chimeric hepatitis B virus (HBV) particles containing PUUV N protein polypeptide (Koletzki et al., 1999). These chimeric HBVs expressing PUUV N protein polypeptide induced a protective immune response in bank voles, the natural reservoir of the PUUV (Ulrich et al., 1999). Another study demonstrated the immunogenic efficacy of HBV core particles carrying the N protein polypeptide of the DOBV, HNTV, or PUUV in a mice model (McClain et al., 2000). These chimeric particles induced a high titer of cross-reactive antibodies (Geldmacher, Skrastina, et al., 2004a, 2004b).

DNA vaccine: DNA vaccines have multiple advantages over inactivated vaccines. They are safe, as they are replication defective. They are also non-virulent and fail to produce clinical symptoms of the disease. As early as 1992, the HNTV DNA vaccine expressing N and G proteins was developed using the vaccinia virus as a vector (Schmaljohn et al., 1992). This vaccine elicited a protective immune response in a hamster model. The same vaccine was later proved protective against HNTV, SEOV, and PUUV (Chu et al., 1995).

Interestingly, anti-HNTV neutralizing antibodies were detected in immunized animals. In contrast, there were no antibodies to the SEOV virus. In clinical trials phase I, neutralizing antibodies were demonstrated in immunized individuals. However, previous exposure to the vaccinia virus appears to interfere with the efficacy of developing neutralizing antibodies in volunteers (McClain et al., 2000).

DNA vaccines appear to be immunogenic and induce neutralizing antibody responses. For example, two DNA vaccines, HTNV and PUUV, were tested in phase I clinical trials (Boudreau et al., 2012). Both vaccines elicited neutralizing antibodies; however, only about half of the vaccinated were seropositive. DNA vaccine against SEOV induced antibody response in Syrian hamsters and protected against infection (Hooper et al., 2001). Rhesus monkey immunization with another DNA vaccine, coding for HNTV and ANDV M segment genome, was shown to induce neutralizing antibodies (Hooper et al., 2006). Neutralizing antibodies can bind to envelop proteins and prevent viral entry (Klasse & Sattentau, 2002; Pantophlet & Burton, 2006). This reduces virus infectivity and prevents dissemination. The ability to elicit neutralizing antibodies is an established benchmark for assessing vaccine efficacy.

Subunit vaccines: Orthohantavirus Gn/Gc and N proteins could elicit a strong humoral immune response (Dantas et al., 1986; Park & Kim, 2008; Pettersson et al., 2014). Gn/Gc proteins could induce neutralizing antibody response (Rissanen et al., 2021), while N protein activates non-neutralizing antibodies (Lundkvist & Niklasson, 1992). Additionally, the N protein stimulates the T cell immune response (Elgh et al., 1998; Wang et al., 2011). N protein was shown to induce the cross-reacting immune response (de Carvalho Nicacio et al., 2002; Van Epps et al., 1999). Similarly, recombinant DOBV N protein-induced antibodies cross-react with PUUV and HNTV in mice (Geldmacher, Schmaler, et al., 2004a, 2004b). In another study, immunization with SEOV recombinant N protein induced high-titer antibody (Schmidt et al., 2005). Recently, the efficacy of eliciting humoral and T cell immune response by delivery of PUUV Gn/Gc and N protein using microvesicles was demonstrated (Shkair et al., 2022). However, the efficacy of these recombinant proteins' protection against lethal infection remains to be determined (Kruger et al., 2011).

2.10 Impact of Interventions on HFRS Outbreak During COVID-19 Pandemic

In December 2019, cases of an unidentified illness were reported in Wuhan, Hubei Province, China. As a result of the increased infection rate and severe outcome, the illness was quickly identified to be caused by a novel coronavirus named severe acute respiratory syndrome coronavirus 2 (SARS-CoV-2) (Spiteri et al., 2020) as it had a genome similar to that of the coronavirus infection that caused the SARS outbreak in 2003 (Gupta et al., 2020). Subsequently, the disease was caused by coronavirus disease 2019 (COVID-19) (Spiteri et al., 2020). The virus rapidly spread worldwide, causing a serious threat to human global health (Mizumoto et al., 2020; Wang et al., 2020), leading to the World Health Organization to declare a pandemic on March 11 2020 ("Baygildina, A.A. Modern ideas about the pathogenesis of hemorrhagic fever with renal syndrome / A.A. Baygildina // Medical Bulletin of Bashkortostan. – 2014. – T.9, No.1. – pp. 98–108,"; Gralinski & Menachery, 2020; Wang et al., 2020).

As a response to the outbreak, many countries developed stringent measures to combat the spread of the virus. In the first cases reported in the provinces of China, including Jiangsu and Hubei Provinces, the government swiftly restricted the movement of people (J. T. Wu et al., 2020a, 2020b, 2020c). On January 22, 2020, Jiangsu Province confirmed the first case of COVID-19; soon after, mainland China warned the world that the new virus was lethal and contingent (Singhal, 2020). The Chinese government developed rapid countermeasures, including lockdowns, travel restrictions and work suspensions to stop the virus's spread (Kurita et al., 2021; Shen et al., 2020).

The European countries, including Finland, France, Germany, Italy, Spain, Sweden, and the UK, reported COVID-19 cases in January 2020. Later, the cases spread throughout Europe, and many countries imposed preventive measures such as the closure of airports, lockdowns, restrictions on the movement of people and suspension of sports and cultural activities (Al-Salem et al., 2021). The spread of the virus continued to rise, and by March 11, the infections were diagnosed worldwide. In collaboration with the WHO, most countries imposed stringent measures to help control the infection. Measures, including the closure of the universities and schools, were put in place, camping and hiking were suspended, and mass gatherings of people were put on hold. Many researchers report that these restrictions effectively controlled the spread of COVID-19 (Choi & Ki, 2020; Ji et al., 2020; "Organization WH. COVID19 STRATEGY UPDATE. 2020;1–18. https://www.who.int/COVID19 STRATEGY UPDATE. Accessed 10 Dec 2020").

However, these measures also influenced the surveillance and spread of other infectious diseases (D. Wu, J. Lu, L. Cao, et al., 2020; D. Wu, J. Lu, Y. Liu, et al., 2020), including natural focal diseases such as HFRS (Jiang et al., 2017). A study in China showed that stringent preventive measures against COVID-19 contributed to a decline in HFRS incidence (Jiang et al., 2017; Xiao et al., 2021). In Europe and Russia, HRFS infections during the COVID-19 outbreak in 2020 were lower than in previous years ("On the state of sanitary and epidemiological well-being of the population in the Russian Federation in 2022: State report. M.: Federal Service for Supervision of Consumer Rights Protection and Human Welfare, 2023. 368 p. https://rospotrebnadzor.ru/upload/iblock/b50/t4kqksh4b12a2iwjnha29922vu7naki5/GD-SEB.pdf,"; "Surveillance Atlas of Infectious Diseases. [online source]. URL: http://atlas.ecdc.europa.eu/public/index.aspx,"). However, in Thailand, it was found that social distancing led to an increase in dengue cases (Lim et al., 2020). Therefore, the impacts of COVID-19 interventions on the spread of HFRS infections led to the reduction of the infections, but it was inconsistent on other diseases such as dengue.

However, there are limitations in this finding, as HFRS is associated with specific territories. The impact of interventions on HFRS during COVID-19 varies across regions, making it challenging to assert a consistent and uniform impact, with a two-fold decrease in case numbers observed globally. Also, some individuals remained undiagnosed with HFRS as a result of the overwhelming healthcare system during the pandemic.

2.11 Conclusions

Currently, more than 20 species of orthohantaviruses are known to spread through a vast territory of the Old World. Moreover, there are occasional reports of new species. In particular, novel orthohantavirus serotypes have been isolated from small animals inhabiting India and Thailand, and two species were found in Africa. These data provide evidence for the possible existence of new genotypes of orthohantaviruses in the Old World.

Orthohantavirus infection is an endemic zoonosis worldwide. Several serotypes, such as HNTV, PUUV, DOBV, and SEOV, were identified as causing HFRS. PUUV and DOBV have been identified as causing the disease in Europe, including Russia. HNTV causes human health problems in China, South Korea, and Japan, while SEOV is observed worldwide. China remains the most active HFRS epidemic region, where 90% of all orthohantavirus infections diagnosed worldwide are documented.

Clinically, HFRS is characterized by acute kidney injury and increased vascular permeability. There are limited specific treatment options. Therefore, the most effective approach for HFRS management is to prevent infection. HFRS management remains challenging due to limited therapeutic options targeting orthohantavirus entry and replication. Therefore, the treatment protocol is mainly symptomatic. In this view, preventing orthohantavirus infection appears essential to control outbreaks. The only vaccine approved for preventing orthohantavirus infection is Hantavax, which could protect against HNTV and SEOV, the orthohantaviruses endemic in Asia. These vaccines could induce long-term immune response with antibodies detected 33 months post-immunization.

The emergence of orthohantavirus infection could impact the healthcare system in many countries, which have limited experience in diagnosing and treating emerging infections. Therefore, awareness of the circulation of orthohantaviruses and associated healthcare burdens is essential for developing prevention measures. One approach could be integrating screening small mammals for orthohantavirus antibodies and antigens using ELISA or PCR methods into epidemiological surveys. Also, serological testing of febrile patients for anti-ortho Hantavirus IgM could facilitate early diagnosis of orthohantavirus infection in non-endemic countries. Additionally, an analysis of the seroprevalence of the human population could provide a better understanding of the prevalence of orthohantavirus infection, especially in non-endemic regions.

Acknowledgements This work has been supported by the Kazan Federal University Strategic Academic Leadership Program (PRIORITY-2030).

References

(HFRS)—, C. f. D. C. a. P. H. F. w. R. S. *Hantavirus Available online:* https://www.cdc.gov/hantavirus/hfrs/index.html#:~:text=Suggested%20Reading-,What%20is%20hemorrhagic%20fever%20with%20renal%20syndrome%3F,hemorrhagic%20fever%2C%20and%20nephropathia%20epidemica *(15.09.2022).*

Acuna, R., Cifuentes-Munoz, N., Marquez, C. L., Bulling, M., Klingstrom, J., Mancini, R., Lozach, P. Y., & Tischler, N. D. (2014). Hantavirus Gn and Gc glycoproteins self-assemble into virus-like particles. *Journal of Virology, 88*(4), 2344–2348. https://doi.org/10.1128/JVI.03118-13

Al-Salem, W., Moraga, P., Ghazi, H., Madad, S., & Hotez, P. J. (2021). The emergence and transmission of COVID-19 in European countries, 2019–2020: A comprehensive review of timelines, cases and containment. *International Health, 13*(5), 383–398. https://doi.org/10.1093/inthealth/ihab037

Ali, H. S., Drewes, S., Weber de Melo, V., Schlegel, M., Freise, J., Groschup, M. H., Heckel, G., & Ulrich, R. G. (2015). Complete genome of a Puumala virus strain from Central Europe. *Virus Genes, 50*(2), 292–298. https://doi.org/10.1007/s11262-014-1157-6

Antoine, M., Langlois, M. E., Bres, E., Rabeyrin, M., Reynes, J. M., & Deeb, A. (2021). Imported haemorrhagic fever with renal syndrome caused by Dobrava-Belgrade hantavirus in France. *Clinical Kidney Journal, 14*(3), 1014–1016. https://doi.org/10.1093/ckj/sfaa006

Antonen, J., Leppanen, I., Tenhunen, J., Arvola, P., Makela, S., Vaheri, A., & Mustonen, J. (2013). A severe case of Puumala hantavirus infection successfully treated with bradykinin receptor antagonist icatibant. *Scand Journal of Infectious Diseases, 45*(6), 494–496. https://doi.org/10.3109/00365548.2012.755268

Arai, S., Gu, S. H., Baek, L. J., Tabara, K., Bennett, S. N., Oh, H. S., Takada, N., Kang, H. J., Tanaka-Taya, K., Morikawa, S., Okabe, N., Yanagihara, R., & Song, J. W. (2012). Divergent ancestral lineages of newfound hantaviruses harbored by phylogenetically related crocidurine shrew species in Korea. *Virology, 424*(2), 99–105. https://doi.org/10.1016/j.virol.2011.11.013

Arai, S., Kikuchi, F., Bawm, S., Son, N. T., Lin, K. S., Tu, V. T., Aoki, K., Tsuchiya, K., Tanaka-Taya, K., Morikawa, S., Oishi, K., & Yanagihara, R. (2019). Molecular Phylogeny of Mobatviruses (Hantaviridae) in Myanmar and Vietnam. *Viruses, 11*(3). https://doi.org/10.3390/v11030228

Arai, S., Nguyen, S. T., Boldgiv, B., Fukui, D., Araki, K., Dang, C. N., Ohdachi, S. D., Nguyen, N. X., Pham, T. D., Boldbaatar, B., Satoh, H., Yoshikawa, Y., Morikawa, S., Tanaka-Taya, K., Yanagihara, R., & Oishi, K. (2013). Novel bat-borne hantavirus, Vietnam. *Emerging Infectious Diseases, 19*(7), 1159–1161. https://doi.org/10.3201/eid1907.121549

Arai, S., Ohdachi, S. D., Asakawa, M., Kang, H. J., Mocz, G., Arikawa, J., Okabe, N., & Yanagihara, R. (2008). Molecular phylogeny of a newfound hantavirus in the Japanese shrew mole (Urotrichus talpoides). *Proceedings of the National Academy of Sciences of the United States of America, 105*(42), 16296–16301. https://doi.org/10.1073/pnas.0808942105

Arai, S., Taniguchi, S., Aoki, K., Yoshikawa, Y., Kyuwa, S., Tanaka-Taya, K., Masangkay, J. S., Omatsu, T., Puentespina, R., Jr., Watanabe, S., Alviola, P., Alvarez, J., Eres, E., Cosico, E., Quibod, M., Morikawa, S., Yanagihara, R., & Oishi, K. (2016). Molecular phylogeny of a genetically divergent hantavirus harbored by the Geoffroy's rousette (Rousettus amplexicaudatus), a frugivorous bat species in the Philippines. *Infection, Genetics and Evolution, 45*, 26–32. https://doi.org/10.1016/j.meegid.2016.08.008

Asikainen, K., Hanninen, T., Henttonen, H., Niemimaa, J., Laakkonen, J., Andersen, H. K., Bille, N., Leirs, H., Vaheri, A., & Plyusnin, A. (2000). Molecular evolution of puumala hantavirus in Fennoscandia: Phylogenetic analysis of strains from two recolonization routes, Karelia and Denmark. *Journal of General Virology, 81*(Pt 12), 2833–2841. https://doi.org/10.1099/0022-1317-81-12-2833

Aude Lalis. (2020). The first identification of Tula Hantavirus in Iran. *Malaria Control & Elimination, 9*.

Avsic-Zupanc, T., Nemirov, K., Petrovec, M., Trilar, T., Poljak, M., Vaheri, A., & Plyusnin, A. (2000). Genetic analysis of wild-type Dobrava hantavirus in Slovenia: Co-existence of two distinct genetic lineages within the same natural focus. *Journal of General Virology, 81*(Pt 7), 1747–1755. https://doi.org/10.1099/0022-1317-81-7-1747

Avsic-Zupanc, T., Xiao, S. Y., Stojanovic, R., Gligic, A., van der Groen, G., & LeDuc, J. W. (1992). Characterization of Dobrava virus: A Hantavirus from Slovenia. *Yugoslavia. Journal of Medical Virology, 38*(2), 132–137. https://doi.org/10.1002/jmv.1890380211

Baygildina, A. A. (2014). Modern ideas about the pathogenesis of hemorrhagic fever with renal syndrome / A.A. Baygildina. *Medical Bulletin of Bashkortostan, T.9*(1), 98–108.

Bennett, S. N., Gu, S. H., Kang, H. J., Arai, S., & Yanagihara, R. (2014). Reconstructing the evolutionary origins and phylogeography of hantaviruses. *Trends in Microbiology, 22*(8), 473–482. https://doi.org/10.1016/j.tim.2014.04.008

Bergstedt Oscarsson, K., Brorstad, A., Baudin, M., Lindberg, A., Forssen, A., Evander, M., Eriksson, M., & Ahlm, C. (2016). Human Puumala hantavirus infection in northern Sweden; increased seroprevalence and association to risk and health factors. *BMC Infectious Diseases, 16*(1), 566. https://doi.org/10.1186/s12879-016-1879-2

Bi, Z., Formenty, P. B., & Roth, C. E. (2008). Hantavirus infection: A review and global update. *Journal of Infection in Developing Countries, 2*(1), 3–23. https://doi.org/10.3855/jidc.317

Binder, F., Reiche, S., Roman-Sosa, G., Saathoff, M., Ryll, R., Trimpert, J., Kunec, D., Hoper, D., & Ulrich, R. G. (2020). Isolation and characterization of new Puumala orthohantavirus strains from Germany. *Virus Genes, 56*(4), 448–460. https://doi.org/10.1007/s11262-020-01755-3

Boudreau, E. F., Josleyn, M., Ullman, D., Fisher, D., Dalrymple, L., Sellers-Myers, K., Loudon, P., Rusnak, J., Rivard, R., Schmaljohn, C., & Hooper, J. W. (2012). A Phase 1 clinical trial of Hantaan virus and Puumala virus M-segment DNA vaccines for hemorrhagic fever with renal syndrome. *Vaccine, 30*(11), 1951–1958. https://doi.org/10.1016/j.vaccine.2012.01.024

Brummer-Korvenkontio, M., Manni, T., Ukkonen, S., & Vaheri, A. (1986). Detection of hemagglutination-inhibiting antibodies in patients with nephropathia epidemica and Korean hemorrhagic fever by using Puumala virus cell culture antigen. *Journal of Infectious Diseases, 153*(5), 997–998. https://doi.org/10.1093/infdis/153.5.997-a

Brummer-Korvenkontio, M., Vaheri, A., Hovi, T., von Bonsdorff, C. H., Vuorimies, J., Manni, T., Penttinen, K., Oker-Blom, N., & Lahdevirta, J. (1980). Nephropathia epidemica: Detection of antigen in bank voles and serologic diagnosis of human infection. *Journal of Infectious Diseases, 141*(2), 131–134. https://doi.org/10.1093/infdis/141.2.131

Cao, S., Ma, J., Cheng, C., Ju, W., & Wang, Y. (2016). Genetic characterization of hantaviruses isolated from rodents in the port cities of Heilongjiang, China, in 2014. *BMC Veterinary Research, 12*, 69. https://doi.org/10.1186/s12917-016-0695-7

Carey, D. E., Reuben, R., Panicker, K. N., Shope, R. E., & Myers, R. M. (1971). Thottapalayam virus: a presumptive arbovirus isolated from a shrew in India. *Indian Journal of Medical Research, 59*(11), 1758–1760. https://www.ncbi.nlm.nih.gov/pubmed/5169031

Casals, J., Henderson, B. E., Hoogstraal, H., Johnson, K. M., & Shelokov, A. (1970). A review of Soviet viral hemorrhagic fevers, 1969. *Journal of Infectious Diseases, 122*(5), 437–453. https://doi.org/10.1093/infdis/122.5.437

Centers for Disease Control and Prevention Cleaning Up after Rodents|Rodents|CDC. Availa-ble online: https://www.cdc.gov/rodents/prevent_infestations/clean_up.html#:~:text=Clean%20up%20rodent%20urine%20and,or%20droppings%20and%20cleaning%20product (15.09.2022).

Centers for Disease Control and Prevention Facts about Hantaviruses. What You Need to Know to Prevent the Disease Pulmonary Syndrome (HPS). Available online: https://www.cdc.gov/hantavirus/pdf/hps_brochure.pdf (23.08.2022).

Centers for Disease Control and Prevention Technical/Clinical Information: HPS Treatment—Hantavirus. Available online: https://www.cdc.gov/hantavirus/technical/hps/treatment.html (12.07.2022).).

Chandy, S., Abraham, S., & Sridharan, G. (2008). Hantaviruses: An emerging public health threat in India? *A Review. Journal of Biosciences, 33*(4), 495–504. https://doi.org/10.1007/s12038-008-0068-x

Chandy, S., Mitra, S., Sathish, N., Vijayakumar, T. S., Abraham, O. C., Jesudason, M. V., Abraham, P., Yoshimatsu, K., Arikawa, J., & Sridharan, G. (2005). A pilot study for serological evidence of hantavirus infection in human population in south India. *Indian Journal of Medical Research, 122*(3), 211–215. https://www.ncbi.nlm.nih.gov/pubmed/16251777

Chappell, J. G., Tsoleridis, T., Onianwa, O., Drake, G., Ashpole, I., Dobbs, P., Edema, W., Kumi-Ansah, F., Bennett, M., Tarlinton, R. E., Ball, J. K., & McClure, C. P. (2020). Retrieval of the complete coding sequence of the UK-endemic tatenale orthohantavirus reveals extensive strain variation and supports its classification as a novel species. *Viruses, 12*(4). https://doi.org/10.3390/v12040454

Chen, H. X., & Qiu, F. X. (1993). Epidemiologic surveillance on the hemorrhagic fever with renal syndrome in China. *Chinese Medical Journal (Engl), 106*(11), 857–863. https://www.ncbi.nlm.nih.gov/pubmed/7908258

Chen, H. X., Luo, Z. Z., & Zhang, J. J. (2002). Hantavirus vaccine efficacy evaluation working group. Large scale field evaluation on vaccines of hemorrhagic fever with renal syndrome in China. *Chinese Journal of Epidemiology, 23*, 145–147.

Cheng, L. F., Wang, F., Zhang, L., Yu, L., Ye, W., Liu, Z. Y., Ying, Q. K., Wu, X. A., Xu, Z. K., & Zhang, F. L. (2016). Incorporation of GM-CSF or CD40L enhances the immunogenicity of Hantaan virus-like particles. *Frontiers in Cellular and Infection Microbiology, 6*, 185. https://doi.org/10.3389/fcimb.2016.00185

Chin, C., Chiueh, T. S., Yang, W. C., Yang, T. H., Shih, C. M., Lin, H. T., Lin, K. C., Lien, J. C., Tsai, T. F., Ruo, S. L., Nichol, S. T., Ksiazek, T. G., Rollin, P. E., Peters, C. J., Wu, T. N., & Shen, C. Y. (2000). Hantavirus infection in Taiwan: The experience of a geographically unique area. *Journal of Medical Virology, 60*(2), 237–247. https://doi.org/10.1002/(sici)1096-9071(200002)60:2%3c237::aid-jmv21%3e3.0.co;2-b

Cho, H. W., & Howard, C. R. (1999). Antibody responses in humans to an inactivated hantavirus vaccine (Hantavax). *Vaccine, 17*(20–21), 2569–2575. https://doi.org/10.1016/s0264-410x(99)00057-2

Cho, H. W., Howard, C. R., & Lee, H. W. (2002). Review of an inactivated vaccine against hantaviruses. *Intervirology, 45*(4–6), 328–333. https://doi.org/10.1159/000067925

Choi, K. H. (2012). Viral polymerases. *Advances in Experimental Medicine and Biology, 726*, 267–304. https://doi.org/10.1007/978-1-4614-0980-9_12

Choi, S., & Ki, M. (2020). Estimating the reproductive number and the outbreak size of COVID-19 in Korea. *Epidemiol Health, 42*, Article e2020011. https://doi.org/10.4178/epih.e2020011

Chu, Y. K., Jennings, G. B., & Schmaljohn, C. S. (1995). A vaccinia virus-vectored Hantaan virus vaccine protects hamsters from challenge with Hantaan and Seoul viruses but not Puumala virus. *Journal of Virology, 69*(10), 6417–6423. https://doi.org/10.1128/JVI.69.10.6417-6423.1995

Chu, Y. K., Gligic, A., Tomanovic, S., Bozovjc, B., Obradovic, M., Woo, Y. D., An, C. N., Kim, H., Jiang, Y. S., Park, S. C., et al. (1999). A field efficacy trial of inactivated Hantaan Virus Vaccine (Hantavax(TM)) against Hemorrhagic Fever with Renal Syndrome (HFRS) in the Endemic Areas of Yugoslavia from 1996 to 1998. *Journal of the Korean Society of Virology, 29*, 55–64.

Clement, J., Maes, P., Muthusethupathi, M., Nainan, G., & van Ranst, M. (2006). First evidence of fatal hantavirus nephropathy in India, mimicking leptospirosis. *Nephrology Dialysis Transplantation, 21*(3), 826–827. https://doi.org/10.1093/ndt/gfi334

Connolly-Andersen, A. M., Rasmuson, J., Oman, M., & Ahlm, C. (2018). Mesenteric Vein Thrombosis following platelet transfusion in a patient with Hemorrhagic Fever with Renal Syndrome: A case report. *TH Open, 2*(3), e261–e264. https://doi.org/10.1055/s-0038-1669456

Dantas, J. R., Jr., Okuno, Y., Asada, H., Tamura, M., Takahashi, M., Tanishita, O., Takahashi, Y., Kurata, T., & Yamanishi, K. (1986). Characterization of glycoproteins of viruses causing hemorrhagic fever with renal syndrome (HFRS) using monoclonal antibodies. *Virology, 151*(2), 379–384. https://doi.org/10.1016/0042-6822(86)90058-9

Daud, N. H., Kariwa, H., Tanikawa, Y., Nakamura, I., Seto, T., Miyashita, D., Yoshii, K., Nakauchi, M., Yoshimatsu, K., Arikawa, J., & Takashima, I. (2007). Mode of infection of Hokkaido virus (Genus Hantavirus) among grey red-backed voles, Myodes rufocanus, in Hokkaido. *Japan. Microbiology and Immunology, 51*(11), 1081–1090. https://doi.org/10.1111/j.1348-0421.2007.tb04003.x

de Carvalho Nicacio, C., Valle, G. D., & M., Padula, P., Bjorling, E., Plyusnin, A., & Lundkvist, A. (2002). Cross-protection against challenge with Puumala virus after immunization with nucleocapsid proteins from different hantaviruses. *Journal of Virology, 76*(13), 6669–6677. https://doi.org/10.1128/jvi.76.13.6669-6677.2002

de Oliveira, R. C., Guterres, A., Fernandes, J., D'Andrea, P. S., Bonvicino, C. R., & de Lemos, E. R. (2014). HantaVirus Researchervoirs: Current status with an emphasis on data from Brazil. *Viruses, 6*(5), 1929–1973. https://doi.org/10.3390/v6051929

de Vries, A., Vennema, H., Bekker, D. L., Maas, M., Adema, J., Opsteegh, M., van der Giessen, J. W. B., & Reusken, C. (2016). Characterization of Puumala hantavirus in bank voles from two regions in the Netherlands where human cases occurred. *Journal of General Virology, 97*(7), 1500–1510. https://doi.org/10.1099/jgv.0.000481

Dearing, M. D., & Dizney, L. (2010). Ecology of hantavirus in a changing world. *Annals of the New York Academy of Sciences, 1195*, 99–112. https://doi.org/10.1111/j.1749-6632.2010.05452.x

Dheerasekara, K., Sumathipala, S., & Muthugala, R. (2020). Hantavirus infections-treatment and prevention. *Curr Treat Options Infectious Diseases, 12*(4), 410–421. https://doi.org/10.1007/s40506-020-00236-3

Dong, G. M., Han, L., An, Q., Liu, W. X., Kong, Y., & Yang, L. H. (2005). Immunization effect of purified bivalent vaccine to haemorrhagic fever with renal syndrome manufactured from primary cultured hamster kidney cells. *Chinese Medical Journal (Engl), 118*(9), 766–768. https://www.ncbi.nlm.nih.gov/pubmed/15899141

Dong, Y., Ma, T., Zhang, X., Ying, Q., Han, M., Zhang, M., Yang, R., Li, Y., Wang, F., Liu, R., & Wu, X. (2019). Incorporation of CD40 ligand or granulocyte-macrophage colony stimulating factor into Hantaan virus (HTNV) virus-like particles significantly enhances the long-term immunity potency against HTNV infection. *Journal of Medical Microbiology, 68*(3), 480–492. https://doi.org/10.1099/jmm.0.000897

Dunst, R., Mettang, T., & Kuhlmann, U. (1998). Severe thrombocytopenia and response to corticosteroids in a case of nephropathia epidemica. *American Journal of Kidney Diseases, 31*(1), 116–120. https://doi.org/10.1053/ajkd.1998.v31.pm9428461

Dzagurova, T. K., Siniugina, A. A., Ishmukhametov, A. A., Egorova, M. S., Kurashova, S. S., Balovneva, M. V., Deviatkin, A. A., Tkachenko, P. E., Leonovich, O. A., & Tkachenko, E. A.

(2020). Pre-clinical studies of inactivated polyvalent HFRS vaccine. *Frontiers in Cellular and Infection Microbiology, 10*, Article 545372. https://doi.org/10.3389/fcimb.2020.545372

Easterbrook, J. D., & Klein, S. L. (2008). Corticosteroids modulate Seoul virus infection, regulatory T-cell responses and matrix metalloprotease 9 expression in male, but not female, Norway rats. *Journal of General Virology, 89*(Pt 11), 2723–2730. https://doi.org/10.1099/vir.0.2008/03715-0

Elgh, F., Linderholm, M., Wadell, G., Tarnvik, A., & Juto, P. (1998). Development of humoral cross-reactivity to the nucleocapsid protein of heterologous hantaviruses in nephropathia epidemica. *FEMS Immunology and Medical Microbiology, 22*(4), 309–315. https://doi.org/10.1111/j.1574-695X.1998.tb01220.x

Elwell, M. R., Ward, G. S., Tingpalapong, M., & LeDuc, J. W. (1985). Serologic evidence of Hantaan-like virus in rodents and man in Thailand. *Southeast Asian Journal of Tropical Medicine Public Health, 16*(3), 349–354. https://www.ncbi.nlm.nih.gov/pubmed/3938073

Escutenaire, S., Chalon, P., Heyman, P., Van der Auwera, G., van der Groen, G., Verhagen, R., Thomas, I., Karelle-Bui, L., Vaheri, A., Pastoret, P. P., & Plyusnin, A. (2001). Genetic characterization of Puumala hantavirus strains from Belgium: Evidence for a distinct phylogenetic lineage. *Virus Research, 74*(1–2), 1–15. https://doi.org/10.1016/s0168-1702(00)00224-0

Escutenaire, S., & Pastoret, P. P. (2001). [Hantavirus infection epidemiology in Belgium]. *Bulletin et memoires de l'Academie royale de medecine de Belgique, 156*(1–2), 137–144; discussion 144–136. https://www.ncbi.nlm.nih.gov/pubmed/11697188 (Epidemiologie de l'infection par hantavirus en Belgique.)

Fang, L. Z., Zhao, L., Wen, H. L., Zhang, Z. T., Liu, J. W., He, S. T., Xue, Z. F., Ma, D. Q., Zhang, X. S., Zhang, Y., & Yu, X. J. (2015). Reservoir host expansion of hantavirus. *China. Emerging Infectious Diseases, 21*(1), 170–171. https://doi.org/10.3201/eid2101.140960

Fougeroux, C., Goksoyr, L., Idorn, M., Soroka, V., Myeni, S. K., Dagil, R., Janitzek, C. M., Sogaard, M., Aves, K. L., Horsted, E. W., Erdogan, S. M., Gustavsson, T., Dorosz, J., Clemmensen, S., Fredsgaard, L., Thrane, S., Vidal-Calvo, E. E., Khalife, P., Hulen, T. M., … Sander, A. F. (2021). Capsid-like particles decorated with the SARS-CoV-2 receptor-binding domain elicit strong virus neutralization activity. *Nature Communications, 12*(1), 324. https://doi.org/10.1038/s41467-020-20251-8

Furuta, Y., Komeno, T., & Nakamura, T. (2017). Favipiravir (T-705), a broad spectrum inhibitor of viral RNA polymerase. *Proceedings of the Japan Academy, Series B, Physical and Biological Sciences, 93*(7), 449–463. https://doi.org/10.2183/pjab.93.027

Garanina, S. B., Platonov, A. E., Zhuravlev, V. I., Murashkina, A. N., Yakimenko, V. V., Korneev, A. G., & Shipulin, G. A. (2009). Genetic diversity and geographic distribution of hantaviruses in Russia. *Zoonoses and Public Health, 56*(6–7), 297–309. https://doi.org/10.1111/j.1863-2378.2008.01210.x

Ge, X. Y., Yang, W. H., Pan, H., Zhou, J. H., Han, X., Zhu, G. J., Desmond, J. S., Daszak, P., Shi, Z. L., & Zhang, Y. Z. (2016). Fugong virus, a novel hantavirus harbored by the small oriental vole (Eothenomys eleusis) in China. *Virology of Journal, 13*, 27. https://doi.org/10.1186/s12985-016-0483-9

Geldmacher, A., Schmaler, M., Kruger, D. H., & Ulrich, R. (2004a). Yeast-expressed hantavirus Dobrava nucleocapsid protein induces a strong, long-lasting, and highly cross-reactive immune response in mice. *Viral Immunology, 17*(1), 115–122. https://doi.org/10.1089/088282404322875511

Geldmacher, A., Skrastina, D., Petrovskis, I., Borisova, G., Berriman, J. A., Roseman, A. M., Crowther, R. A., Fischer, J., Musema, S., Gelderblom, H. R., Lundkvist, A., Renhofa, R., Ose, V., Kruger, D. H., Pumpens, P., & Ulrich, R. (2004b). An amino-terminal segment of hantavirus nucleocapsid protein presented on hepatitis B virus core particles induces a strong and highly cross-reactive antibody response in mice. *Virology, 323*(1), 108–119. https://doi.org/10.1016/j.virol.2004.02.022

GenBank. https://www.ncbi.nlm.nih.gov/nuccore/NC_055632.1 (Retrieved on 20th January 2024).

Gralinski, L. E., & Menachery, V. D. (2020). Return of the Coronavirus: 2019-nCoV. Viruses, 12(2). https://doi.org/10.3390/v12020135

Gu, S. H., Lim, B. K., Kadjo, B., Arai, S., Kim, J. A., Nicolas, V., Lalis, A., Denys, C., Cook, J. A., Dominguez, S. R., Holmes, K. V., Urushadze, L., Sidamonidze, K., Putkaradze, D., Kuzmin, I. V., Kosoy, M. Y., Song, J. W., & Yanagihara, R. (2014). Molecular phylogeny of hantaviruses harbored by insectivorous bats in Cote d'Ivoire and Vietnam. *Viruses, 6*(5), 1897–1910. https://doi.org/10.3390/v6051897

Gu, S. H., Nicolas, V., Lalis, A., Sathirapongsasuti, N., & Yanagihara, R. (2013). Complete genome sequence and molecular phylogeny of a newfound hantavirus harbored by the Doucet's musk shrew (Crocidura douceti) in Guinea. *Infection, Genetics and Evolution, 20*, 118–123. https://doi.org/10.1016/j.meegid.2013.08.016

Guang, M. Y., Liu, G. Z., & Cosgriff, T. M. (1989). Hemorrhage in hemorrhagic fever with renal syndrome in China. *Rev Infectious Diseases, 11*(Suppl 4), S884-890. https://doi.org/10.1093/clinids/11.supplement_4.s844

Guénet, Jean Louis, Annie Orth and François Bonhomme. "Origins and Phylogenetic Relationships of the Laboratory Mouse." (2012).

Guo, W. P., Lin, X. D., Wang, W., Tian, J. H., Cong, M. L., Zhang, H. L., Wang, M. R., Zhou, R. H., Wang, J. B., Li, M. H., Xu, J., Holmes, E. C., & Zhang, Y. Z. (2013). Phylogeny and origins of hantaviruses harbored by bats, insectivores, and rodents. *PLoS Pathogens, 9*(2), Article e1003159. https://doi.org/10.1371/journal.ppat.1003159

Gupta, D., Sahoo, A. K., & Singh, A. (2020). Ivermectin: Potential candidate for the treatment of Covid 19. *Brazil Journal on Infectious Diseases, 24*(4), 369–371. https://doi.org/10.1016/j.bjid.2020.06.002

Hall, P. R., Hjelle, B., Brown, D. C., Ye, C., Bondu-Hawkins, V., Kilpatrick, K. A., & Larson, R. S. (2008). Multivalent presentation of antihantavirus peptides on nanoparticles enhances infection blockade. *Antimicrobial Agents and Chemotherapy, 52*(6), 2079–2088. https://doi.org/10.1128/AAC.01415-07

Hall, P. R., Leitao, A., Ye, C., Kilpatrick, K., Hjelle, B., Oprea, T. I., & Larson, R. S. (2010). Small molecule inhibitors of hantavirus infection. *Bioorganic & Medicinal Chemistry Letters, 20*(23), 7085–7091. https://doi.org/10.1016/j.bmcl.2010.09.092

Hautala, T., Sironen, T., Vapalahti, O., Paakko, E., Sarkioja, T., Salmela, P. I., Vaheri, A., Plyusnin, A., & Kauma, H. (2002). Hypophyseal hemorrhage and panhypopituitarism during Puumala Virus Infection: Magnetic Resonance Imaging and detection of viral antigen in the hypophysis. *Clinical Infectious Diseases, 35*(1), 96–101. https://doi.org/10.1086/340859

Holmes, E. C., & Zhang, Y. Z. (2015). The evolution and emergence of hantaviruses. *Current Opinion in Virology, 10*, 27–33. https://doi.org/10.1016/j.coviro.2014.12.007

Hooper, J. W., Custer, D. M., Smith, J., & Wahl-Jensen, V. (2006). Hantaan/Andes virus DNA vaccine elicits a broadly cross-reactive neutralizing antibody response in nonhuman primates. *Virology, 347*(1), 208–216. https://doi.org/10.1016/j.virol.2005.11.035

Hooper, J. W., Custer, D. M., Thompson, E., & Schmaljohn, C. S. (2001). DNA vaccination with the Hantaan virus M gene protects Hamsters against three of four HFRS hantaviruses and elicits a high-titer neutralizing antibody response in Rhesus monkeys. *Journal of Virology, 75*(18), 8469–8477. https://doi.org/10.1128/jvi.75.18.8469-8477.2001

Huggins, J. W., Hsiang, C. M., Cosgriff, T. M., Guang, M. Y., Smith, J. I., Wu, Z. O., LeDuc, J. W., Zheng, Z. M., Meegan, J. M., Wang, Q. N., et al. (1991). Prospective, double-blind, concurrent, placebo-controlled clinical trial of intravenous ribavirin therapy of hemorrhagic fever with renal syndrome. *Journal of Infectious Diseases, 164*(6), 1119–1127. https://doi.org/10.1093/infdis/164.6.1119

Hussein, I., Haseeb, A., & Haque, A. (2011). *MA Mir recent advances in Hantavirus molecular biology and disease*. Advances in applied 2011.

ICTV Current ICTV taxonomy release. Available online: https://ictv.global/taxonomy (Retrieved on 8 August 2022).

Jameson, L., Taori, S., Atkinson, B., Levick, P., Featherstone, C., Van Der Burgt, G., McCarthy, N., Hart, J., Osborne, J., & Walsh, A. (2013). Pet rats as a source of hantavirus in England and Wales, 2013. *Eurosurveillance, 18*(9), 20415.

Ji, T., Chen, H. L., Xu, J., Wu, L. N., Li, J. J., Chen, K., & Qin, G. (2020). Lockdown contained the spread of 2019 Novel Coronavirus Disease in Huangshi City, China: Early epidemiological findings. *Clin Infectious Diseases, 71*(6), 1454–1460. https://doi.org/10.1093/cid/ciaa390

Jiang, H., Du, H., Wang, L. M., Wang, P. Z., & Bai, X. F. (2016). Hemorrhagic fever with renal syndrome: pathogenesis and clinical picture. *Frontiers in Cellular and Infection Microbiology, 6*, 1. https://doi.org/10.3389/fcimb.2016.00001

Jiang, H., Zheng, X., Wang, L., Du, H., Wang, P., & Bai, X. (2017). Hantavirus infection: A global zoonotic challenge. *Virol Sin, 32*(1), 32–43. https://doi.org/10.1007/s12250-016-3899-x

Jiang, J. F., Zhang, W. Y., Wu, X. M., Zhang, P. H., & Cao, W. C. (2007). Soochong virus and Amur virus might be the same entities of hantavirus. *Journal of Medical Virology, 79*(11), 1792–1795. https://doi.org/10.1002/jmv.20957

Johnson, K. M. (2001). Hantaviruses: History and overview. *Curr Top Microbiology and Immunology, 256*, 1–14. https://doi.org/10.1007/978-3-642-56753-7_1

Jonsson, C. B., Figueiredo, L. T., & Vapalahti, O. (2010). A global perspective on hantavirus ecology, epidemiology, and disease. *Clinical Microbiology Reviews, 23*(2), 412–441. https://doi.org/10.1128/CMR.00062-09

Jung, J., Ko, S. J., Oh, H. S., Moon, S. M., Song, J. W., & Huh, K. (2018). Protective effectiveness of inactivated Hantavirus Vaccine Against Hemorrhagic Fever With Renal Syndrome. *Journal of Infectious Diseases, 217*(9), 1417–1420. https://doi.org/10.1093/infdis/jiy037

Jung, Y. T., & Kim, G. R. (1995). Genomic characterization of M and S RNA segments of hantaviruses isolated from bats. *Acta Virologica, 39*(4), 231–233. https://www.ncbi.nlm.nih.gov/pubmed/8825306

Kabwe, E., Davidyuk, Y., Shamsutdinov, A., Garanina, E., Martynova, E., Kitaeva, K., Malisheni, M., Isaeva, G., Savitskaya, T., Urbanowicz, R. A., Morzunov, S., Katongo, C., Rizvanov, A., & Khaiboullina, S. (2020). Orthohantaviruses, emerging zoonotic pathogens. *Pathogens, 9*(9). https://doi.org/10.3390/pathogens9090775

Kariwa, H., Yoshimatsu, K., & Arikawa, J. (2007a). Hantavirus infection in East Asia. *Comparative Immunology, Microbiology Infectious Diseases, 30*(5–6), 341–356. https://doi.org/10.1016/j.cimid.2007.05.011

Kariwa, H., Yoshimatsu, K., & Arikawa, J. (2007b). Hantavirus infection in east Asia. *Comparative Immunology, Microbiology and Infectious Diseases., 30*(5–6), 341–356.

Khalil, H., Hornfeldt, B., Evander, M., Magnusson, M., Olsson, G., & Ecke, F. (2014). Dynamics and drivers of hantavirus prevalence in rodent populations. *Vector Borne and Zoonotic Diseases, 14*(8), 537–551. https://doi.org/10.1089/vbz.2013.1562

Kikuchi, F., Arai, S., Hejduk, J., Hayashi, A., Markowski, J., Markowski, M., Rychlik, L., Khodzinskyi, V., Kamiya, H., Mizutani, T., Suzuki, M., Sikorska, B., Liberski, P. P., & Yanagihara, R. (2023). Phylogeny of Shrew- and Mole-Borne Hantaviruses in Poland and Ukraine. *Viruses, 15*(4). https://doi.org/10.3390/v15040881

Kikuchi, F., Senoo, K., Arai, S., Tsuchiya, K., Son, N. T., Motokawa, M., Ranorosoa, M. C., Bawm, S., Lin, K. S., Suzuki, H., Unno, A., Nakata, K., Harada, M., Tanaka-Taya, K., Morikawa, S., Suzuki, M., Mizutani, T., & Yanagihara, R. (2021). Rodent-Borne Orthohantaviruses in Vietnam. *Madagascar and Japan. Viruses, 13*(7). https://doi.org/10.3390/v13071343

Kim, G. R., Lee, Y. T., & Park, C. H. (1994). A new natural reservoir of hantavirus: Isolation of hantaviruses from lung tissues of bats. *Archives of Virology, 134*(1–2), 85–95. https://doi.org/10.1007/BF01379109

Kim, J. A., Kim, W. K., No, J. S., Lee, S. H., Lee, S. Y., Kim, J. H., Kho, J. H., Lee, D., Song, D. H., Gu, S. H., Jeong, S. T., Park, M. S., Kim, H. C., Klein, T. A., & Song, J. W. (2016). Genetic diversity and reassortment of Hantaan Virus Tripartite RNA Genomes in nature, the Republic of Korea. *PLoS Neglected Tropical Diseases, 10*(6), Article e0004650. https://doi.org/10.1371/journal.pntd.0004650

Klasse, P. J., & Sattentau, Q. J. (2002). Occupancy and mechanism in antibody-mediated neutralization of animal viruses. *Journal of General Virology, 83*(Pt 9), 2091–2108. https://doi.org/10.1099/0022-1317-83-9-2091

Klempa, B. (2018). Reassortment events in the evolution of Hantaviruses. *Virus Genes, 54*(5), 638–646. https://doi.org/10.1007/s11262-018-1590-z

Klempa, B., Avsic-Zupanc, T., Clement, J., Dzagurova, T. K., Henttonen, H., Heyman, P., Jakab, F., Kruger, D. H., Maes, P., Papa, A., Tkachenko, E. A., Ulrich, R. G., Vapalahti, O., & Vaheri, A. (2013). Complex evolution and epidemiology of Dobrava-Belgrade hantavirus: Definition of genotypes and their characteristics. *Archives of Virology, 158*(3), 521–529. https://doi.org/10.1007/s00705-012-1514-5

Klempa, B., Witkowski, P. T., Popugaeva, E., Auste, B., Koivogui, L., Fichet-Calvet, E., Strecker, T., Ter Meulen, J., & Kruger, D. H. (2012). Sangassou virus, the first hantavirus isolate from Africa, displays genetic and functional properties distinct from those of other murinae-associated hantaviruses. *Journal of Virology, 86*(7), 3819–3827. https://doi.org/10.1128/JVI.05879-11

Koletzki, D., Biel, S. S., Meisel, H., Nugel, E., Gelderblom, H. R., Kruger, D. H., & Ulrich, R. (1999). HBV core particles allow the insertion and surface exposure of the entire potentially protective region of Puumala hantavirus nucleocapsid protein. *Biological Chemistry, 380*(3), 325–333. https://doi.org/10.1515/BC.1999.044

Krautkramer, E., & Zeier, M. (2014). Old World hantaviruses: Aspects of pathogenesis and clinical course of acute renal failure. *Virus Research, 187*, 59–64. https://doi.org/10.1016/j.virusres.2013.12.043

Kruger, D. H., Figueiredo, L. T., Song, J. W., & Klempa, B. (2015). Hantaviruses–globally emerging pathogens. *Journal of Clinical Virology, 64*, 128–136. https://doi.org/10.1016/j.jcv.2014.08.033

Kruger, D. H., Schonrich, G., & Klempa, B. (2011). Human pathogenic hantaviruses and prevention of infection. *Human Vaccines, 7*(6), 685–693. https://doi.org/10.4161/hv.7.6.15197

Kruger, D. H., Ulrich, R., & Lundkvist, A. A. (2001). Hantavirus infections and their prevention. *Microbes and Infection, 3*(13), 1129–1144. https://doi.org/10.1016/s1286-4579(01)01474-5

Kuhn, J. H., & Schmaljohn, C. S. (2023). A brief history of Bunyaviral Family Hantaviridae. *Diseases, 11*(1). https://doi.org/10.3390/diseases11010038

Kukkonen, S. K., Vaheri, A., & Plyusnin, A. (2005). L protein, the RNA-dependent RNA polymerase of hantaviruses. *Archives of Virology, 150*(3), 533–556. https://doi.org/10.1007/s00705-004-0414-8

Kurita, J., Sugawara, T., & Ohkusa, Y. (2021). Estimated effectiveness of school closure and voluntary event cancellation as COVID-19 countermeasures in Japan. *Journal of Infection Chemother, 27*(1), 62–64. https://doi.org/10.1016/j.jiac.2020.08.012

Kutanan, W., Kampuansai, J., Brunelli, A., Ghirotto, S., Pittayaporn, P., Ruangchai, S., Schroder, R., Macholdt, E., Srikummool, M., Kangwanpong, D., Hubner, A., Arias, L., & Stoneking, M. (2018). New insights from Thailand into the maternal genetic history of Mainland Southeast Asia. *European Journal of Human Genetics, 26*(6), 898–911. https://doi.org/10.1038/s41431-018-0113-7

Laenen, L., Vergote, V., Calisher, C. H., Klempa, B., Klingstrom, J., Kuhn, J. H., & Maes, P. (2019). Hantaviridae: Current classification and future perspectives. *Viruses, 11*(9). https://doi.org/10.3390/v11090788

Laenen, L., Vergote, V., Kafetzopoulou, L. E., Wawina, T. B., Vassou, D., Cook, J. A., Hugot, J. P., Deboutte, W., Kang, H. J., Witkowski, P. T., Koppen-Rung, P., Kruger, D. H., Lickova, M., Stang, A., Strieskova, L., Szemes, T., Markowski, J., Hejduk, J., Kafetzopoulos, D., … Maes, P. (2018). A Novel Hantavirus of the European Mole, Bruges Virus, is involved in frequent Nova Virus coinfections. *Genome Biology and Evolution, 10*(1), 45–55. https://doi.org/10.1093/gbe/evx268

Laine, O., Leppanen, I., Koskela, S., Antonen, J., Makela, S., Sinisalo, M., Vaheri, A., & Mustonen, J. (2015). Severe Puumala virus infection in a patient with a lymphoproliferative disease treated with icatibant. *Infectious Diseases (Lond), 47*(2), 107–111. https://doi.org/10.3109/00365548.2014.969304

Latus, J., Kitterer, D., Segerer, S., Artunc, F., Alscher, M. D., & Braun, N. (2015). Severe thrombocytopenia in hantavirus-induced nephropathia epidemica. *Infection, 43*(1), 83–87. https://doi.org/10.1007/s15010-014-0699-9

Lee, H. W., Baek, L. J., & Johnson, K. M. (1982). Isolation of Hantaan virus, the etiologic agent of Korean hemorrhagic fever, from wild urban rats. *Journal of Infectious Diseases, 146*(5), 638–644. https://doi.org/10.1093/infdis/146.5.638

Lee, H. W., Lee, P. W., & Johnson, K. M. (1978). Isolation of the etiologic agent of Korean Hemorrhagic fever. *Journal of Infectious Diseases, 137*(3), 298–308. https://doi.org/10.1093/infdis/137.3.298

Lee, S. H., Kim, W. K., No, J. S., Kim, J. A., Kim, J. I., Gu, S. H., Kim, H. C., Klein, T. A., Park, M. S., & Song, J. W. (2017). Dynamic circulation and genetic exchange of a Shrew-borne Hantavirus, Imjin virus, in the Republic of Korea. *Scientific Reports, 7*, 44369. https://doi.org/10.1038/srep44369

Leopardi, S., Drzewniokova, P., Baggieri, M., Marchi, A., Bucci, P., Bregoli, M., De Benedictis, P., Gobbo, F., Bellinati, L., Citterio, C., Monne, I., Pastori, A., Zamperin, G., Palumbo, E., Festa, F., Castellan, M., Zorzan, M., D'Ugo, E., Zucca, P., Terregino, C., & Magurano, F. (2022). Identification of Dobrava-Belgrade Virus in Apodemus flavicollis from North-Eastern Italy during Enhanced Mortality. *Viruses, 14*(6). https://doi.org/10.3390/v14061241

Li, Z., Zeng, H., Wang, Y., Zhang, Y., Cheng, L., Zhang, F., Lei, Y., Jin, B., Ma, Y., & Chen, L. (2017). The assessment of Hantaan virus-specific antibody responses after the immunization program for hemorrhagic fever with renal syndrome in northwest China. *Human Vaccines Immunother, 13*(4), 802–807. https://doi.org/10.1080/21645515.2016.1253645

Lim, J. T., Dickens, B. S. L., Chew, L. Z. X., Choo, E. L. W., Koo, J. R., Aik, J., Ng, L. C., & Cook, A. R. (2020). Impact of sars-cov-2 interventions on dengue transmission. *PLoS Neglected Tropical Diseases, 14*(10), Article e0008719. https://doi.org/10.1371/journal.pntd.0008719

Linderholm, M., & Elgh, F. (2001). Clinical characteristics of hantavirus infections on the Eurasian continent. *Curr Top Microbiology and Immunology, 256*, 135–151. https://doi.org/10.1007/978-3-642-56753-7_8

Ling, J., Sironen, T., Voutilainen, L., Hepojoki, S., Niemimaa, J., Isoviita, V. M., Vaheri, A., Henttonen, H., & Vapalahti, O. (2014). Hantaviruses in Finnish soricomorphs: Evidence for two distinct hantaviruses carried by Sorex araneus suggesting ancient host-switch. *Infection, Genetics and Evolution, 27*, 51–61. https://doi.org/10.1016/j.meegid.2014.06.023

Ling, J., Smura, T., Tamarit, D., Huitu, O., Voutilainen, L., Henttonen, H., Vaheri, A., Vapalahti, O., & Sironen, T. (2018). Evolution and postglacial colonization of Seewis hantavirus with Sorex araneus in Finland. *Infection, Genetics and Evolution, 57*, 88–97. https://doi.org/10.1016/j.meegid.2017.11.010

Ling, J., Verner-Carlsson, J., Eriksson, P., Plyusnina, A., Lohmus, M., Jarhult, J. D., van de Goot, F., Plyusnin, A., Lundkvist, A., & Sironen, T. (2019). Genetic analyses of Seoul hantavirus genome recovered from rats (Rattus norvegicus) in the Netherlands unveils diverse routes of spread into Europe. *Journal of Medical Virology, 91*(5), 724–730. https://doi.org/10.1002/jmv.25390

Liu, R., Ma, H., Shu, J., Zhang, Q., Han, M., Liu, Z., Jin, X., Zhang, F., & Wu, X. (2019). Vaccines and Therapeutics Against Hantaviruses. *Frontiers in Microbiology, 10*, 2989. https://doi.org/10.3389/fmicb.2019.02989

Lober, C., Anheier, B., Lindow, S., Klenk, H. D., & Feldmann, H. (2001). The Hantaan virus glycoprotein precursor is cleaved at the conserved pentapeptide WAASA. *Virology, 289*(2), 224–229. https://doi.org/10.1006/viro.2001.1171

Lokugamage, K., Kariwa, H., Hayasaka, D., Cui, B. Z., Iwasaki, T., Lokugamage, N., Ivanov, L. I., Volkov, V. I., Demenev, V. A., Slonova, R., Kompanets, G., Kushnaryova, T., Kurata, T., Maeda, K., Araki, K., Mizutani, T., Yoshimatsu, K., Arikawa, J., & Takashima, I. (2002). Genetic characterization of hantaviruses transmitted by the Korean field mouse (Apodemus peninsulae). *Far East Russia. Emerging Infectious Diseases, 8*(8), 768–776. https://doi.org/10.3201/eid0808.010494

Lundkvist, A., & Niklasson, B. (1992). Bank vole monoclonal antibodies against Puumala virus envelope glycoproteins: Identification of epitopes involved in neutralization. *Archives of Virology, 126*(1–4), 93–105. https://doi.org/10.1007/BF01309687

Maes, P., Clement, J., & Van Ranst, M. (2009). Recent approaches in hantavirus vaccine development. *Expert Review of Vaccines, 8*(1), 67–76. https://doi.org/10.1586/14760584.8.1.67
Malinin, O. V., & Platonov, A. E. (2017). Insufficient efficacy and safety of intravenous ribavirin in treatment of haemorrhagic fever with renal syndrome caused by Puumala virus. *Infectious Diseases (Lond), 49*(7), 514–520. https://doi.org/10.1080/23744235.2017.1293841
Mayor, J., Engler, O., & Rothenberger, S. (2021). Antiviral Efficacy of Ribavirin and Favipiravir against Hantaan Virus. *Microorganisms, 9*(6). https://doi.org/10.3390/microorganisms9061306
McClain, D. J., Summers, P. L., Harrison, S. A., Schmaljohn, A. L., & Schmaljohn, C. S. (2000). Clinical evaluation of a vaccinia-vectored Hantaan virus vaccine. *Journal of Medical Virology, 60*(1), 77–85. https://doi.org/10.1002/(sici)1096-9071(200001)60:1%3c77::aid-jmv13%3e3.0.co;2-s
McCormick, J. B., Sasso, D. R., Palmer, E. L., & Kiley, M. P. (1982). Morphological identification of the agent of Korean haemorrhagic fever (Hantaan virus)as a member of the Bunyaviridae. *Lancet, 1*(8275), 765–768. https://doi.org/10.1016/s0140-6736(82)91812-8
Meheretu, Y., Cizkova, D., Tesikova, J., Welegerima, K., Tomas, Z., Kidane, D., Girmay, K., Schmidt-Chanasit, J., Bryja, J., Gunther, S., Bryjova, A., Leirs, H., & Gouy de Bellocq, J. (2012). High diversity of RNA viruses in rodents. *Ethiopia. Emerging Infectious Diseases, 18*(12), 2047–2050. https://doi.org/10.3201/eid1812.120596
Meheretu, Y., Stanley, W. T., Craig, E. W., Gouy de Bellocq, J., Bryja, J., Leirs, H., Pahlmann, M., & Gunther, S. (2019). Tigray Orthohantavirus infects two related rodent species adapted to different elevations in Ethiopia. *Vector Borne and Zoonotic Diseases, 19*(12), 950–953. https://doi.org/10.1089/vbz.2019.2452
Milholland, M. T., Castro-Arellano, I., Suzan, G., Garcia-Pena, G. E., Lee, T. E., Jr., Rohde, R. E., Alonso Aguirre, A., & Mills, J. N. (2018). Global diversity and distribution of Hantaviruses and their hosts. *EcoHealth, 15*(1), 163–208. https://doi.org/10.1007/s10393-017-1305-2
Mills, J. N. (2005). Regulation of rodent-borne viruses in the natural host: implications for human disease. *Archives of Virology Suppl*(19), 45–57. https://doi.org/10.1007/3-211-29981-5_5
Mir, M. A. (2010). Hantaviruses. *Clinics in Laboratory Medicine, 30*(1), 67–91. https://doi.org/10.1016/j.cll.2010.01.004
Mizumoto, K., Kagaya, K., & Chowell, G. (2020). Early epidemiological assessment of the transmission potential and virulence of coronavirus disease 2019 (COVID-19) in Wuhan City, China, January-February, 2020. *BMC Medicine, 18*(1), 217. https://doi.org/10.1186/s12916-020-01691-x
Muyangwa, M., Martynova, E. V., Khaiboullina, S. F., Morzunov, S. P., & Rizvanov, A. A. (2015). Hantaviral proteins: Structure, functions, and role in Hantavirus Infection. *Frontiers in Microbiology, 6*, 1326. https://doi.org/10.3389/fmicb.2015.01326
Myhrman, G. (1951). Nephropathia epidemica a new infectious disease in northern Scandinavia. *Acta Medica Scandinavica, 140*(1), 52–56. https://doi.org/10.1111/j.0954-6820.1951.tb10155.x
Noack, D., Goeijenbier, M., Reusken, C., Koopmans, M. P. G., & Rockx, B. H. G. (2020). Orthohantavirus pathogenesis and cell tropism. *Frontiers in Cellular and Infection Microbiology, 10*, 399. https://doi.org/10.3389/fcimb.2020.00399
Ohlopkova, O. V., Stolbunova, K. A., Popov, I. V., Popov, I. V., Kabwe, E., Davidyuk, Y. N., Stepanyuk, M. A., Moshkin, A. D., Kononova, Y. V., Lukbanova, E. A., Ermakov, A. M., Chikindas, M. L., Sobolev, I. A., Khaiboullina, S. F., & Shestopalov, A. M. (2024). Detection of Brno loanvirus (Loanvirus brunaense) in common noctule bats (Nyctalus noctula) in Southern Russia. *Brazilian Journal of Microbiology*. https://doi.org/10.1007/s42770-024-01587-5
Olsson, G. E., White, N., Ahlm, C., Elgh, F., Verlemyr, A. C., Juto, P., & Palo, R. T. (2002). Demographic factors associated with hantavirus infection in bank voles (Clethrionomys glareolus). *Emerging Infectious Diseases, 8*(9), 924–929. https://doi.org/10.3201/eid0809.020037
On the state of sanitary and epidemiological well-being of the population in the Russian Federation in 2022: State report. M.: Federal Service for Supervision of Consumer Rights Protection and Human Welfare, 2023. 368 p. https://rospotrebnadzor.ru/upload/iblock/b50/t4kqksh4b12a2iwjnha29922vu7naki5/GD-SEB.pdf.

Organization WH. COVID19 STRATEGY UPDATE. 2020;1–18. https:// www. who. int/ COVID19 STRATEGY UPDATE. Retrieved 10 Dec 2020.

PAHO/WHO Hantavirus. Available online: https://www3.paho.org/hq/index.php?option=com_content&view=article&id=14911:hantavirus&Itemid=40721&lang=en#:~:text=Hantavirus%20(HV)%20is%20an%20emerging,of%20respiratory%20distress%20and%20hypotension (13.10.2022).

Pantophlet, R., & Burton, D. R. (2006). GP120: Target for neutralizing HIV-1 antibodies. *Annual Review of Immunology, 24*, 739–769. https://doi.org/10.1146/annurev.immunol.24.021605.090557

Park, K., Kim, C. S., & Moon, K. T. (2004). Protective effectiveness of hantavirus vaccine. *Emerging Infectious Diseases, 10*(12), 2218–2220. https://doi.org/10.3201/eid1012.040684

Park, K., Kim, W. K., Lee, S. H., Kim, J., Lee, J., Cho, S., Lee, G. Y., No, J. S., Lee, K. H., & Song, J. W. (2021). A novel genotype of Hantaan orthohantavirus harbored by Apodemus agrarius chejuensis as a potential etiologic agent of hemorrhagic fever with renal syndrome in Republic of Korea. *PLoS Neglected Tropical Diseases, 15*(5), Article e0009400. https://doi.org/10.1371/journal.pntd.0009400

Park, S. M., & Kim, J. (2008). A soluble and heat-resistant form of hantavirus nucleocapsid protein for the serodiagnosis of HFRS. *Journal of Virological Methods, 147*(1), 1–9. https://doi.org/10.1016/j.jviromet.2007.08.001

Pettersson, L., Thunberg, T., Rocklov, J., Klingstrom, J., Evander, M., & Ahlm, C. (2014). Viral load and humoral immune response in association with disease severity in Puumala hantavirus-infected patients–implications for treatment. *Clinical Microbiology & Infection, 20*(3), 235–241. https://doi.org/10.1111/1469-0691.12259

Pljusnin, A., & Elliott, R. M. (2011). *Bunyaviridae: Molecular and cellular biology*. Caister Academic Press.

Plyusnin, A., & Morzunov, S. (2001). Virus evolution and genetic diversity of Hantaviruses and their rodent hosts. Hantaviruses, 47–75.

Plyusnin, A., & Sironen, T. (2014). Evolution of Hantaviruses: Co-speciation with reservoir hosts for more than 100 MYR. *Virus Researchearch, 187*, 22–26.

Plyusnin, A., Vapalahti, O., Lundkvist, A., Henttonen, H., & Vaheri, A. (1996). Newly recognised hantavirus in Siberian lemmings. *Lancet, 347*(9018), 1835. https://doi.org/10.1016/s0140-6736(96)91655-4

Plyusnina, A., Ibrahim, I. N., & Plyusnin, A. (2009). A newly recognized hantavirus in the Asian house rat (Rattus tanezumi) in Indonesia. *Journal of General Virology, 90*(Pt 1), 205–209. https://doi.org/10.1099/vir.0.006155-0

Poor, A. Cricetidae World Rats and Mice, Voles, Hamsters, and Relatives Available online: https://animaldiversity.org/accounts/Cricetidae/.

Povalishina, T. (1965). On the influence of the human activity upon the existence and detection of natural foci of haemorrhagic fever with a renal syndrome. B. Rasick^ and K. Heyberger [ed.] Theoretical questions of natural foci of diseases. Czechoslovak Academy of Sciences.

Radosa, L., Schlegel, M., Gebauer, P., Ansorge, H., Heroldova, M., Janova, E., Stanko, M., Mosansky, L., Fricova, J., Pejcoch, M., Suchomel, J., Purchart, L., Groschup, M. H., Kruger, D. H., Ulrich, R. G., & Klempa, B. (2013). Detection of shrew-borne hantavirus in Eurasian pygmy shrew (Sorex minutus) in Central Europe. *Infection, Genetics and Evolution, 19*, 403–410. https://doi.org/10.1016/j.meegid.2013.04.008

Raharinosy, V., Olive, M. M., Andriamiarimanana, F. M., Andriamandimby, S. F., Ravalohery, J. P., Andriamamonjy, S., Filippone, C., Rakoto, D. A. D., Telfer, S., & Heraud, J. M. (2018). Geographical distribution and relative risk of Anjozorobe virus (Thailand orthohantavirus) infection in black rats (Rattus rattus) in Madagascar. *Virology of Journal, 15*(1), 83. https://doi.org/10.1186/s12985-018-0992-9

Razzauti, M., Plyusnina, A., Henttonen, H., & Plyusnin, A. (2008). Accumulation of point mutations and reassortment of genomic RNA segments are involved in the microevolution of Puumala hantavirus in a bank vole (Myodes glareolus) population. *Journal of General Virology, 89*(Pt 7), 1649–1660. https://doi.org/10.1099/vir.0.2008/001248-0

Razzauti, M., Plyusnina, A., Henttonen, H., & Plyusnin, A. (2013). Microevolution of Puumala hantavirus during a complete population cycle of its host, the bank vole (Myodes glareolus). *PLoS ONE, 8*(5), Article e64447. https://doi.org/10.1371/journal.pone.0064447

Razzauti, M., Plyusnina, A., Niemimaa, J., Henttonen, H., & Plyusnin, A. (2012). Co-circulation of two Puumala hantavirus lineages in Latvia: A Russian lineage described previously and a novel Latvian lineage. *Journal of Medical Virology, 84*(2), 314–318. https://doi.org/10.1002/jmv.22263

Reusken, C., & Heyman, P. (2013). Factors driving hantavirus emergence in Europe. *Current Opinion in Virology, 3*(1), 92–99. https://doi.org/10.1016/j.coviro.2013.01.002

Rey, G.-C. A. (2021). The surface glycoproteins of Hantaviruses. *Current Opinion in Virology, 50*, 87–94.

Reynes, J. M., Razafindralambo, N. K., Lacoste, V., Olive, M. M., Barivelo, T. A., Soarimalala, V., Heraud, J. M., & Lavergne, A. (2014). Anjozorobe hantavirus, a new genetic variant of Thailand virus detected in rodents from Madagascar. *Vector Borne and Zoonotic Diseases, 14*(3), 212–219. https://doi.org/10.1089/vbz.2013.1359

Rhen, T., & Cidlowski, J. A. (2005). Antiinflammatory action of glucocorticoids–new mechanisms for old drugs. *New England Journal of Medicine, 353*(16), 1711–1723. https://doi.org/10.1056/NEJMra050541

Rissanen, I., Krumm, S. A., Stass, R., Whitaker, A., Voss, J. E., Bruce, E. A., Rothenberger, S., Kunz, S., Burton, D. R., Huiskonen, J. T., Botten, J. W., Bowden, T. A., & Doores, K. J. (2021). Structural basis for a neutralizing antibody response elicited by a Recombinant Hantaan Virus Gn Immunogen. *mBio, 12*(4), e0253120. https://doi.org/10.1128/mBio.02531-20

Rizvanov, A. A., Khaiboullina, S. F., & St Jeor, S. (2004). Development of reassortant viruses between pathogenic hantavirus strains. *Virology, 327*(2), 225–232. https://doi.org/10.1016/j.virol.2004.07.012

Rodriguez, L. L., Owens, J. H., Peters, C. J., & Nichol, S. T. (1998). Genetic reassortment among viruses causing Hantavirus Pulmonary Syndrome. *Virology, 242*(1), 99–106.

Schlegel, M., Kindler, E., Essbauer, S. S., Wolf, R., Thiel, J., Groschup, M. H., Heckel, G., Oehme, R. M., & Ulrich, R. G. (2012). Tula virus infections in the Eurasian water vole in Central Europe. *Vector Borne and Zoonotic Diseases, 12*(6), 503–513. https://doi.org/10.1089/vbz.2011.0784

Schmaljohn, C. S. (2012). Vaccines for hantaviruses: Progress and issues. *Expert Review of Vaccines, 11*(5), 511–513. https://doi.org/10.1586/erv.12.15

Schmaljohn, C. S., Hasty, S. E., & Dalrymple, J. M. (1992). Preparation of candidate vaccinia-vectored vaccines for haemorrhagic fever with renal syndrome. *Vaccine, 10*(1), 10–13. https://doi.org/10.1016/0264-410x(92)90412-d

Schmaljohn, C. S., Hasty, S. E., Harrison, S. A., & Dalrymple, J. M. (1983). Characterization of Hantaan virions, the prototype virus of hemorrhagic fever with renal syndrome. *Journal of Infectious Diseases, 148*(6), 1005–1012. https://doi.org/10.1093/infdis/148.6.1005

Schmidt, J., Jandrig, B., Klempa, B., Yoshimatsu, K., Arikawa, J., Meisel, H., Niedrig, M., Pitra, C., Kruger, D. H., & Ulrich, R. (2005). Nucleocapsid protein of cell culture-adapted Seoul virus strain 80–39: Analysis of its encoding sequence, expression in yeast and immuno-reactivity. *Virus Genes, 30*(1), 37–48. https://doi.org/10.1007/s11262-004-4580-2

Sehgal, A., Mehta, S., Sahay, K., Martynova, E., Rizvanov, A., Baranwal, M., Chandy, S., Khaiboullina, S., Kabwe, E., & Davidyuk, Y. (2023). Hemorrhagic Fever with Renal Syndrome in Asia: History, pathogenesis, diagnosis, treatment, and prevention. *Viruses, 15*(2). https://doi.org/10.3390/v15020561

Seitsonen, E., Hynninen, M., Kolho, E., Kallio-Kokko, H., & Pettila, V. (2006). Corticosteroids combined with continuous veno-venous hemodiafiltration for treatment of hantavirus pulmonary syndrome caused by Puumala virus infection. *Eur J Clin Microbiol Infectious Diseases, 25*(4), 261–266. https://doi.org/10.1007/s10096-006-0117-z

Severson, W. E., Schmaljohn, C. S., Javadian, A., & Jonsson, C. B. (2003). Ribavirin causes error catastrophe during Hantaan virus replication. *Journal of Virology, 77*(1), 481–488. https://doi.org/10.1128/jvi.77.1.481-488.2003

Shastri, B., Kofman, A., Hennenfent, A., Klena, J. D., Nicol, S., Graziano, J. C., Morales-Betoulle, M., Cannon, D., Maradiaga, A., Tran, A., & Ramdeen, S. K. (2019). Domestically Acquired Seoul Virus Causing Hemophagocytic Lymphohistiocytosis-Washington, DC, 2018. *Open Forum Infectious Diseases, 6*(10), ofz404. https://doi.org/10.1093/ofid/ofz404

Shen, J., Duan, H., Zhang, B., Wang, J., Ji, J. S., Wang, J., Pan, L., Wang, X., Zhao, K., Ying, B., Tang, S., Zhang, J., Liang, C., Sun, H., Lv, Y., Li, Y., Li, T., Li, L., Liu, H., … Shi, X. (2020). Prevention and control of COVID-19 in public transportation: Experience from China. *Environmental Pollution, 266*(Pt 2), Article 115291. https://doi.org/10.1016/j.envpol.2020.115291

Shkair, L., Garanina, E. E., Martynova, E. V., Kolesnikova, A. I., Arkhipova, S. S., Titova, A. A., Rizvanov, A. A., & Khaiboullina, S. F. (2022). Immunogenic properties of MVs containing structural Hantaviral proteins: An original study. *Pharmaceutics, 14*(1). https://doi.org/10.3390/pharmaceutics14010093

Sibold, C., Meisel, H., Kruger, D. H., Labuda, M., Lysy, J., Kozuch, O., Pejcoch, M., Vaheri, A., & Plyusnin, A. (1999). Recombination in Tula hantavirus evolution: Analysis of genetic lineages from Slovakia. *Journal of Virology, 73*(1), 667–675. https://doi.org/10.1128/JVI.73.1.667-675.1999

Singh, S., Numan, A., Sharma, D., Shukla, R., Alexander, A., Jain, G. K., Ahmad, F. J., & Kesharwani, P. (2022). Epidemiology, virology and clinical aspects of hantavirus infections: An overview. *International Journal Environ Health Res, 32*(8), 1815–1826. https://doi.org/10.1080/09603123.2021.1917527

Singhal, T. (2020). A Review of Coronavirus Disease-2019 (COVID-19). *Indian Journal of Pediatrics, 87*(4), 281–286. https://doi.org/10.1007/s12098-020-03263-6

Sironen, T., Vaheri, A., & Plyusnin, A. (2001). Molecular evolution of Puumala hantavirus. *Journal of Virology, 75*(23), 11803–11810. https://doi.org/10.1128/JVI.75.23.11803-11810.2001

Smadel, J. E. (1953). Epidemic hemorrhagic fever. *American Journal of Public Health and the Nations Health, 43*(10), 1327–1330.

Smorodintsev, A. A., Chudakov, V., & Churilov, A. (1959). Haemorrhagic Nephroso-Nephritis. *Haemorrhagic Nephroso-Nephritis.*

Sohn, Y. M., Rho, H. O., Park, M. S., Kim, J. S., & Summers, P. L. (2001). Primary humoral immune responses to formalin inactivated hemorrhxsagic fever with renal syndrome vaccine (Hantavax): Consideration of active immunization in South Korea. *Yonsei Medical Journal, 42*(3), 278–284. https://doi.org/10.3349/ymj.2001.42.3.278

Song, G. (1999). Epidemiological progresses of hemorrhagic fever with renal syndrome in China. *Chinese Medical Journal (Engl), 112*(5), 472–477. https://www.ncbi.nlm.nih.gov/pubmed/11593522

Song, J. W., Baek, L. J., Schmaljohn, C. S., & Yanagihara, R. (2007a). Thottapalayam virus, a prototype shrewborne hantavirus. *Emerging Infectious Diseases, 13*(7), 980–985. https://doi.org/10.3201/eid1307.070031

Song, J. W., Kang, H. J., Song, K. J., Truong, T. T., Bennett, S. N., Arai, S., Truong, N. U., & Yanagihara, R. (2007b). Newfound hantavirus in Chinese mole shrew. *Vietnam. Emerging Infectious Diseases, 13*(11), 1784–1787. https://doi.org/10.3201/eid1311.070492

Song, J. W., Song, K. J., Baek, L. J., Frost, B., Poncz, M., & Park, K. (2005). In vivo characterization of the integrin beta3 as a receptor for Hantaan virus cellular entry. *Experimental & Molecular Medicine, 37*(2), 121–127. https://doi.org/10.1038/emm.2005.16

Song, J. Y., Jeong, H. W., Yun, J. W., Lee, J., Woo, H. J., Bae, J. Y., Park, M. S., Choi, W. S., Park, D. W., Noh, J. Y., Cheong, H. J., & Kim, W. J. (2020). Immunogenicity and safety of a modified three-dose priming and booster schedule for the Hantaan virus vaccine (Hantavax): A multi-center phase III clinical trial in healthy adults. *Vaccine, 38*(50), 8016–8023. https://doi.org/10.1016/j.vaccine.2020.10.035

Song, J. Y., Woo, H. J., Cheong, H. J., Noh, J. Y., Baek, L. J., & Kim, W. J. (2016). Long-term immunogenicity and safety of inactivated Hantaan virus vaccine (Hantavax) in healthy adults. *Vaccine, 34*(10), 1289–1295. https://doi.org/10.1016/j.vaccine.2016.01.031

Souza, W. M., Bello, G., Amarilla, A. A., Alfonso, H. L., Aquino, V. H., & Figueiredo, L. T. (2014). Phylogeography and evolutionary history of rodent-borne hantaviruses. *Infection, Genetics and Evolution, 21*, 198–204. https://doi.org/10.1016/j.meegid.2013.11.015

Spiteri, G., Fielding, J., Diercke, M., Campese, C., Enouf, V., Gaymard, A., Bella, A., Sognamiglio, P., Sierra Moros, M. J., Riutort, A. N., Demina, Y. V., Mahieu, R., Broas, M., Bengner, M., Buda, S., Schilling, J., Filleul, L., Lepoutre, A., Saura, C., Mailles, A., Levy-Bruhl, D., Coignard, B., Bernard-Stoecklin, S., Behillil, S., van der Werf, S., Valette, M., Lina, B., Riccardo, F., Nicastri, E., Casas, I., Larrauri, A., Salom Castell, M., Pozo, F., Maksyutov, R. A., Martin, C., Van Ranst, M., Bossuyt, N., Siira, L., Sane, J., Tegmark-Wisell, K., Palmerus, M., Broberg, E. K., Beaute, J., Jorgensen, P., Bundle, N., Pereyaslov, D., Adlhoch, C., Pukkila, J., Pebody, R., Olsen, S., & Ciancio, B. C. (2020). First cases of coronavirus disease 2019 (COVID-19) in the WHO European Region, 24 January to 21 February 2020. *Eurosurveillance, 25*(9). https://doi.org/10.2807/1560-7917.ES.2020.25.9.2000178

Steer, A. (1955). Pathology of hemorrhagic fever: a comparison of the findings; 1951 and 1952. *The American Journal of Pathology, 31*(2), 201–221. https://www.ncbi.nlm.nih.gov/pubmed/14350062

Strakova, P., Dufkova, L., Sirmarova, J., Salat, J., Bartonicka, T., Klempa, B., Pfaff, F., Hoper, D., Hoffmann, B., Ulrich, R. G., & Ruzek, D. (2017). Novel hantavirus identified in European bat species Nyctalus noctula. *Infection, Genetics and Evolution, 48*, 127–130. https://doi.org/10.1016/j.meegid.2016.12.025

Sumibcay, L., Kadjo, B., Gu, S. H., Kang, H. J., Lim, B. K., Cook, J. A., Song, J. W., & Yanagihara, R. (2012). Divergent lineage of a novel hantavirus in the banana pipistrelle (Neoromicia nanus) in Cote d'Ivoire. *Virology of Journal, 9*, 34. https://doi.org/10.1186/1743-422X-9-34

Surveillance Atlas of Infectious Diseases. [online source]. http://atlas.ecdc.europa.eu/public/index.aspx.

Taller, A. M., Xiao, S. Y., Godec, M. S., Gligic, A., Avsic-Zupanc, T., Goldfarb, L. G., Yanagihara, R., & Asher, D. M. (1993). Belgrade virus, a cause of hemorrhagic fever with renal syndrome in the Balkans, is closely related to Dobrava virus of field mice. *Journal of Infectious Diseases, 168*(3), 750–753. https://doi.org/10.1093/infdis/168.3.750

Taylor, S. L., Wahl-Jensen, V., Copeland, A. M., Jahrling, P. B., & Schmaljohn, C. S. (2013). Endothelial cell permeability during hantavirus infection involves factor XII-dependent increased activation of the kallikrein-kinin system. *PLoS Pathogens, 9*(7), Article e1003470. https://doi.org/10.1371/journal.ppat.1003470

Tian, H., & Stenseth, N. C. (2019). The ecological dynamics of hantavirus diseases: From environmental variability to disease prevention largely based on data from China. *PLoS Neglected Tropical Diseases, 13*(2), Article e0006901. https://doi.org/10.1371/journal.pntd.0006901

Tian, H., Yu, P., Bjornstad, O. N., Cazelles, B., Yang, J., Tan, H., Huang, S., Cui, Y., Dong, L., Ma, C., Ma, C., Zhou, S., Laine, M., Wu, X., Zhang, Y., Wang, J., Yang, R., Stenseth, N. C., & Xu, B. (2017). Anthropogenically driven environmental changes shift the ecological dynamics of hemorrhagic fever with renal syndrome. *PLoS Pathogens, 13*(1), Article e1006198. https://doi.org/10.1371/journal.ppat.1006198

Tkachenko, E. A., Dzagurova, T. K., & Tkachenko, P. E. (2014). Current status of Hantavirus vaccines development. In *Novel technologies for vaccine development* (pp. 113–151). Springer.

Tkachenko, E. A., Ishmukhametov, A. A., Dzagurova, T. K., Bernshtein, A. D., Morozov, V. G., Siniugina, A. A., Kurashova, S. S., Balkina, A. S., Tkachenko, P. E., Kruger, D. H., & Klempa, B. (2019). Hemorrhagic Fever with Renal Syndrome. *Russia. Emerging Infectious Diseases, 25*(12), 2325–2328. https://doi.org/10.3201/eid2512.181649

Ulrich, R., Koletzki, D., Lachmann, S., Lundkvist, A., Zankl, A., Kazaks, A., Kurth, A., Gelderblom, H. R., Borisova, G., Meisel, H., & Kruger, D. H. (1999). New chimaeric hepatitis B virus core particles carrying hantavirus (serotype Puumala) epitopes: Immunogenicity and protection against virus challenge. *Journal of Biotechnology, 73*(2–3), 141–153. https://doi.org/10.1016/s0168-1656(99)00117-0

Vaheri, A., Henttonen, H., Voutilainen, L., Mustonen, J., Sironen, T., & Vapalahti, O. (2013). Hantavirus infections in Europe and their impact on public health. *Reviews in Medical Virology, 23*(1), 35–49. https://doi.org/10.1002/rmv.1722

Vaheri, A., Vapalahti, O., & Plyusnin, A. (2008). How to diagnose hantavirus infections and detect them in rodents and insectivores. *Reviews in Medical Virology, 18*(4), 277–288. https://doi.org/10.1002/rmv.581

Van Epps, H. L., Schmaljohn, C. S., & Ennis, F. A. (1999). Human memory cytotoxic T-lymphocyte (CTL) responses to Hantaan virus infection: Identification of virus-specific and cross-reactive CD8(+) CTL epitopes on nucleocapsid protein. *Journal of Virology, 73*(7), 5301–5308. https://doi.org/10.1128/JVI.73.7.5301-5308.1999

Vial, P. A., Valdivieso, F., Calvo, M., Rioseco, M. L., Riquelme, R., Araneda, A., Tomicic, V., Graf, J., Paredes, L., Florenzano, M., Bidart, T., Cuiza, A., Marco, C., Hjelle, B., Ye, C., Hanfelt-Goade, D., Vial, C., Rivera, J. C., Delgado, I., Mertz, G. J., & Hantavirus Study Group in, C. (2015). A non-randomized multicentre trial of human immune plasma for treatment of hantavirus cardiopulmonary syndrome caused by Andes virus. *Antiviral Therapy, 20*(4), 377–386. https://doi.org/10.3851/IMP2875

Vial, P. A., Valdivieso, F., Ferres, M., Riquelme, R., Rioseco, M. L., Calvo, M., Castillo, C., Diaz, R., Scholz, L., Cuiza, A., Belmar, E., Hernandez, C., Martinez, J., Lee, S. J., Mertz, G. J., & Hantavirus Study Group in, C. (2013). High-dose intravenous methylprednisolone for hantavirus cardiopulmonary syndrome in Chile: A double-blind, randomized controlled clinical trial. *Clin Infectious Diseases, 57*(7), 943–951. https://doi.org/10.1093/cid/cit394

Wagenknecht, H.-A. (2009). Book review. *Protein Science, 13*, 3331–3332. https://doi.org/10.1110/ps.041082704

Wang, C. Q., Gao, J. H., Li, M., Guo, W. P., Lu, M. Q., Wang, W., Hu, M. X., Li, M. H., Yang, J., Liang, H. J., Tian, X. F., Holmes, E. C., & Zhang, Y. Z. (2014). Co-circulation of Hantaan, Kenkeme, and Khabarovsk Hantaviruses in Bolshoy Ussuriysky Island, China. *Virus Research, 191*, 51–58. https://doi.org/10.1016/j.virusres.2014.07.021

Wang, D., Hu, B., Hu, C., Zhu, F., Liu, X., Zhang, J., Wang, B., Xiang, H., Cheng, Z., Xiong, Y., Zhao, Y., Li, Y., Wang, X., & Peng, Z. (2020). Clinical characteristics of 138 hospitalized patients with 2019 Novel Coronavirus-Infected Pneumonia in Wuhan. *China. JAMA, 323*(11), 1061–1069. https://doi.org/10.1001/jama.2020.1585

Wang, H., Yoshimatsu, K., Ebihara, H., Ogino, M., Araki, K., Kariwa, H., Wang, Z., Luo, Z., Li, D., Hang, C., & Arikawa, J. (2000a). Genetic diversity of hantaviruses isolated in china and characterization of novel hantaviruses isolated from Niviventer confucianus and Rattus rattus. *Virology, 278*(2), 332–345. https://doi.org/10.1006/viro.2000.0630

Wang, H., Yoshimatsu, K., Ebihara, H., Ogino, M., Araki, K., Kariwa, H., & Arikawa, J. (2000b). Genetic diversity of hantaviruses isolated in China and characterization of novel hantaviruses isolated from Niviventer confucianus and Rattus rattus. *Virology, 278*(2), 332–345.

Wang, J. J., Wei, Z. Z., Wei, J., Ma, C. A., Dong, J. H., Lu, X. L., Zheng, Y., Yu, P. B., Qu, J. H., & Dong, L. F. (2012). [Long term epidemiological effects of vaccination on hemorrhagical fever with renal syndrome (HFRS) in Shaanxi provincial HFRS epidemic areas]. *Zhonghua Liu Xing Bing Xue Za Zhi, 33*(3), 309–312. https://www.ncbi.nlm.nih.gov/pubmed/22613385

Wang, M., Wang, J., Wang, T., Li, J., Hui, L., & Ha, X. (2013). Thrombocytopenia as a predictor of severe acute kidney injury in patients with Hantaan virus infections. *PLoS ONE, 8*(1), Article e53236. https://doi.org/10.1371/journal.pone.0053236

Wang, M., Zhu, Y., Wang, J., Lv, T., & Jin, B. (2011). Identification of three novel CTL epitopes within nucleocapsid protein of Hantaan virus. *Viral Immunology, 24*(6), 449–454. https://doi.org/10.1089/vim.2011.0026

Watson, D. C., Sargianou, M., Papa, A., Chra, P., Starakis, I., & Panos, G. (2014). Epidemiology of Hantavirus infections in humans: A comprehensive, global overview. *Critical Reviews in Microbiology, 40*(3), 261–272. https://doi.org/10.3109/1040841X.2013.783555

Weiss, S., Sudi, L. E., Dux, A., Mangu, C. D., Ntinginya, N. E., Shirima, G. M., Kondgen, S., Schubert, G., Witkowski, P. T., Muyembe, J. J., Ahuka, S., Klempa, B., Leendertz, F. H., & Kruger, D. H. (2022). Kiwira Virus, a Newfound Hantavirus discovered in free-tailed Bats (Molossidae) in East and Central Africa. *Viruses, 14*(11). https://doi.org/10.3390/v14112368

Weiss, S., Witkowski, P. T., Auste, B., Nowak, K., Weber, N., Fahr, J., Mombouli, J. V., Wolfe, N. D., Drexler, J. F., Drosten, C., Klempa, B., Leendertz, F. H., & Kruger, D. H. (2012). Hantavirus in bat, Sierra Leone. *Emerging Infectious Diseases, 18*(1), 159–161. https://doi.org/10.3201/eid1801.111026

Witkowski, P. T., Drexler, J. F., Kallies, R., Lickova, M., Bokorova, S., Maganga, G. D., Szemes, T., Leroy, E. M., Kruger, D. H., Drosten, C., & Klempa, B. (2016). Phylogenetic analysis of a newfound bat-borne hantavirus supports a laurasiatherian host association for ancestral mammalian hantaviruses. *Infection, Genetics and Evolution, 41*, 113–119. https://doi.org/10.1016/j.meegid.2016.03.036

Wu, D., Lu, J., Cao, L., Ma, X., Liu, Q., Liu, Y., & Zhang, Z. (2020a). Positive effects of COVID-19 control measures on pneumonia prevention. *International Journal Infectious Diseases, 96*, 548–549. https://doi.org/10.1016/j.ijid.2020.05.069

Wu, D., Lu, J., Liu, Y., Zhang, Z., & Luo, L. (2020b). Positive effects of COVID-19 control measures on influenza prevention. *International Journal Infectious Diseases, 95*, 345–346. https://doi.org/10.1016/j.ijid.2020.04.009

Wu, J. T., Leung, K., & Leung, G. M. (2020c). Nowcasting and forecasting the potential domestic and international spread of the 2019-nCoV outbreak originating in Wuhan, China: A modelling study. *Lancet, 395*(10225), 689–697. https://doi.org/10.1016/S0140-6736(20)30260-9

Xiao, Y., Li, Y., Li, Y., Yu, C., Bai, Y., Wang, L., & Wang, Y. (2021). Estimating the long-term epidemiological trends and seasonality of Hemorrhagic Fever with Renal Syndrome in China. *Infection and Drug Resistance, 14*, 3849–3862. https://doi.org/10.2147/IDR.S325787

Xu, L., Wu, J., He, B., Qin, S., Xia, L., Qin, M., Li, N., & Tu, C. (2015). Novel hantavirus identified in black-bearded tomb bats, China. *Infection, Genetics and Evolution, 31*, 158–160. https://doi.org/10.1016/j.meegid.2015.01.018

Xu, R., Yang, X. Y., Yang, D. F., Zou, C. Y., Gong, P. L., & Zeng, F. D. (2009). Phase I evaluation of the safety and pharmacokinetics of a single-dose intravenous injection of a murine monoclonal antibody against Hantaan virus in healthy volunteers. *Antimicrobial Agents and Chemotherapy, 53*(12), 5055–5059. https://doi.org/10.1128/AAC.00728-09

Xu, Z., Wei, L., Wang, L., Wang, H., & Jiang, S. (2002). The in vitro and in vivo protective activity of monoclonal antibodies directed against Hantaan virus: Potential application for immunotherapy and passive immunization. *Biochemical and Biophysical Research Communications, 298*(4), 552–558. https://doi.org/10.1016/s0006-291x(02)02491-9

Yamanishi, K., Tanishita, O., Tamura, M., Asada, H., Kondo, K., Takagi, M., Yoshida, I., Konobe, T., & Fukai, K. (1988). Development of inactivated vaccine against virus causing haemorrhagic fever with renal syndrome. *Vaccine, 6*(3), 278–282. https://doi.org/10.1016/0264-410x(88)90224-1

Yanagihara, R., Gu, S. H., Arai, S., Kang, H. J., & Song, J. W. (2014). Hantaviruses: Rediscovery and new beginnings. *Virus Research, 187*, 6–14. https://doi.org/10.1016/j.virusres.2013.12.038

Yashina, L. N., Abramov, S. A., Zhigalin, A. V., Smetannikova, N. A., Dupal, T. A., Krivopalov, A. V., Kikuchi, F., Senoo, K., Arai, S., Mizutani, T., Suzuki, M., Cook, J. A., & Yanagihara, R. (2021). Geographic distribution and phylogeny of Soricine Shrew-Borne Seewis Virus and Altai Virus in Russia. *Viruses, 13*(7). https://doi.org/10.3390/v13071286

Yashina, L. N., Panov, V. V., Abramov, S. A., Smetannikova, N. A., Luchnikova, E. M., Dupal, T. A., Krivopalov, A. V., Arai, S., & Yanagihara, R. (2022). Academ Virus, a Novel Hantavirus in the Siberian Mole (Talpa altaica) from Russia. *Viruses, 14*(2). https://doi.org/10.3390/v14020309

Yi, Y., Park, H., & Jung, J. (2018). Effectiveness of inactivated hantavirus vaccine on the disease severity of hemorrhagic fever with renal syndrome. *Kidney Research and Clinical Practice, 37*(4), 366–372. https://doi.org/10.23876/j.krcp.18.0044

Ying, X., Lai, X., Jin, X., Cai, L., & Li, X. (2020). Continuous renal replacement therapy rescues severe haemorrhagic fever with renal syndrome in pregnancy: A case report. *BMC Infectious Diseases, 20*(1), 920. https://doi.org/10.1186/s12879-020-05638-8

Zana, B., Kemenesi, G., Buzas, D., Csorba, G., Gorfol, T., Khan, F. A. A., Tahir, N., Zeghbib, S., Madai, M., Papp, H., Foldes, F., Urban, P., Herczeg, R., Toth, G. E., & Jakab, F. (2019). Molecular Identification of a Novel Hantavirus in Malaysian Bronze Tube-Nosed Bats (Murina aenea). *Viruses, 11*(10). https://doi.org/10.3390/v11100887

Zeller, H. G., Karabatsos, N., Calisher, C. H., Digoutte, J. P., Cropp, C. B., Murphy, F. A., & Shope, R. E. (1989). Electron microscopic and antigenic studies of uncharacterized viruses. II. Evidence suggesting the placement of viruses in the family Bunyaviridae. *Archives of Virology, 108*(3–4), 211–227. https://doi.org/10.1007/BF01310935

Zhang, X. K., Takashima, I., & Hashimoto, N. (1989). Characteristics of passive immunity against hantavirus infection in rats. *Archives of Virology, 105*(3–4), 235–246. https://doi.org/10.1007/BF01311360

Zhang, Y., Yuan, J., Yang, X., Zhou, J., Yang, W., Peng, C., Zhang, H. L., & Shi, Z. (2011). A novel hantavirus detected in Yunnan red-backed vole (Eothenomys miletus) in China. *Journal of General Virology, 92*(Pt 6), 1454–1457. https://doi.org/10.1099/vir.0.030122-0

Zhang, Y. Z. (2014). Discovery of hantaviruses in bats and insectivores and the evolution of the genus Hantavirus. *Virus Research, 187*, 15–21. https://doi.org/10.1016/j.virusres.2013.12.035

Zhang, Y. Z., Xiao, D. L., Wang, Y., Wang, H. X., Sun, L., Tao, X. X., & Qu, Y. G. (2004). [The epidemic characteristics and preventive measures of hemorrhagic fever with syndromes in China]. *Zhonghua Liu Xing Bing Xue Za Zhi, 25*(6), 466–469. https://www.ncbi.nlm.nih.gov/pubmed/15231118

Zhang, Y. Z., Zou, Y., Fu, Z. F., & Plyusnin, A. (2010). Hantavirus infections in humans and animals. *China. Emerging Infectious Diseases, 16*(8), 1195–1203. https://doi.org/10.3201/eid1608.090470

Zheng, Y., Zhou, B. Y., Wei, J., Xu, Y., Dong, J. H., Guan, L. Y., Ma, P., Yu, P. B., & Wang, J. J. (2018). Persistence of immune responses to vaccine against haemorrhagic fever with renal syndrome in healthy adults aged 16–60 years: Results from an open-label2-year follow-up study. *Infectious Diseases (Lond), 50*(1), 21–26. https://doi.org/10.1080/23744235.2017.1353704

Zou, L. X., & Sun, L. (2020). Analysis of Hemorrhagic Fever with Renal Syndrome using Wavelet Tools in Mainland China, 2004–2019. *Frontiers in Public Health, 8*, Article 571984. https://doi.org/10.3389/fpubh.2020.571984

Zou, Y., Wang, J. B., Gaowa, H. S., Yao, L. S., Hu, G. W., Li, M. H., Chen, H. X., Plyusnin, A., Shao, R., & Zhang, Y. Z. (2008). Isolation and genetic characterization of hantaviruses carried by Microtus voles in China. *Journal of Medical Virology, 80*(4), 680–688. https://doi.org/10.1002/jmv.21119

Part II
Outbreak Prone Diseases

Chapter 3
Epidemiology of Cholera Epidemic in Southern Africa Region

Peter Suwirakwenda Nyasulu, Jacques Tamuzi, Gideon Kofi Gelegbe, and Fingani Annie Mphande

Abstract Persistent issues like urbanization, rapid population expansion, and natural disasters caused by climate change provide a significant risk of cholera epidemics in low- and middle-income countries. The cholera pandemic that impacted numerous nations in Southern Africa from 2022 to 2023 lasted a long time and continues to harm the region, putting further burden on people and healthcare systems. Despite the lack of agreement on future climate change in Southern Africa, there appears to be agreement on increased variability in climate extremes, including regionally diverse drought, and precipitation changes. This must be prioritized in future drought and precipitation planning in Southern Africa to ensure that activities remain effective in the face of climate change-inducing cholera epidemics. Cholera prediction models will benefit from including nutrient influx, phytoplankton and zooplankton blooms, human cholera vulnerability in Southern Africa, and other climate variables to detect outbreaks early. It necessitates a comprehensive and whole-of-society strategy at the local, national, and regional levels to do additional research on cholera pandemic gaps and potential scenarios related with climate change that could induce cholera epidemics in Southern Africa.

Keywords Cholera · Epidemics · Climate change · Gaps · Southern Africa

P. S. Nyasulu (✉)
Division of Epidemiology and Biostatistics, Faculty of Medicine and Health Sciences, Stellenbosch University, Cape Town, South Africa
e-mail: pnyasulu@sun.ac.za

J. Tamuzi
Division of Epidemiology and Biostatistics, Faculty of Health Sciences, School of Public Health, University of the Witwatersrand, Johannesburg, South Africa

G. K. Gelegbe
Department of Biochemistry and Molecular Medicine, School of Medicine, University for Development Studies, Tamale, Ghana

F. A. Mphande
Faculty of Medicine, King Mongkut's Institute of Technology Ladkrabang, Bangkok, Thailand

F. Mphande and P. Nyasulu (eds.), *Evaluating Outbreak Potential of Infections in Tropical Climates*, https://doi.org/10.1007/978-981-95-0618-7_3

List of Abbreviations

COVID-19	Severe acute respiratory syndrome Corona virus 2
DRC	The Democratic Republic of Congo
SDG	United Nations Sustainable Development Goals

3.1 Introduction and Disease Burden

Cholera is an ancient disease labeled the disease of poverty due to its tendency to thrive in poor socioeconomic conditions (Mengel et al., 2014). Over 200 serogroups of V. cholerae have been identified, though only two namely O1 and O139 cause outbreaks (Schwartz et al., 2019). Following years of decline, cholera has now resurged despite modern advances in infectious disease control and prevention. Globally, it is estimated that there are 1.3–4 million cholera cases and 21,000–143,000 cholera-related deaths each year (Ali et al., 2015). Since 2021, the world has been experiencing intense and protracted cholera outbreaks. In 2021 alone, 23 countries reported cholera outbreaks, a Figure which rose to 30 in 2022 (Harris, 2023). Some of these countries are not cholera-endemic and had previously not reported cholera cases for up to 30 years (Khoury, 2023). These recent Cholera outbreaks have been associated with high case fatality rates. In 2021, the average global Cholera CFR was reported as 1.9% (2.9% in Africa), which is significantly higher above the threshold level (1%) and the highest Figure seen in more than a decade (Cholera—Malawi, 2023). Cholera spatial epidemiology is the study of the spread and control of the disease spatial pattern and epidemics. Previous studies have shown that multifactorial causation such as human behavior, ecology and other infectious risk factors influence the disease outbreaks (Rasam et al., 2014).

Persistent challenges such as urbanization, rapid population growth, and natural disasters due to climate change threaten to maintain the high-risk of cholera outbreaks in low- and middle-income countries (LMICs) (Mengel et al., 2014). The cholera epidemic that affected multiple countries in Southern Africa in 2022–2023 persisted for a long duration and continues to impact the region, placing additional strain on communities and healthcare facilities (UNICEF, 2024) (Table 3.1). The number of countries reporting cases of cholera increased between 2021 and 2023 coinciding with the COVID-19 pandemic, and gradually dropped in 2024 to similar levels as 2021 (Fig. 3.1). Urbanization, rapid population growth, natural disasters and climate change related effects remain the major contributing factors in countries reporting cases (Fig. 3.1).

Between 2021 and 2023, cholera cases were reported from 14 African countries (Table 3.1). The highest number of cumulative cholera cases were reported from Malawi, followed by the Democratic Republic of Congo (DRC) and Mozambique. Apart from COVID-19, Malawi and Mozambique had experienced the longest lived tropical cyclone in history, Cyclone Freddy in 2022, which brought massive

Table 3.1 Cholera cases in African countries between January 2022 and May 2023 cholera cases

Country	Total number of cholera cases	Total number of deaths
Malawi	58,456	1,755
DRC	35,599	381
Mozambique	29,280	131
Nigeria	24,831	624
Cameroon	16,034	343
Kenya	9,863	157
Ethiopia	5,036	84
South Sudan	980	2
Zimbabwe	593	18
Zambia	481	11
Burundi	365	3
United Republic of Tanzania	82	3
South Africa	8	0
Eswatini	2	0

Source https://www.arcgis.com/apps/dashboards/8a0bb70fc8ae41d285d47797465b817a

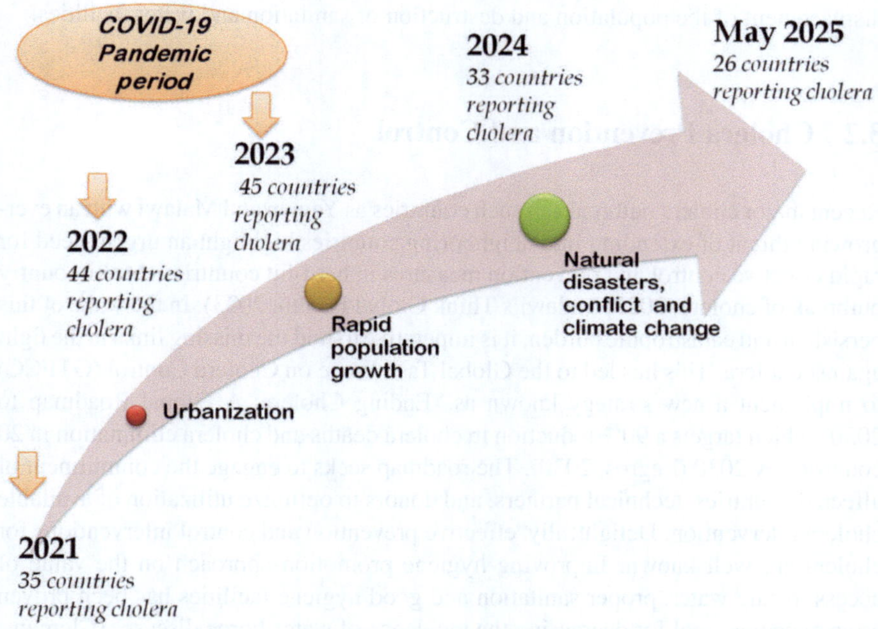

Fig. 3.1 Number of countries reporting cholera cases between 2021 and 2025. *Source* WHO https://www.who.int/emergencies/situations/cholera-upsurge

devastation in the respective countries and a surge in cholera cases (Adriano et al., 2023).

From January 2022 to December 2023, Southern African countries including Malawi (58, 456 cases and 1,755 deaths), Mozambique (29, 280 cases and 131 deaths), Zimbabwe (491 cases and 18 cases), South Africa (11 cases and 1 death), and Eswatini (2 cases and 0 death) experienced prolonged cholera outbreaks (WHO, 2023). Malawi is experiencing its worst cholera outbreak in the past two decades (Cholera—Malawi, 2023; Gavi, 2023). Cholera has been endemic in Malawi since 1998 with seasonal occurrence (Perez-Saez et al., 2022). However, the current cholera outbreak has spanned through all seasons. The current outbreak was declared by the Ministry of Health of Malawi on 3rd March, 2022 (Cholera—Malawi, 2023). It has lasted over a year causing a cumulative total cases of nearly 60,000 and over 1,500 deaths, with an alarming case fatality rate of 3.1% which is more than three times the emergency threshold (Malawi Cholera Flash Appeal, 2023) as of 25 April, 2023. Cholera cases and deaths have been reported in all 29 districts in the country, making it the biggest active cholera outbreak in Africa (Multi-country outbreak of cholera, 2023). The Malawi Government declared cholera a public health emergency on 5th December, 2023 (UNICEF Malawi, 2023; Action Against Cholera, 2023; Wise, 2023). The impact of the outbreak in the Southern region of Malawi has been compounded by the effects of the tropical storm, Cyclone Freddy that caused displacement of the population and destruction of sanitation and water facilities.

3.2 Cholera Prevention and Control

Recent major cholera outbreaks in such countries as Yemen and Malawi with an ever-growing threat of extending into neighboring countries highlight an urgent need for rapid effective control and prevention measures in hard-hit countries (Multi-country outbreak of cholera, 2023; Malawi's Think Global Health, 2023). In the wake of this persistent and catastrophic burden, it is imperative to find the missing links in the fight against cholera. This has led to the Global Task Force on Cholera Control (GTFCC) to implement a new strategy known as "Ending Cholera: A Global Roadmap to 2030" which targets a 90% reduction in cholera deaths and cholera elimination in 20 countries by 2030 (Legros, 2030). The roadmap seeks to engage the commitment of affected countries, technical partners, and donors to optimize utilization of available cholera intervention. Delightfully, effective prevention and control interventions for cholera are well known. Improving hygiene promotion approach on the value of access to safe water, proper sanitation and good hygiene facilities has been proven as an expedient tool for decreasing the incidence of water-borne diseases (Clemens, 2011; PubMed, 2023; Kaponda et al., 2019). Across multiple contexts, vaccine has been demonstrated to be safe and offering good protection to children and adults, with limited protection offered to young children (Shaikh et al., 2020; Ng′ombe et al., 2022). Cholera vaccine is considered a short-term intervention that provides ample time to plan for longer term cholera elimination interventions including universal global access to Water, sanitation, and hygiene (WASH) (Vaccine Stockpile, 2017).

There are three cholera vaccines pre-qualified by the WHO, namely Dukoral, Shanchol, and Euvichol (Wierzba, 2019). However, they only render immunogenicity that lasts up to 5 years in adults and 3 years in children. In a previous study done among high-risk population of fishermen in Malawi, a reactive vaccine had over 80% effectiveness at 3 months post vaccination (Song et al., 2021). An added benefit was that it was shown to be a cost-effective intervention relative to the Malawi gross domestic product per capita (Ilboudo et al., 2021).

The Global Roadmap through its strategic axes recommends multi-sectoral approach that is fortified with effective coordination in the fight to prevent cholera outbreaks. The biggest challenge, however still remains adapting the available interventions to local contexts to sufficiently address the gaps in cholera control and prevention (Legros, 2030; Roadmap, 2023). With limited resources in low and middle countries it is important to establish the geographical areas, populations and interventions that need to be given the highest priority. This would help channel resources to areas most in need.

Identification of contextually appropriate indicators for cholera hotspots mapping in Malawi and actual hotspot mapping would aid prioritizing interest to areas that bear the greatest burden in Malawi. This would inspire adequate preparedness, strengthening surveillance system, and acting before outbreaks become immensely unmanageable. In so doing, Malawi would drift back on the path toward eliminating cholera as a public health problem and reducing mortality by 2030.

This global roadmap will guide policymakers in designing and implementing the much-needed national cholera control plan. This will ensure optimal delivery of the vaccine and HP Approaches, suitable monitoring of their progress as well as sustained commitment to eliminate cholera. Ultimately, this will accelerate the process of achieving the 2030 Global Roadmap, thereby ensuring Universal Health Coverage. This will have a direct positive boost toward realizing such Sustainable Development Goals (SDGs) including SDG3 "good health and wellbeing" (SDG3) and "clean water and sanitation" (SDG6) (Morton et al., 2017; Bangert et al., 2017). Furthermore, it will support the country's realization of other related SDGS including reducing poverty (SDG1), reducing hunger (SDG2) and improving economic growth (SDG9) (Morton et al., 2017).

The cholera epidemic that affected multiple countries in Eastern and Southern Africa in 2023 persists and continues to impact the region, placing additional strain on communities and healthcare facilities. Since 2023, 13 countries in the region have battled one of the worst cholera outbreaks to hit the region in years, and as of 15 January, 2024, more than 200,000 cases, including over 3000 deaths, have been reported. In addition, the impact of climate change, worsened by phenomena such as El Niño, further underscores the urgency of the situation (UNICEF, 2024). As we extend our unwavering support to ongoing government initiatives in ensuring clean water supply, safe sanitation, implementing vaccinations, and working with communities, among other critical interventions, a comprehensive response that not only addresses the immediate health crisis but also considers the broader implications for children in the region is vital (UNICEF, 2024).

3.3 Transmission and Climate Change in Southern Africa

Multiple factors may explain the resurgence and transmission of cholera in Southern African countries. Southern Africa is located in the subtropical region and is known to have warm temperatures that are optimal for the proliferation of infectious disease agents such as Vibrio cholerae (Hunter, 2003; Mendelsohn & Dawson, 2008; Dudley et al., 2015). Some researchers have made links between geographical locations and climate conditions and the proliferation of V. cholerae pathogens (Bompangue Nkoko et al., 2011). Data emanating from the use of climate models, satellite data, and known patterns in the spread of disease show that with warmer temperatures and increased rainfall, cholera spreads more readily inland, especially in areas of denser populations (WHO, 2024). Climate change significantly threatens human health, manifesting through increasingly frequent and severe weather events such as storms, extreme heat, floods, droughts, and wildfires (WHO, 2024). It influences the spread and incidence of cholera in the Southern Africa through several interconnected pathways, worsening existing vulnerabilities and creating new challenges for public health (WHO, 2024). El Nino is a global phenomenon defined by abnormal warming of the Pacific Ocean, which causes dramatic changes in meteorological conditions around the world. El Nino is a global phenomenon defined by abnormal warming of the Pacific Ocean, which causes dramatic changes in meteorological conditions around the world. Its enormous impact on climate patterns is closely associated with cholera epidemics in Southern Africa (WHO, 2024). Flooding can contaminate water supplies with V. cholerae and impair sanitary systems, producing favorable conditions for disease transmission. During the 2015–2016 El Nino, Mozambique experienced catastrophic flooding, which resulted in mass displacement. The crowded and unclean environment in temporary camps contributed to the spread of cholera (WHO, 2024). The El Niño event, which generates phytoplacton and zooplankton blooms due to the confluence of rain and nutrients from land into the warm SST, could explain the geographically dispersed cholera epidemics since a significant "infectious dose" of V. cholerae may have originated from river overflow (Colwell & Huq, 1994; Christaki et al., 2020).

Two hypotheses evolved to explain how cholera spread in the African Great Lakes Region (AGLR), which is distant from the coastal marine settings that are thought to represent V. cholerae's native biotope. The first theory suggests that some cholera strains may persist in AGLR lakes. Weather factors, such as seasonal rainfall and

El Niño warm episodes, may increase plankton growth and V. cholerae multiplication, comparable to cholera epidemiology. Climatic changes have caused biological adjustments to the lakes. The temperature of the AGLR has grown during the last three decades (Bompangue Nkoko et al., 2011; Hecky et al., 1994; Vollmer et al., 2005; O'Reilly et al., 2003). Algal community structure has also changed; for instance, the reported Lake Tanganyika cyanobacteria-chrysophytes-chlorophytes community of 1975 was replaced by a cyanobacteria-chlorophytes-diatom community (Bompangue Nkoko et al., 2011; Cocquyt & Vyverman, 2005). These environmental changes, which were observed in Lakes Victoria, Malawi (another African Great Lake, also known as Lake Nyasa), and Tanganyika, could have affected the dynamics of cholera (Bompangue Nkoko et al., 2011). Cholera outbreaks in Lake Chilwa, Malawi, close the border with Mozambique, may also be investigated to explain these hypotheses (Khonje et al., 2012). These hypotheses, when taken in light of climate change in Southern Africa, may increase the risk of cholera in the region. Furthermore, it was stated that 100% of Malawi's shallow wells were feces-contaminated, particularly during the rainy season. The drinking water was obtained from potentially unsafe sources (unprotected wells, rivers, and lakes) (Shariff et al., 2024; Gaffga et al., 2007). Furthermore, it is stated that one-third (32%) of Malawi's clean water sources are not operational at any given moment due to failure and inadequate maintenance (Shariff et al., 2024; Gaffga et al., 2007). Poor sanitation in Zimbabwe was regarded to be a major contributing factor to the cholera outbreak, with a pit latrine density of one per 10,000 persons in refugee camps. Cyclone Idai devastated Mozambique in March 2019, inflicting widespread floods and destruction. In the aftermath, Mozambique witnessed a significant cholera outbreak, with over 4,000 recorded cases and numerous deaths (WHO, 2024). Rising temperatures associated with climate change contribute to the spread of Vibrio cholerae in aquatic environments. Droughts reduce the availability of clean water, forcing people to rely on contaminated water sources, which increases the risk of cholera outbreaks (WHO, 2024). In Zambia, protracted drought conditions have resulted in severe water scarcity, affecting 6.5 million people and aggravating cholera outbreaks. Higher temperatures promote the survival and spread of V. cholerae (WHO, 2024). These environmental challenges, directly and indirectly, impact public health, heightening the risks of fatalities, the prevalence of non-communicable diseases, and the emergence and spread of infectious diseases (WHO, 2024). Cholera, a disease that rapidly spreads in areas lacking clean water, poses an immediate and pressing threat (WHO, 2024). Poor sanitation exacerbates its severity, a problem further intensified by climate change-altering precipitation patterns. This underscores the need for swift and decisive action to address the crisis (WHO, 2024). However, there is little information available on the ecology of cholera outbreaks, particularly in terms of environmental determinants and reservoirs in Southern Africa. Such information is critical to the development of effective methods for cholera prevention and control both now and in the future.

3.4 Human Cholera Susceptibility in Southern Africa

According to Southern Africa Development Community (SADC), only 61 percent of the region's population currently has access to safe drinking water, and only two out of every five people have access to adequate sanitation (Oxfam/ile, 2024). Extreme weather events, such as storms, cyclones, and floods, exacerbate vulnerability by destroying WASH infrastructure and creating barriers to adequate water and sanitation in Southern Africa. Repairing damaged water infrastructure is a costly endeavor, and the majority of facilities destroyed during Tropical Storm Ana and Cyclone Gombe are still in disrepair, leaving people who previously had access to clean water without safe supplies and increasing their cholera risk. Following the two storms, several public and private latrines collapsed, putting further strain on the existing, already inadequate facilities. Governments and agencies in the region require rapid funds to quickly execute programs and projects that will enhance people's cleanliness and access to clean water, as these two aspects are critical in the fight against cholera spread. People living with human immunodeficiency virus (HIV) are estimated at 20.8 million [19.2 million–23.0 million] and 450 000 [360 000–580 000] in eastern and southern Africa (UNAIDS, 2024). The HIV-1 and Vibrio cholerae epidemics currently share a large geographic overlap in Southern Africa. Environmental factors such as temperature and water availability, as well as natural disasters like floods and earthquakes, can all have an impact on cholera distribution and prevalence by interrupting sanitation systems. WASH initiatives are commonly used to control epidemics. In regions where cholera is endemic, HIV infection increases individual susceptibility to cholera (Nkoane & Adefolalu, 2024). Among microbial factors studied, HIV infection was noted in Mozambique to be associated with a higher occurrence of cholera (Seidlein et al., 2008), and features of the gut microbiome have been linked with the rate of recovery from cholera, though the risk of cholera imparted by the gut microbiome remains to be elucidated (Hsiao et al., 2014). Other case reports suggest that HIV-infected individuals may have longer duration of excretion of V. cholerae, with the pathogen detected in stools 6 months after initial diarrheal illness (Utsalo et al., 1999). Alternatively, HIV-infected patients may be more likely to develop symptomatic disease when exposed to V. cholerae. HIV preferentially infects gut-associated lymphoid tissue and impairs gastrointestinal mucosal immunity (Mehandru et al., 2004). This reduced mucosal immunity may make HIV-infected individuals more vulnerable to V.cholerae. However, more investigations exploring a causal connection between HIV and symptomatic cholera are necessary (Sévère et al., 2016). Vaccination with oral cholera vaccines (OCV) is an effective way to reduce the high cholera incidence when deployed in combination with improved WASH facilities (Sinyange et al., 2018). The observed immunogenicity was dependent on the serotype, the number of CD4 + T cells, and the viral load, therefore these factors should be considered when creating and deploying a vaccine for this vulnerable population (Luchen et al., 2021). Poverty exacerbates the cholera outbreak. People living in poverty are usually forced to rely on unsafe water sources and have limited access to medical treatment. Malnutrition, widespread in Southern African countries, reduces immunity and increases vulnerability to cholera (Cholera—Malawi, 2023). Furthermore, the economic impact of cholera on households can be severe, with affected families incurring significant out-of-pocket expenses for treatment and missed income due to illness. When all of these factors are considered together, it is possible that the vulnerability to cholera in Southern Africa may be increased during periods of severe drought, seasonal rainfall, and warm episodes caused by El Niño.

3.5 Recent Spatial Epidemiology

The year 2022 witnessed a global upsurge in cholera cases, indicating that the situation in Southern Africa was not isolated. This trend persisted into 2023 (Table 3.1). However, what sets apart the 2023 scenario is the unexpected and concerning occurrence of cholera outbreaks in not only the endemic countries (Malawi, Mozambique, Zimbabwe) but also in South Africa. Particularly alarming are the large-scale outbreaks in Malawi and Mozambique, which deviate from the typical endemic pattern. Epidemic cholera hypothesis in combination with temperature and precipitation have been associated with spatial distribution of cholera transmission and susceptibility as described above, Southern Africa may be viewed as a high-risk region actually and in future. The hotspot analysis from data collected from the WHO (WHO, 2023) showed that Mozambique, Malawi, Zimbabwe, and Zambia remained high spot with 95%CI. However, due to high migration dynamics across Southern Africa, cholera epidemics may spread in other regional countries (Wendel, 2015). Despite a lack of consensus on future climate change in Southern Africa, there does appear to be an agreement on an increased variability in climate extremes, with spatially heterogeneous drought and precipitation changes. This needs to be at the forefront of future drought and precipitation planning to make sure actions remain effective under climate change in Southern Africa. Cholera prediction models will benefit from the inclusion of nutrient influx and phytoplankton and zooplankton blooms, human cholera susceptibility in Southern Africa, in addition to other climatic variables for the early detection of outbreaks.

3.6 Integrated Surveillance and One Health

Genomic microbial surveillance and cross-border collaborations have a key role to play in identifying new cholera introductions, areas prone to cholera importation, and the main routes of cholera circulation in Southern Africa (Smith et al., 2023). Southern African countries should establish policy share data cholera as described in the global strategic preparedness, readiness and response plan for cholera (WHO, 2023). This includes coordination, collaborative surveillance, community protection, Safe and scalable care, countermeasures, and research in Southern Africa (WHO,

2023). All of these elements are essential to better understanding cholera epidemiology in Southern Africa. Accordingly, to effectively control the spread of cholera, the SADC recommended that the member states develop and implement a collaborative, multi-sectoral and transdisciplinary response plan incorporating climatic effects on cholera re-emergence scenarios (Africa, 2024). Southern African countries should make several efforts to mitigate the spread and impacts of cholera in their countries, including cholera as one of their priority diseases, requiring public health surveillance and response and developing guidelines to support the implementation of multi-sectoral cholera prevention and control plans and strategies (Kaseya et al., 2024). As the hard-fought gains and progress remain uncontained due to the continued adversities of climate change, the limited capacities of the health systems and the lack of resilience to climate effects (Kaseya et al., 2024), it demands a holistic and whole-of-society approach at the local, national, and regional levels to conduct more research on possible scenario associated with climate change that may trigger cholera epidemics in Southern Africa. Southern Africa should also emphasize a policy of cholera vaccination in endemic areas, prior to the cholera season. Fishing communities are at increased risk of contracting cholera and are also facing specific consequences due to the crisis. Fishing communities—especially men and boys—are at particularly high-risk as they use lake waters as a source of drinking water (including while fishing) and for defecation, cooking, and bathing, including while fishing, according to a study based on the OCV campaign in these communities in Southern Africa (OCHA, 2023).

3.7 Gaps and Way Forward

In the review, multiple gaps that could explain cholera resurgence in Southern Africa have been unraveled and discussed. The lack of access to safe drinking water in Southern Africa is one of the major contributing factors to cholera outbreaks within the region. Erratic rainfall patterns with climate change as a possible contributing factor have resulted in droughts contributing to lack of access to safe drinking water. Apart from climate, change governance and limited or lack of policies to manage cholera especially in endemic countries have contributed to prolonged outbreaks in endemic countries (Table 3.2).

Policies can only be implemented if communities are aware of these policies and have the capacity to implement these policies. It is therefore crucial for strong governance in cholera endemic areas to ensure that policies are implemented at household, community, and national level. By creating awareness at all levels including the factors that drive the community spread of cholera and ways to stop the spread within communities could assist in reducing the number of cholera cases and deaths in endemic countries. Managing the impact of climate change within countries could and working with communities to better adapt to these changes and find ways to reduce the spread of cholera within this setting is essential (Fig. 3.2).

Table 3.2 Cholera gaps, hypothesis and way forwards in Southern Africa

Gaps	Way forward
Lack of access to safe drinking water in Southern Africa	Southern African nations should work hard to strengthen their clean drinking water policies
Susceptibility of cholera in high HIV burden countries under climate change	Further research is needed to determine the susceptibility of cholera in high HIV load areas to climatic change
WASH associated to climate change	A mathematical model with geographic simulations to design the impact of severe drought and precipitation on WASH
Lack of effective policy on cholera cross-border transmission control	Draft a cross-border control guideline for Southern Africa during cholera outbreaks
Gaps in governance and Policy on preparedness, readiness and response plan for cholera	Rigorous application of the WHO guideline on preparedness, readiness and response plan for cholera
The role of phytoplankton and zooplankton blooms from southern African lakes, rivers, and wells inducing cholera epidemics	Ecological research should be carried out in Southern African lakes, rivers, and wells
Gaps in scenario and simulation including the severity of El Nino and drought affecting Southern Africa and its severity in inducing cholera outbreaks	Mathematical model using geospatial simulation to predict potential cholera outbreak scenarios linked to climate change
Different environmental determinants and reservoir of cholera in Southern Africa	Ecological and experimental studies determining potential environmental determinants and reservoirs in Southern Africa

3.8 Conclusion

Climate change including drought and El Nino compromising water access, sanitation provision, rising temperatures, and increased rainfall were identified as crucial factors contributing to endemic cholera incidence in Southern Africa. Regardless of the hurdles, understanding the patterns in the association between environmental factors and endemic cholera in Southern Africa is critical for outbreak prevention and mitigation. Southern Africa should make more efforts to prevent cholera epidemics now by increasing WASH in the region and conducting more research on mathematical models, particularly geospatial modeling, to determine possible cholera epidemic scenarios associated to climate change.

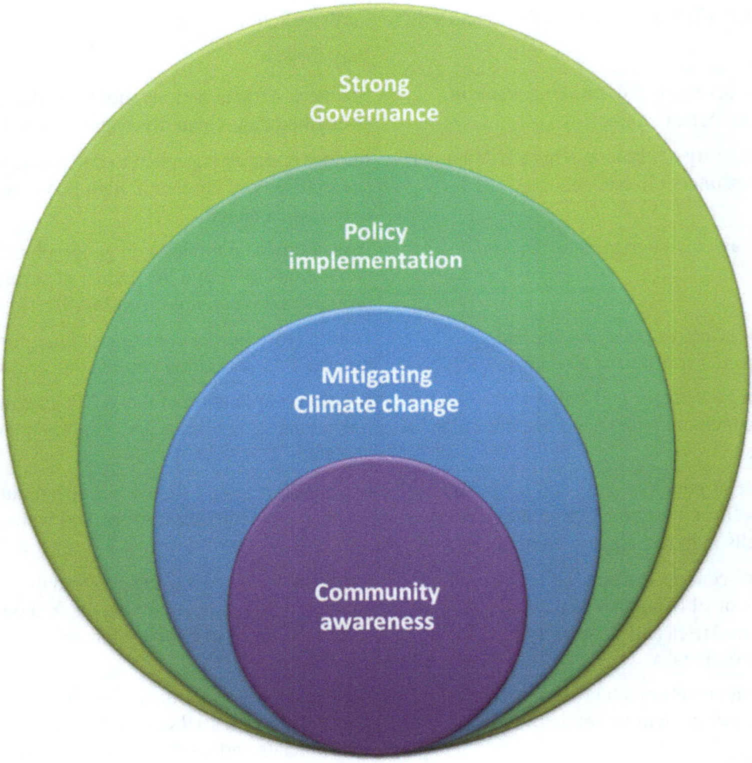

Fig. 3.2 The fight against cholera requires a multi-sectoral approach with strong governance as the overarching support system that can successfully develop and implement policies at all levels, adapting to changes brought about by climate change and its associated effects that enhance cholera transmission

References

Action against cholera | UNICEF Malawi [Internet]. 2023 [cited 2023 May 2]. https://www.unicef.org/malawi/reports/action-against-cholera

Adriano, L. F., Nazir, A., & Uwishema, O. (2023). The devastating effect of cyclone Freddy amidst the deadliest cholera outbreak in Malawi: A double burden for an already weak healthcare system-short communication. *Annals of Medicine and Surgery, 16;85*(7), 3761–3763. https://doi.org/10.1097/MS9.0000000000000961. PMID: 37427161; PMCID: PMC10328608.

Africa CDC. (2024, February). Ommuniqué from Africa CDC on the Southern Africa Development Community (SADC) Extra Ordinary Virtual Summit of Heads of State and Government on the Cholera situation in the region [Internet]. https://africacdc.org/news-item/communique-from-africa-cdc-on-the-southern-africa-development-community-sadc-extra-ordinary-virtual-summit-of-heads-of-state-and-government-on-the-cholera-situation-in-the-region/

Ali, M., Nelson, A. R., Lopez, A. L., & Sack, D. A. (2015, June 4). Updated global burden of cholera in endemic countries. In J. V. Remais, (Ed.) *PLoS Negl Tropical Diseases, 9*(6). e0003832.

Bangert, M., Molyneux, D. H., Lindsay, S. W., Fitzpatrick, C., & Engels, D. (2017, Apr 4). The cross-cutting contribution of the end of neglected tropical diseases to the sustainable development goals. *Infectious Diseases of Poverty, 6*(1), 73.

Bompangue Nkoko, D., Giraudoux, P., Plisnier, P. D., Tinda, A. M., Piarroux, M., & Sudre, B., et al. (2011, Nov). Dynamics of cholera outbreaks in Great Lakes region of Africa, 1978–2008. *Emerging Infectious Diseases, 17*(11), 2026–2034.

Cholera—Malawi [Internet]. (cited 2023, May 2). https://www.who.int/emergencies/disease-outbreak-news/item/2022-DON435

Christaki, E., Dimitriou, P., Pantavou, K., & Nikolopoulos, G. K. (2020). The impact of climate change on cholera: A review on the global status and future challenges. *Atmosphere, 11*(5), 449.

Clemens, J. D. (2011, May 24). Vaccines in the time of cholera. *Proceedings of the National academy of Sciences of the United States of America, 108*(21), 8529–8530.

Cocquyt, C., & Vyverman, W. (2005). Phytoplankton in Lake Tanganyika: A comparison of community composition and biomass off Kigoma with previous studies 27 years ago. *Journal of Great Lakes Research., 31*(4), 535–546.

Colwell, R. R., & Huq, A. (1994, December 15). Environmental reservoir of vibrio cholerae: The causative agent of cholera. *Annals of the New York Academy of Sciences, 740*, 44–54.

Deployments from the oral cholera vaccine stockpile. (2017, Aug 11). 2013–2017. *Weekly Epidemiological Record, 92*(32), 437–442.

Dudley, J. P., Hoberg, E. P., Jenkins, E. J., & Parkinson, A. J. (2015, Dec). Climate change in the North American Arctic: A one health perspective. *EcoHealth, 12*(4), 713–725.

Gaffga, N. H., Tauxe, R. V., & Mintz, E. D. (2007). Cholera: A new homeland in Africa? *American Journal of Tropical Medicine and Hygiene., 77*(4), 705.

Harris, E. (2023, Apr 25). WHO warns "very high" global risk as cholera cases spread. *JAMA, 329*(16), 1340.

Hecky, R., Bugenyi, F., Ochumba, P., Talling, J., Mugidde, R., & Gophen, M., et al. (1994). Deoxygenation of the deep water of Lake Victoria. *East Africa Limnology and oceanography, 39*(6), 1476–1481.

Hsiao, A., Ahmed, A. S., Subramanian, S., Griffin, N. W., Drewry, L. L., & Petri, W. A., et al. (2014). Members of the human gut microbiota involved in recovery from Vibrio cholerae infection. *Nature, 515*(7527), 423–426.

Hunter, P. R. (2003). Climate change and waterborne and vector-borne disease. *Journal of Applied Microbiology, 94*(Suppl), 37S-46S.

Ilboudo, P. G., Mengel, M. A., Gessner, B. D., Ngwira, B., Cavailler, P., & Le Gargasson, J. B. (2021, Mar). Cost-effectiveness of a reactive oral cholera immunization campaign using Shanchol^{TM} in Malawi. *Cost Eff Resour Alloc, 10*(19), 17.

Kaponda, P., Muthukrishnan, S., Barber, R., & Holm, R. H. (2019, Nov 1). Drinking water quality and human dimensions of cholera patients to inform evidence-based prevention investment in Karonga District. *Malawi. Water Supply., 19*(7), 2079–2087.

Kaseya, J., Dereje, N., Tajudeen, R., Ngongo, A. N., Ndembi, N., & Fallah, M. P. (2024, March 7). Climate change and malaria, dengue and cholera outbreaks in Africa: A call for concerted actions. *BMJ Global Health, 9*(3).

Khonje, A., Metcalf, C. A., Diggle, E., Mlozowa, D., Jere, C., & Akesson, A., et al. (2012, Jun). Cholera outbreak in districts around Lake Chilwa, Malawi: Lessons learned. *Malawi Medical Journal, 24*(2), 29–33.

Khoury, P. (2023, Jan). Cholera is back but the world is looking away. *BMJ, 19*(380), Article p141.

Legros, D. D. (2030). Ending cholera : A global roadmap to 2030.

Luchen, C. C., Mwaba, J., Ng'ombe, H., Alabi, P. I. O., Simuyandi, M., & Chilyabanyama, O. N., et al. (2021). Effect of HIV status and retinol on immunogenicity to oral cholera vaccine in adult population living in an endemic area of Lukanga Swamps, Zambia. *PLoS One, 16*(12), e0260552.

Malawi Cholera Flash Appeal. (2023, February–June). Malawi | ReliefWeb [Internet], [cited 2023 May 2]. https://reliefweb.int/report/malawi/malawi-cholera-flash-appeal-2023-february-june-2023

Malawi's Cholera Outbreak Could Spill Over into Neighboring Countries | Think Global Health [Internet]. Council on Foreign Relations. [cited 2023 May 3]. https://www.thinkglobalhealth.org/article/malawis-cholera-outbreak-could-spill-over-neighboring-countries

Malawi's worst cholera epidemic in decades sparks massive demand for vaccines | Gavi, the vaccine alliance [Internet], [cited 2023 May 2]. https://www.gavi.org/vaccineswork/malawis-worst-cholera-epidemic-decades-sparks-massive-demand-vaccines-stocks-run

Mehandru, S., Poles, M. A., Tenner-Racz, K., Horowitz, A., Hurley, A., & Hogan, C., et al. (2004, Sep 20). Primary HIV-1 infection is associated with preferential depletion of CD4+ T lymphocytes from effector sites in the gastrointestinal tract. *Journal of Experimental Medicine, 200*(6), 761–770.

Mendelsohn, J., & Dawson, T. (2008, Mar). Climate and cholera in KwaZulu-Natal, South Africa: The role of environmental factors and implications for epidemic preparedness. *International Journal of Hygiene and Environmental Health, 211*(1–2), 156–162.

Mengel, M. A, Delrieu, I., Heyerdahl, L., & Gessner B. D. (2014). Cholera outbreaks in Africa. In G. B. Nair, Y. Takeda, (Eds.), *Cholera outbreaks* [Internet] (Current topics in microbiology and immunology, Vol. 379, pp. 117–144). Springer Berlin Heidelberg [cited 2023 May 2]. https://link.springer.com/10.1007/82_2014_369

Morton, S., Pencheon, D., & Squires, N. (2017, Oct). Sustainable Development Goals (SDGs), and their implementation. *British Medical Bulletin, 24*, 1–10.

Multi-country outbreak of cholera, external situation report #1–28 March 2023 [Internet]. [cited 2023 May 2]. https://www.who.int/publications/m/item/multi-country-outbreak-of-cholera--external-situation-report--1---28-march-2023

Ng′ombe, H., Simuyandi, M., Mwaba, J., Luchen, C. C., Alabi, P., & Chilyabanyama, O. N., et al. (2022, January 5). Immunogenicity and waning immunity from the oral cholera vaccine (Shanchol^{TM}) in adults residing in Lukanga swamps of Zambia. In R. Borrow, (Ed.), *PLoS ONE, 17*(1). e0262239.

Nkoane, M. A., & Adefolalu, A. O. (2024). Rapid-onset diarrhoea in HIV patient: The importance of suspecting cholera in non-endemic areas. *Southern African Journal of Infectious Diseases., 39*(1), 619.

OCHA. (2023, June). Malawi cholera flash appeal 2023 (February–June 2023) [Internet], [cited 2025 Mar 5]. https://www.unocha.org/publications/report/malawi/malawi-cholera-flash-appeal-2023-february-june-2023

O'Reilly, C. M., Alin, S. R., Plisnier, P. D., Cohen, A. S., & McKee, B. A. (2003). Climate change decreases aquatic ecosystem productivity of Lake Tanganyika. *Africa. Nature., 424*(6950), 766–768.

Oxfam/ile. (2024, December). Southern African countries struggling with cholera outbreak [Internet], [cited 2025 Mar 3]. https://www.rural21.com/english/news/detail/article/southern-african-countries-struggling-with-cholera-outbreak.html

Perez-Saez, J., Lessler, J., Lee, E. C., Luquero, F. J., Malembaka, E. B., & Finger, F., et al. (2022, Jun). The seasonality of cholera in Sub-Saharan Africa: A statistical modelling study. *The Lancet Global Health., 10*(6), e831–e839.

Rasam, A., Ghazali, R., Noor, A., Mohd, W., Hamid, J., & Bazlan, M., et al. (2014). Spatial epidemiological techniques in cholera mapping and analysis towards a local scale predictive modelling. In *IOP Publishing*. p. 012095.

Responding to the cholera outbreak in Malawi | UNICEF Malawi [Internet]. [cited 2023 May 2]. https://www.unicef.org/malawi/responding-cholera-outbreak-malawi

Roadmap 2030—Global Task Force on Cholera Control [Internet]. [cited 2023 May 2]. https://www.gtfcc.org/about-cholera/roadmap-2030/

Schwartz, K., Hammerl, J. A., Göllner, C., & Strauch, E. (2019, April 12). Environmental and clinical strains of vibrio cholerae Non-O1, Non-O139 from Germany possess similar virulence gene profiles. *Frontier in Microbiology, 10*, 733.

Sévère, K., Anglade, S. B., Bertil, C., Duncan, A., Joseph, P., & Deroncenay, A., et al. (2016, Nov 2). Clinical features of human immunodeficiency virus-infected patients presenting with cholera in Port-au-Prince. *Haiti: American Journal of Tropical Medicine and Hygiene, 95*(5), 999–1003.

Shaikh, H., Lynch, J., Kim, J., & Excler, J. L. (2020, Feb). Current and future cholera vaccines. *Vaccine, 29*(38), A118–A126.

Shariff, S., Kantawala, B., Siddiq, A., Oseili, T., Nazir, A., & Uwishema, O. (2024). Cholera outbreak in Malawi: Empirical assessment and lessons learnt. *IJS Global Health., 7*(3), Article e0262.

Sinyange, N., Brunkard, J. M., Kapata, N., Mazaba, M. L., Musonda, K. G., & Hamoonga, R., et al. (2018, May 18). Cholera Epidemic—Lusaka, Zambia, October 2017–May 2018. *MMWR: Morbidity and Mortality Weekly Report, 67*(19), 556–559.

Smith, A. M., Sekwadi, P., Erasmus, L. K., Lee, C. C., Stroika, S. G., & Ndzabandzaba, S., et al. (2023, Aug). Imported cholera cases, South Africa, 2023. *Emerging Infectious Diseases, 29*(8), 1687–1690.

Social capital, collective action and access to water in rural Kenya—PubMed [Internet]. [cited 2023 Apr 26]. https://pubmed.ncbi.nlm.nih.gov/25181474/

Song, K. R., Lim, J. K., Park, S. E., Saluja, T., Cho, S. I., & Wartel, T. A., et al. (2021, Dec 15). Oral cholera vaccine efficacy and effectiveness. *Vaccines (Basel), 9*(12), 1482.

UNAIDS. (2024). Eastern and Southern Africa-regional profile [Internet], [cited 2025 Mar 5]. https://www.unaids.org/sites/default/files/media_asset/2024-unaids-global-aids-update-eastern-southern-africa_en.pdf

UNICEF. (2024, January). As cholera cases continue to rise in parts of Southern Africa, UNICEF calls for increased focus on children in the cholera response [Internet], [cited 2025 Mar 3]. https://www.unicef.org/press-releases/cholera-cases-continue-rise-parts-southern-africa-unicef-calls-increased-focus

Utsalo, S. J., Eko, F. O., Umoh, F., & Asindi, A. A. (1999, Apr). Faecal excretion of Vibrio cholerae during convalescence of cholera patients in Calabar, Nigeria. *European Journal of Epidemiol, 15*(4), 379–381.

Vollmer, M. K., Bootsma, H. A., Hecky, R. E., Patterson, G., Halfman, J. D., Edmond, J. M., et al. (2005). Deep-water warming trend in Lake Malawi. *East Africa. Limnology and oceanography., 50*(2), 727–732.

von Seidlein, L., Wang, X. Y., Macuamule, A., Mondlane, C., Puri, M., & Hendriksen, I., et al. (2008, May). Is HIV infection associated with an increased risk for cholera? Findings from a case-control study in Mozambique. *Tropical Medicine & International Health, 13*(5), 683–688.

Wendel, J. (2015). Climate change predicted to worsen spread of cholera. *Eos Trans AGU*.

WHO. (2023, April). Cholera Africa [Internet], [cited 2024 Mar 5]. https://www.arcgis.com/apps/dashboards/8a0bb70fc8ae41d285d47797465b817a

WHO. (2023). Global strategic preparedness, readiness and response plan for cholera [Internet], [cited 2025 Mar 6]. https://cdn.who.int/media/docs/default-source/documents/emergencies/global-cholera-sprrp-v7-2023-05-19_cleared.pdf?sfvrsn=7b5f7ced_1&download=true

WHO/Africa. (2024). Understanding the link between climate change and cholera in Africa. [Internet], [cited 2025 Mar 5]. https://files.aho.afro.who.int/afahobckpcontainer/production/files/Analytical_Brief_on_Climate_Change_and_Cholera_in_the_African_Region.pdf

Wierzba, T. F. (2019, Jun 3). Oral cholera vaccines and their impact on the global burden of disease. *Human Vaccines & Immunotherapeutics, 15*(6), 1294–1301.

Wise, J. (2023, Feb). Cholera: Malawi is in grip of its deadliest outbreak. *BMJ, 9*(380), Article p. 328.

Chapter 4
Co-infection; A Neglected Health Condition in Northern Ghana in the Wake of COVID-19

Gideon Kofi Helegbe, Paul Armah Aryee, and Peter Suwirakwenda Nyasulu

Abstract During the upsurge of COVID-19 infection, a lot of attention was shifted away from other common infections of public health interest such as malaria, hepatitis B, TB, HIV, etc. The prominence given to COVID-19 also resulted in the near breakout of yellow fever disease in the Savannah Region of Ghana. With the COVID-19 restrictions, many individuals stayed home with these common conditions (malaria, hepatitis B, TB, HIV, etc.), thus, recording low prevalences at the hospitals, encouraging self-medication, and enabling co-infections to thrive. It became apparent that the COVID-19 pandemic exposed the level of preparedness of Ghana as a nation in addressing public health issues in real-time. This chapter will focus on the prevalence, consequences, and management of several key infectious diseases in Ghana with particular reference to co-infections common in northern Ghana. Co-infections are a significant public health concern, especially in low-resource contexts such as Ghana where several infectious agents affect a single host simultaneously.

Keywords COVID-19 · Hepatitis B · TB · HIV · Co-infection · Ghana

---

G. K. Helegbe (✉)
Department of Biochemistry and Molecular Medicine, School of Medicine, University for Development Studies, Tamale, Ghana
e-mail: ghelegbe@uds.edu.gh

P. A. Aryee
Department of Nutritional Sciences, School of Allied Health Sciences, University for Development Studies, Tamale, Ghana

P. S. Nyasulu
Faculty of Health Sciences, School of Public Health, University of the Witwatersrand, Johannesburg, South Africa

F. Mphande and P. Nyasulu (eds.), *Evaluating Outbreak Potential of Infections in Tropical Climates*, https://doi.org/10.1007/978-981-95-0618-7_4

List of Abbreviations

ART	Antiretroviral therapy
COVID-19	Corona virus disease-2019 (SARS-CoV 2)
HIV	Human immunodeficiency virus
TB	Tuberculosis
PMTCT	Prevention of Mother to child transmission of HIV
GMIS	Ghana Malaria Indicator Survey
ITN	Insecticide treated nets
LLINs	Long-lasting Insecticidal Nets
SMC	Seasonal Malaria Chemoprevention
RDTs	Rapid Diagnostic Tests
ACTs	Artemisinin based combination therapies
NTCP	National Tuberculosis Control
GHS	Ghana Health Service

4.1 Epidemiology and Transmission of Key Infectious Diseases in Ghana

Hepatitis B, HIV, malaria, and tuberculosis (TB) are the common prevailing diseases in West African countries and this chapter will focus on these four infectious diseases. In addition to occurring separately, Hepatitis B, HIV, Malaria, and TB often overlap among patients thereby complicating diagnostic processes and dispensation of care or medicines.

4.1.1 HIV in Ghana

HIV continues to be a critical public health concern in Ghana, despite the efforts and considerable progress through interventions like antiretroviral therapy (ART). Since the first case reported in 1986, Ghana has taken measures on testing, treatment, and public awareness to curb the epidemic. The prevalence of HIV in Ghana mirrors challenges which can be linked to sociocultural practices, gender inequality, and health system inefficiencies (Boah et al., 2023; UNAIDS, 2023a).

Meanwhile, around 330,000 people, including 18,000 children, are living with HIV in Ghana. The prevalence rate in adults is 1.5%, with women showing 2.0%, higher compared to men's 1.0% (UNAIDS, 2023b). This gender disparity is attributed to factors such as gender-based violence, inequitable healthcare access, and lower levels of HIV knowledge among women (Asamoah et al., 2017). The Northern Region has one of the lowest HIV prevalence rates in Ghana, reflecting rural lifestyles and

Table 4.1 Some risk factors associated with HIV transmission

Risk factor	Activity	Risk population
Low condom use	High risk sexual activity is just 25.8% among adults, with lower rates among women (UNAIDS, 2023)	Adults
Socio-cultural practices	Practices such as polygamy, stigma, and discrimination hinder access to testing and treatment (Boah et al., 2023)	Adults, Adolescents, children
Vertical transmission	Despite 90% coverage of PMTCT programs, gaps remain, leading to 12.6% vertical transmission (UNAIDS, 2023)	Adults, adolescents, children

fewer high-risk behaviors compared to urban regions (Boah et al., 2023). However, limited healthcare access and cultural barriers still pose challenges to HIV control efforts. Several risk factors have been associated with HIV transmission including, low condom use, socio-cultural practices and vertical transmission (Table 4.1).

HIV affects mostly adults aged 15 years and above, who account for 320,000 cases. Women represent a significant majority, highlighting gender disparities in access to care and prevention. For children (0–14 years), an estimated 18,000 live with HIV, underscoring the need for enhanced PMTCT interventions (Croxford et al., 2017; UNAIDS, 2023). The introduction of ART in 2003 significantly changed the trajectory of the HIV epidemic in Ghana. The prevalence and AIDS related deaths rose sharply, with limited access to treatment. HIV incidence declined from 3.38 per 1,000 people in 1990 to 0.94 per 1,000 in 2020, and AIDS related deaths dropped by 4% annually after 2004 (Boah et al., 2023). ART also improved survival, leading to a stabilization of HIV prevalence despite reductions in new infections (Zaidi et al., 2013).

ART has transformed HIV from a fatal disease to a manageable chronic condition. While prevalence initially increased due to prolonged survival, ART now contributes to reduced mortality and incidence. Nevertheless, gaps in access to care, stigma, and inequities in treatment persist (Mills et al., 2011; UNAIDS, 2023). HIV management in Ghana has seen significant advancements, particularly after the introduction of ART. However, persistent challenges require sustained efforts, including addressing stigma, increasing ART coverage, and improving prevention strategies.

4.1.2 *Malaria in Ghana*

Malaria is one of the most significant public health concerns in Ghana, accounting for a large proportion of outpatient visits and hospital admissions annually. Despite years of interventions and measures to reduce its prevalence, malaria remains endemic, with high transmission rates in all regions, especially among vulnerable populations such as children under five years and pregnant women (World Health Organization [WHO], 2023b; Ghana Health Service, 2022a). Efforts to combat malaria in Ghana have focused on preventive measures, early diagnosis, and treatment through a multisectoral approach.

The prevalence of malaria in Ghana varies by region, influenced by climate, environmental conditions, and socioeconomic factors. According to the Ghana Malaria Indicator Survey (GMIS), 2022, malaria prevalence by microscopy in children aged 6–59 months was approximately 20%, showing regional differences, with the highest burden in the northern and forest zones. This represents a decline from 27% recorded in 2019, indicating gradual progress in malaria control (GMIS, 2022). In the Northern Region of Ghana, malaria remains hyperendemic. The region's high prevalence is driven by environmental conditions conducive to mosquito breeding, such as bushy areas, exposed refuse dumps, and stagnant water. Poverty, limited access to healthcare, and low use of preventive measures like insecticide treated nets (ITNs) exacerbate the problem in this region (Ghana Health Service, 2022a).

Several factors contribute to the persistence of malaria in Ghana including environmental conditions, behavioral practices, socioeconomic inequalities and drug resistance (Table 4.2).

Children under five years are the most vulnerable group, accounting for the majority of malaria cases and deaths. Pregnant women are also highly susceptible due to reduced immunity during pregnancy. In 2022, malaria prevalence among children under five in Ghana was higher than in older age groups, underscoring the need for targeted interventions (GMIS, 2022; WHO, 2023a). Over the years, Ghana has achieved notable progress in malaria control, attributed to: Introduction of ITNs and Long-lasting Insecticidal Nets (LLINs).These have significantly reduced malaria incidence by providing physical and chemical barriers against mosquitoes. Seasonal Malaria Chemoprevention (SMC), and Rapid Diagnostic Tests (RDTs) have improved early detection and treatment, reducing malaria related complications (Ghana Health Service, 2022a).

Table 4.2 Factors contributing to persistence of malaria in Ghana

Factor	Consequences
Environmental conditions	The tropical climate and rainy seasons support the breeding of Anopheles mosquitoes, the primary malaria vectors (WHO, 2023)
Behavioral practices	Low ITN usage and inconsistent adherence to malaria prevention programs weaken efforts to curb transmission (GMIS, 2022)
Socioeconomic inequalities	Poverty and inadequate access to healthcare facilities leave many communities vulnerable to the disease
Drug resistance	Emerging resistance to antimalarial drugs, especially in Plasmodium falciparum, poses a growing challenge (WHO, 2023)

Before the widespread implementation of malaria control interventions, the disease was responsible for substantial morbidity and mortality in Ghana. The introduction of ITNs, LLINs, and artemisinin based combination therapies (ACTs) has reduced malaria related deaths significantly. From 2010 to 2020, malaria mortality rates have declined by over 60%, highlighting the impact of sustained intervention programs (WHO, 2023a). Nevertheless, challenges persist, including the uneven distribution of resources, insecticide resistance, and gaps in community education. Efforts must focus on scaling up effective interventions and addressing emerging threats to sustain the progress made.

4.1.3 Tuberculosis in Ghana

Tuberculosis (TB) continues to be a significant public health concern in Ghana, with the disease burden exacerbated by socioeconomic factors, healthcare system challenges, and its link to HIV. Although Ghana has made strides in TB prevention and treatment, gaps in diagnosis, treatment coverage, and awareness persist. Efforts to control TB are spearheaded by the National Tuberculosis Control Programme (NTCP), which aligns with global strategies such as the WHO's End TB Strategy (World Health Organization [WHO], 2023b; Ghana Health Service [GHS], 2022b). Ghana records an estimated TB incidence of 152 cases per 100,000 people annually. Adults aged 15–49, particularly men, bear the greatest disease burden. Urban areas experience higher transmission due to overcrowding and poor living conditions, while rural regions struggle with limited access to healthcare services and underreporting (WHO, 2023b; NTCP, 2022). Despite these challenges, TB treatment success rates have improved, reaching 86% in 2021, a testament to efforts like Directly Observed Treatment, Short Course (DOTS) and expanded case detection (Friedland et al., 2020).

The Northern Region has lower reported TB prevalence compared to urban centers but suffers from significant under diagnosis. The shortage of diagnostic tools such as GeneXpert machines, stigma, and poor health seeking behaviors among rural populations contribute to undetected cases (NTCP, 2022). These challenges highlight the need for targeted interventions in the region, including mobile diagnostic services and community-based education (Alhassan et al., 2020). Several interlinked factors contribute to TB transmission and progression in Ghana (Table 4.3).

The disease predominantly affects economically active adults aged 15–49, making TB not only a health issue but al2022bso an economic burden. Children are also vulnerable, particularly those exposed to untreated TB cases in households. TB meningitis and other severe forms remain common among undiagnosed children (GHS, 2022b; Friedland et al., 2020).

Several initiatives have contributed to Ghana's progress in reducing TB prevalence and mortality:

Table 4.3 Factors contributing to TB transmission in Ghana

Factor	Consequence
HIV Co-infection	TB is the leading cause of death among people living with HIV (PLHIV), with 20% of TB cases associated with HIV (UNAIDS, 2023)
Socioeconomic disparities	Poverty, overcrowding, and malnutrition elevate TB vulnerability in underserved communities (WHO, 2023)
Delayed diagnosis	Cultural stigma and misconceptions about TB hinder timely detection and treatment (Alhassan et al., 2020)
Drug resistance	Multidrug resistant TB (MDRTB) poses an increasing threat, requiring more resources and complex treatments (Friedland et al., 2020)

- GeneXpert Machines: These diagnostics have improved TB detection, including MDRTB.
- Integrated HIV/TB Care: Coordinated care for TB and HIV patients has reduced mortality among coinfected individuals (UNAIDS, 2023).
- Community Engagement: Public health campaigns and partnerships with community leaders have enhanced TB awareness and reduced stigma (Alhassan et al., 2020).
- Despite progress, several barriers hinder Ghana's efforts to eliminate TB:
- Stigma and Myths: TB's association with HIV fosters discrimination and fear, discouraging individuals from seeking diagnosis or treatment.
- Drug Resistance: MDRTB cases require more expensive, prolonged treatment regimens, posing a financial burden on the health system (WHO, 2023b).
- Funding Gaps: Limited resources for TB programs restrict the scale of interventions, including diagnostic and treatment services (Friedland et al., 2020).

To accelerate progress toward TB elimination, Ghana must address these challenges by:

- Expanding access to diagnostics, especially in rural areas.
- Scaling up preventive measures like TB vaccination and chemoprophylaxis.
- Strengthening healthcare systems to ensure uninterrupted drug supply.
- Investing in education to combat stigma and encourage early treatment seeking behavior.

4.2 Impact of HIV, TB, Malaria, and Hepatitis B on Ghanaian Society

HIV, tuberculosis (TB), malaria, and hepatitis B continue to pose significant public health challenges in Ghana, impacting the health, livelihoods, education, and overall socioeconomic development of the country. These diseases not only burden the healthcare system but also deeply affect individuals, families, and communities, ultimately hindering national progress. HIV significantly weakens the immune system, leaving individuals vulnerable to opportunistic infections like TB, which is the leading cause of death among people living with HIV (PLHIV) in Ghana. Malaria, on the other hand, remains the leading cause of morbidity and mortality among children under five and pregnant women, contributing to high infant and maternal death rates. Hepatitis B adds to the burden with its progression to chronic liver diseases such as cirrhosis and hepatocellular carcinoma, which require longterm and expensive care. Together, these diseases strain healthcare systems already grappling with limited resources, diagnostic capacities, and overburdened health personnel (Boah et al., 2023; Ghana Health Service [GHS], 2022b).

The economic toll of these diseases is profound, especially since they primarily affect individuals in the productive age group of 15–49 years. Reduced workforce participation due to illness or death leads to loss of household income and pushes families into poverty. Treatment costs, although subsidized in some cases, remain significant, especially for rural populations that incur additional expenses for diagnostic tests and transportation. This financial strain disproportionately affects low-income households, worsening inequality and limiting access to essential healthcare services. For instance, managing drug-resistant TB and malaria or chronic hepatitis B often requires specialized care, which many cannot afford, further perpetuating cycles of poverty (Friedland et al., 2020; UNAIDS, 2023).

The Impact of these diseases extends to education, particularly for children. Frequent illness or the need to care for sick family members leads to high rates of absenteeism, especially in malaria endemic regions. Stigma associated with diseases like HIV and TB discourages affected children from attending school, creating barriers to education. Furthermore, recurrent illnesses and chronic conditions hinder students' ability to concentrate, reducing their academic performance and long term educational outcomes. This limits their future opportunities and ability to contribute to societal development, perpetuating cycles of underachievement and vulnerability (Croxford et al., 2017; GHS, 2022b).

At the community level, these diseases exacerbate social challenges, including stigma and discrimination. People living with HIV, TB, or hepatitis B often face social exclusion, losing access to employment and community support. This stigma not only discourages individuals from seeking diagnosis and treatment but also facilitates the continued spread of these diseases. Additionally, the intergenerational impact is substantial, as children orphaned by these diseases often face poverty, limited access to education, and poor health outcomes, further destabilizing families and communities (WHO, 2023).

On a national scale, these diseases impose a heavy economic burden. Malaria alone is estimated to cost the Ghanaian economy over $760 million annually, largely due to healthcare expenses and lost productivity. The combined effect of absenteeism, premature deaths, and treatment costs undermines economic growth and development. These diseases also strain national health systems, diverting resources from other critical health issues and revealing gaps in infrastructure and funding. The limited availability of diagnostic tools and treatments, particularly in rural areas, underscores the challenges in achieving universal health coverage (National Tuberculosis Control Programme [NTCP], 2022; Ghana Malaria Indicator Survey [GMIS], 2022).

Despite efforts to address these challenges, significant barriers remain. Weak healthcare infrastructure, inadequate funding, and cultural misconceptions hinder progress. Drug resistance, particularly in TB and malaria cases, poses an emerging threat that requires more resources and innovative treatment strategies. To mitigate these impacts, Ghana must prioritize strengthening its healthcare systems, increasing funding for diagnostic and treatment services, and scaling up preventive measures like vaccinations and public health campaigns. Community engagement and education are also essential to reduce stigma, improve health seeking behavior, and foster a supportive environment for those affected. HIV, TB, malaria, and hepatitis B profoundly affect Ghana's health, economy, education, and social fabric. These diseases undermine individual wellbeing and collective national progress, demanding sustained and integrated efforts to combat their impact. Addressing these challenges will require not only financial investments but also a commitment to equity, innovation, and community centered approaches to health.

4.3 Impact on Public Health

Public health in Ghana has been profoundly affected by the prevalence of hepatitis B, HIV, malaria, and tuberculosis (TB). Each of these diseases carries unique challenges, affecting not only individuals but also families, communities, and the broader socioeconomic framework of the country. Below, the impact of each disease is analyzed in depth.

Hepatitis B

Hepatitis B is a significant public health concern in Ghana, with a prevalence rate of around 12%, particularly among children and rural populations (OforiAsenso & Agyeman, 2016). Chronic hepatitis B is often asymptomatic, leading to late diagnosis and increasing the risk of complications like liver cirrhosis and hepatocellular carcinoma. These conditions account for a significant proportion of liverrelated deaths in the country. The disease is often transmitted from mother to child during childbirth or early childhood, making vaccination critical. Although Ghana introduced the hepatitis B vaccine into its Expanded Programme on Immunization (EPI) in 2002, disparities in vaccine access, particularly in rural areas, hinder its effectiveness.

Hepatitis B's impact extends beyond health. Economically, it imposes a substantial burden on families due to the cost of treatment for advanced liver disease, including antiviral medications and liver transplants, which are often inaccessible to many Ghanaians. Socially, the disease contributes to stigma, which discourages individuals from seeking testing or treatment. Public health programs targeting hepatitis B have emphasized prevention through vaccination, screening, and education, but challenges remain. Improved access to vaccines, routine antenatal screening, and public awareness campaigns are essential to combat the disease and reduce its impact on public health and society.

HIV

HIV continues to have a profound impact on Ghana's public health system, particularly among young adults aged 15–49, who account for the majority of cases (Boah et al., 2023). Despite the introduction of antiretroviral therapy (ART) and increased access to treatment, challenges persist in addressing stigma and ensuring equitable healthcare delivery. HIV significantly weakens the immune system, making individuals vulnerable to opportunistic infections such as tuberculosis. The prevalence of HIV is compounded by factors like poverty, limited access to healthcare in rural areas, and cultural practices that hinder safe sexual health behaviors.

From a health perspective, HIV contributes significantly to morbidity and mortality in Ghana. The disease affects productivity, as individuals in their prime working years are often incapacitated or lose their lives to AIDSrelated complications. The socioeconomic impact is felt at both household and national levels, as families lose breadwinners and healthcare resources are diverted to manage HIVrelated illnesses. Stigma and discrimination remain critical barriers, discouraging individuals from seeking early testing and treatment. Efforts to mitigate the impact of HIV in Ghana have focused on increasing ART coverage, promoting awareness campaigns, and integrating HIV services with maternal and child health programs. However, challenges persist, including inconsistent access to medications and the dual burden of HIV and TB. Achieving sustained progress will require addressing stigma, enhancing healthcare infrastructure, and promoting widespread public education.

Malaria

Malaria remains the most significant public health challenge in Ghana, particularly affecting children under five and pregnant women. According to the Ghana Health Service (2022a), the disease accounts for 40% of outpatient visits and 19% of all deaths. Malaria's cyclical nature, influenced by environmental factors like seasonal rainfall and stagnant water, ensures its persistence in many communities. Control measures such as insecticide treated nets (ITNs), indoor residual spraying, and seasonal malaria chemoprevention have led to some progress, yet gaps in implementation and access remain significant hurdles.

The health Impact of malaria is substantial, causing high morbidity and mortality rates. Pregnant women are particularly vulnerable, as malaria can result in maternal anemia, low birth weight, and infant mortality. Economically, the disease imposes a severe burden on families and the healthcare system. Treatment costs, combined with lost productivity due to illness, strain household incomes and hinder national economic growth. For children, repeated malaria episodes affect school attendance and performance, perpetuating cycles of poverty.

Ongoing efforts to combat malaria in Ghana include expanding access to ITNs, improving diagnostic services, and increasing public awareness. However, the emergence of insecticide resistant mosquitoes and antimalarial drug resistance threatens progress. A multisectoral approach involving robust healthcare systems, environmental management, and community engagement is essential to reduce the public health burden of malaria.

Tuberculosis (TB)

Tuberculosis remains a persistent public health threat in Ghana, particularly among individuals living with HIV. The dual epidemic of TB and HIV significantly complicates treatment and increases mortality rates. The prevalence of TB is exacerbated by factors such as overcrowded living conditions, poverty, and limited access to diagnostic and treatment services (WHO, 2023). The emergence of multidrug resistant TB (MDRTB) further complicates the situation, requiring expensive and prolonged treatment regimens.

The health Impact of TB is profound, with the disease causing chronic respiratory symptoms, weight loss, and fatigue. Untreated TB is highly infectious, contributing to community transmission and straining public health resources. Economically, the disease reduces productivity, as affected individuals are often unable to work during prolonged treatment periods. At the household level, families face significant financial strain due to medical costs and lost income. Public health responses to TB in Ghana have focused on improving diagnostic capacity, expanding access to treatment, and integrating TB and HIV services. However, stigma and misconceptions about the disease remain barriers to early diagnosis and treatment adherence. Strengthening community-based interventions, increasing public awareness, and addressing socioeconomic determinants of health are critical for reducing the burden of TB.

4.3.1 Public Health Initiatives in Ghana

Ghana faces significant health challenges due to infectious diseases like Hepatitis B, HIV, malaria, and tuberculosis (TB), compounded by the growing burden of noncommunicable diseases (NCDs) like diabetes and hypertension. These diseases not only threaten public health but also impede the nation's socio economic development. This section addresses the control strategies, treatment approaches, challenges, and interventions for each disease, alongside lessons learned from other countries.

Hepatitis B

Control and Treatment

Hepatitis B remains a public health challenge in Ghana, with chronic infection prevalence estimated at 12.3% (Schweitzer et al., 2015). Control strategies revolve around vaccination, especially through the Expanded Programme on Immunization (EPI), which has significantly reduced posterchild transmission. Antiviral treatments such as tenofovir and entecavir are used to manage chronic cases, especially among pregnant women to prevent vertical transmission (Martinson et al., 1996). Screening during antenatal care has also improved early detection rates, although gaps remain in coverage and accessibility, particularly in rural areas.

Challenges and Interventions

The lack of awareness about hepatitis B transmission, prevention, and treatment continues to hinder public health efforts. Stigma attached to the disease further discourages individuals from seeking diagnosis or care. Rural populations face additional barriers, including inadequate diagnostic facilities and limited healthcare resources (Ofori Asenso & Agyeman, 2016). To address these challenges, public education campaigns have been intensified, emphasizing preventive measures such as vaccination and safe healthcare practices. Health worker training programs and international partnerships with organizations like WHO and GAVI have enhanced vaccine availability. Expanding diagnostic services and community-based care models is essential to improving hepatitis B management in underserved areas. Lessons from countries like Taiwan, which successfully integrated hepatitis B vaccination into its national immunization program, underscore the importance of sustained funding and widespread public awareness campaigns (Chang et al., 1997).

HIV

Control and Treatment

HIV control in Ghana has improved significantly due to the availability of antiretroviral therapy (ART). The Ghana AIDS Commission and National HIV/AIDS Strategic Plan have prioritized universal access to ART, achieving 74% coverage among people living with HIV (UNAIDS, 2023). Prevention initiatives like voluntary counseling and testing (VCT), prevention of mother to child transmission (PMTCT), and preexposure prophylaxis (PrEP) programs have also contributed to progress.

Challenges and Interventions

Despite these achievements, challenges persist. Stigma and discrimination against people living with HIV (PLWH) remain major barriers to accessing care. Geographic disparities in ART distribution also limit access in rural areas, while funding constraints affect program sustainability (Nketiah Amponsah et al., 2020). In overcoming these challenges, Ghana has strengthened decentralized healthcare delivery, integrating HIV services into primary care facilities. Public education campaigns targeting stigma reduction have been launched alongside efforts to train healthcare workers in HIV management. International collaborations, such as those with PEPFAR and the Global Fund, continue to provide technical and financial support to Ghana's HIV programs (UNAIDS, 2023). South Africa have achieved significant gains by adopting community-based ART distribution models, which Ghana could emulate to enhance rural access.

Malaria

Control and Treatment

Malaria is endemic in Ghana, contributing to 19% of outpatient visits and 22% of hospital admissions in 2022 (NMCP, 2022). Key control measures include the widespread distribution of insecticide treated nets (ITNs), indoor residual spraying (IRS), and intermittent preventive treatment in pregnancy (IPTp). Artemisinin based combination therapies (ACTs) remain the mainstay of malaria treatment, supported by diagnostic tools like rapid diagnostic tests (RDTs) and microscopy.

Challenges and Interventions

The effectiveness of malaria control efforts is hampered by the emergence of insecticide resistance, improper use of ITNs, and limited access to healthcare services in rural regions (Asante et al., 2018). Behavioral and cultural practices also affect compliance with preventive measures. Ghana has strengthened its surveillance systems, enabling real-time detection and response to outbreaks. Public education campaigns promote ITN usage and early treatment seeking behavior. Additionally, Ghana has benefitted from international funding for malaria control, including initiatives supported by the Global Fund and the Roll Back Malaria Partnership. Rwanda's integrated vector management approach, which includes combining ITN use with community driven IRS, offers valuable insights for scaling malaria control efforts in Ghana.

Tuberculosis (TB)

Control and Treatment

TB remains a significant health burden in Ghana, exacerbated by the prevalence of multidrug resistant TB (MDRTB) and its coinfection with HIV. The directly observed treatment short course (DOTS) strategy underpins Ghana's TB control efforts. Recent advances include the introduction of GeneXpert machines, which have improved the timely detection of drug-resistant TB (WHO, 2023b).

Challenges and Interventions

Underdiagnosis and treatment nonadherence are major challenges in TB management. Rural areas face limited diagnostic and treatment facilities, while stigma associated with TB discourages timely healthcare seeking behavior (Owusu Dabo et al., 2018). Additionally, MDRTB cases continue to rise, with insufficient laboratory capacity to detect resistance contributing to the problem. Interventions to address these issues include scaling up diagnostic facilities, decentralizing TB care, and training community health workers to support patients during treatment. Collaboration with international organizations like the Global Fund has bolstered funding for TB programs. Public education campaigns have also been instrumental in combating stigma and improving treatment adherence.

Countries like India have integrated digital adherence technologies, such as 99DOTS, to monitor TB treatment adherence, a model Ghana could adapt to enhance its TB control efforts.

Diabetes and hypertension complicate the management of infectious diseases like TB and HIV. These NCDs increase susceptibility to infections and worsen treatment outcomes (WHO, 2023b). In Ghana, NCD management has been integrated into primary healthcare services to address the dual burden of disease. Expanding access to screening and treatment for NCDs is critical to improving overall health outcomes.

4.4 Management of Co-infections During the COVID-19 Pandemic in Northern Ghana

Northern Ghana presents significant public health concerns due to the high frequency of infectious illnesses such as hepatitis B, HIV, malaria, tuberculosis (TB), Yellow fever and cholera. The onset of the COVID-19 pandemic put a further burden on the healthcare system, complicating the management of these diseases and associated co-infections. This section investigates the prevalence of these diseases, their impact on the population, and the techniques used to control co-infections throughout the pandemic.

a. **Yellow Fever Outbreak in the Savannah Region of Ghana**

During the pandemic, the Savannah Region of Ghana saw a significant rise in yellow fever which presented thorny problems for health care providers and public health officials. The Aedes mosquito transmits yellow fever, which is an epidemic-prone viral hemorrhagic disease, that has historically threatened several places in West Africa including Ghana. Though the government and other global health agencies put in place health strategies aimed at curbing the yellow fever epidemic in Ghana, there are still sporadic outbreaks of the fever among the unvaccinated populations mostly comprised of suspected migrants who are nomadic farmers that come into the country. Knowledge about these nomadic people regarding their perception, attitude, and practices towards yellow fever in Ghana is scanty (Inusah et al., 2023). The limited availability of healthcare resources was a major challenge in managing the yellow fever outbreak. The healthcare system was already under enormous strain as a result of the COVID-19 pandemic, with resources diverted to manage the increase in COVID-19 cases. Hospitals and clinics faced a lack of medical supplies, personnel, and facilities, complicating the response to the yellow fever epidemic. The overlapping symptoms of yellow fever and COVID-19, such as fever and fatigue, put additional strain on diagnostic capabilities.

Vaccination is the most effective way to prevent yellow fever outbreaks. However, during the pandemic, implementing broad vaccination campaigns presented considerable logistical obstacles. Movement limitations, social distancing measures, and concern about COVID-19 transmission hampered the capacity to carry out large-scale vaccination campaigns. Public health officials have to respond by focusing immunization efforts on high-risk areas and demographics. Community engagement and education were crucial in encouraging vaccine uptake during the pandemic.

The use of digital health technologies and mobile health applications facilitated real-time data collection and reporting, allowing health authorities to track the spread of both diseases. To effectively manage the yellow fever outbreak, robust disease surveillance systems were required, which combined yellow fever and COVID-19 monitoring to allow for timely identification and response to new cases. Educating communities about the importance of vaccination and vector control measures, such as eliminating mosquito breeding sites, helped reduce the risk of yellow fever transmission. Involving community leaders and local organizations in health promotion activities ensured culturally sensitive and effective communication. Vector control measures were crucial in mitigating the spread of yellow fever. Public health officials stepped up efforts to minimize mosquito populations through targeted insecticide spraying, distribution of insecticide-treated bed nets, and environmental management. Community members were invited to help eliminate mosquito breeding areas, such as stagnant water sources. The combination of vector control activities with COVID-19 preventive measures, such as encouraging personal protective measures and hygiene behaviors, aided overall disease prevention.

The yellow fever outbreak highlighted the need for strengthening the healthcare system's capacity to respond to multiple infectious disease threats simultaneously. Investments in healthcare infrastructure, including the establishment of dedicated treatment centers and laboratories, were essential. Training healthcare workers on the management of yellow fever and COVID-19 co-infections ensured that patients received appropriate care. The pandemic underscored the importance of building resilient health systems capable of withstanding future public health emergencies. The management of the yellow fever outbreak during the COVID-19 pandemic provided valuable lessons for future public health responses. The importance of maintaining routine immunization services, even during a pandemic, was evident. Strengthening disease surveillance systems and enhancing intersectoral collaboration are critical for effective outbreak response. Investments in healthcare infrastructure, workforce training, and community engagement are necessary to build resilient health systems. The integration of digital health technologies and data-driven approaches can enhance disease monitoring and response capabilities. The yellow fever outbreak in the Savannah Region of Ghana during the COVID-19 pandemic presented significant challenges for public health authorities. Effective management necessitated a complex strategy that includes vaccine programs, integrated disease surveillance, community engagement, vector control measures, and healthcare system strengthening. The event highlighted the need for developing resilient health systems and emphasized the need for continued investments in public health infrastructure and personnel capability (Appawu et al., 2006).

By 2020, yellow fever had risen in prevalence across the continent. Ghana had the highest number of cases per 100,000 people (1267) out of which 10,350 were officially verified (WHO, 2019). According to Nwaiwu et al. (2021), the mortality rate in Ghana ranges from 10 to 17 percent. Up till now, there is no known cure for yellow fever but vaccination has been highlighted as the most effective way to prevent the risk of getting sick or dying from this disease (Angel et al., 2017; Marlow et al., 2016).

b. **Malaria**

A persistent issue confronting the Northern Ghana public health system is malaria, as it leads to significant ill health and deaths, particularly among children below five years and expectant mothers. The efforts to control malaria were made more difficult by the COVID-19 pandemic and these problems were dealt with adaptively so that management of the disease could be done adequately. One of the many effects of COVID-19 on some Malaria intervention programs took place through restrictions in mobility and lockdowns that hindered possible access to insecticide-treated bed nets (ITNs), indoor residual spraying (IRS), and antimalarial medicines (Heuschen et al., 2023).

Routine malaria preventive and treatment programs were disrupted, causing delays in diagnosis and treatment. COVID-19 cases raised the demand on health institutions, diverting resources and attention away from malaria control efforts. Since malaria and COVID-19 share common symptoms, such as fever, this posed diagnostic challenges during the pandemic. Differentiating between the two diseases required efficient diagnostic tools and trained healthcare personnel. The pandemic led to a surge in fever cases, overwhelming healthcare facilities and complicating the diagnostic process. Rapid diagnostic tests (RDTs) for malaria and COVID-19 testing needed to be integrated to ensure timely and accurate diagnosis (Heuschen et al., 2023). Preserving malaria abatement measures throughout the pandemic was imperative. While still following COVID-19 guidelines, public health officers adapted IRS and ITN distribution by applying innovations. Besides providing homes with ITNs, community health workers were also instrumental in sensitizing members of the community to malaria control. Digital platforms and mobile applications facilitated monitoring as well as coordination of preventive initiatives. The COVID-19 pandemic affected antimalarial therapy access through disruption of health services and supply chains (Chanda-Kapata et al., 2022). There have been reports of stockouts in some regions for essential antimalarial drugs or diagnostic kits. Public health officials set up policies aimed at ensuring the availability of these drugs; this included decentralized distribution points and community-based treatments. Patients suffering from malaria received remote consultations and assistance from community health workers and telehealth programs. During the pandemic, integrated community case management (iCCM) of malaria, pneumonia, and diarrhea proved to be successful in treating the disease. By diagnosing and treating malaria cases locally, community health workers relieved the strain on medical facilities. Health education and COVID-19 prevention methods were added to iCCM programs. This strategy reduced the chance of COVID-19 co-infections while ensuring continuity of care for individuals with malaria. The COVID-19 pandemic highlighted the need for strengthening the health system to manage multiple infectious diseases simultaneously. Investments in healthcare infrastructure, training of healthcare workers, and improving supply chain management were essential. Strengthening laboratory capacity for malaria and COVID-19 testing enhanced diagnostic accuracy and disease surveillance (Heuschen et al., 2023). Health information systems were upgraded to facilitate data collection, analysis, and reporting. Community engagement and education were crucial in sustaining malaria control efforts during the pandemic. Public health campaigns raised awareness about the importance of malaria prevention and treatment, even amidst the COVID-19 crisis. Community leaders and local organizations were involved in disseminating health messages and mobilizing community members. Educational materials emphasized the need to seek timely care for malaria symptoms and adhere to preventive measures.

The pandemic ignited novel ideas and studies on malaria prevention. The research done on how COVID-19 impacts malaria transmission and outcomes has given vital insights for effective programs and policy adjustments. Advances in diagnostics equipment, for example, combination RATs for malaria and COVID-19, resulted in an increase in diagnostic efficiency. With the development of data analysis techniques and digital health technologies, illness monitoring significantly improved. The ability to manage malaria during the COVID-19 situation shows the necessity for building strong health systems that can respond to various public health threats. In the long term, there should be continued funding for control programs that address the diagnosis, treatment, and prevention of malaria. To improve general health outcomes measures such as strengthening community health systems as well as integrating malaria service delivery with other medical areas may yield positive results (Heuschen et al., 2023).

Finally, managing malaria during the COVID-19 pandemic in Northern Ghana required a coordinated response and flexible strategies. The pandemic imposed a strain on healthcare resources, complicated testing methods, and stalled malaria control efforts. Nonetheless, malaria services were maintained through innovative techniques of treatment, prevention, community engagement, and health system development. The episode serves as a reminder of the need for solid health systems and ongoing malaria control funding to preserve vulnerable areas and maintain the disease's decline.

c. **TB Infections**

Since 2019, TB has remained the most common cause of death from a single infectious pathogen. Globally, approximately 10.0 million people developed TB disease and there were an estimated 1.2 million TB deaths among people with HIV and an additional 208, 000 deaths among people living with HIV. Adults were responsible for 88% and children, aged < 15 years, for 12% of all persons with TB, in the year 2019 (Chakaya et al., 2021).

Northern Ghana has a high rate of disease burden and mortality from TB, and the COVID-19 pandemic has made managing TB more difficult. The COVID-19 pandemic disrupted TB services, causing delays in diagnosis, treatment interruptions, and decreased access to healthcare facilities. Patients were discouraged from seeking care due to lockdowns, movement restrictions, and fear of COVID-19 transmission. Health facilities were overloaded with COVID-19 cases, diverting resources and attention from TB services. Additionally, the pandemic disrupted supply networks, resulting in shortages of vital TB drugs and testing equipment. The diagnosis approach is made more difficult by the respiratory symptoms that COVID-19 and TB share, such as fever and cough. It took skilled medical professionals and effective diagnostic equipment to distinguish between the two illnesses. The pandemic caused a spike in respiratory infections that overloaded diagnostic centers and made it more difficult to identify TB cases. To guarantee a prompt and precise diagnosis, the integration of COVID-19 and tuberculosis tests was crucial (Alipanah et al., 2018). To effectively address the co-infections, integrated approaches, and robust health systems are needed.

To avoid medication resistance and treatment disruptions during the pandemic, maintaining the continuity of TB treatment was essential. Public health officials put plans in place to guarantee that TB drugs were available, such as community-based treatment programs and decentralized distribution stations. The use of home-based treatment models and multi-month TB medication delivery was implemented to lessen the frequency of hospital visits. Patients with tuberculosis received remote consultations and support from community health workers and telehealth programs. It was essential to implement infection control procedures to stop the spread of COVID-19 and tuberculosis in hospital environments. To guarantee proper isolation and treatment, healthcare facilities adopted methods to segregate COVID-19 and tuberculosis patients. Healthcare professionals received training on infection management and personal protective equipment (PPE) to reduce the danger of co-infection. Training in infection prevention and control was provided to community health workers so they could provide patients with community education and assistance (Afum et al., 2021).

Community engagement and education were essential in raising awareness about TB symptoms and the significance of seeking timely care. Integrating TB and COVID-19 services enhanced the efficiency of healthcare delivery and improved patient outcomes. Dual screening and testing for TB and COVID-19 allowed for timely diagnosis and appropriate management of co-infections. Community health workers played a vital role in TB case detection, treatment adherence support, and health education. House-to-house screening and contact tracing activities were conducted to identify and manage TB cases at the community level (Adusei-Poku et al., 2023). Health information systems were upgraded to capture data on both diseases, facilitating coordinated response efforts. Joint training programs for healthcare workers ensured that they were equipped to manage co-infections effectively. The COVID-19 pandemic highlighted the need for strengthening the health system to manage TB and other infectious diseases. Investments in healthcare infrastructure, training of healthcare workers, and improving supply chain management were essential (Alene et al., 2020). Strengthening laboratory capacity for TB and COVID-19 testing enhanced diagnostic accuracy and disease surveillance. Health information systems were upgraded to facilitate data collection, analysis, and reporting.

The pandemic sparked new ideas and research in the treatment of TB. Research on the effects of COVID-19 on TB outcomes and transmission has yielded important information for programmatic and policy changes. Diagnostic efficiency was increased by advancements in diagnostic instruments, such as combination fast testing for COVID-19 and TB (Adusei-Poku et al., 2023). Data analytics and digital health technologies improved illness surveillance and response plans (Mangtani et al., 2014). The COVID-19 pandemic's experience with treating TB highlights the significance of creating robust health systems that can address a variety of public health risks. It is crucial to maintain funding for TB control initiatives that include diagnosis, treatment, and prevention. Overall health results can be enhanced by fortifying community health systems and incorporating TB services with other medical initiatives. Digital technologies enable enhanced surveillance systems to deliver real-time data for well-informed decision-making. To maintain progress in TB control and accomplish elimination objectives, cooperation at the national, regional, and international levels is essential (Loembe & Nkengesong, 2021). In Northern Ghana, managing TB during the COVID-19 pandemic necessitated coordinated efforts and flexible approaches. The pandemic put a strain on healthcare resources, interrupted TB services, and presented diagnostic issues. On the other hand, the continuation of tuberculosis services was guaranteed by creative strategies in prevention, treatment, community involvement, and health system strengthening. The experience emphasizes the necessity of robust health systems and continuous funding for TB control to safeguard susceptible people and maintain the disease's progress toward eradication.

d. **Hepatitis**

Serious public health crises in northern Ghana are caused by hepatitis, particularly B and C. Management of hepatitis became more difficult during the COVID-19 pandemic, thus making it necessary for integrated approaches into resilient health systems able enough to address co-infections. Hepatitis services were also hindered by the pandemic leading to delays in diagnosis and treatment interruptions alongside reduced options for healthcare facilities. Patients faced with movement restrictions, lockdowns as well as fear of hiding away from access care were further dissuaded from seeking medical attention. Overwhelming cases of COVID-19 at health centers diverted resources meant for hepatitis services from being used on patients needing them. Lastly, supply chains were affected due to the pandemic resulting in a lack or inadequate delivery of important medicines for treating hepatitis-infected individuals (Abesig et al., 2020). The diagnosis approach was complicated by the common symptoms between COVID-19 and hepatitis, such as fever and exhaustion. Only specialists and effective diagnostic equipment could distinguish the two illnesses from each other. The pandemic caused a spike in cases with liver-related symptoms, which overloaded diagnostic centers and made it more difficult to identify instances of hepatitis. It was crucial to combine COVID-19 and hepatitis testing to guarantee prompt and precise diagnosis. During the pandemic, it was essential to continue treating hepatitis to avoid treatment disruptions and consequences connected to the liver. Strategies were put in place by public health authorities to guarantee the supply of hepatitis drugs. These included community-based treatment efforts and decentralized distribution stations. Multi-month dispensing of hepatitis drugs and home-based care models were adopted to reduce the need for frequent health facility visits. Telehealth services and community health workers provide remote consultations and support to hepatitis patients (Abesig et al., 2020).

It was imperative to implement infection control strategies to stop the spread of COVID-19 and hepatitis in hospital environments. To ensure proper isolation and treatment, healthcare facilities established methods to isolate patients with COVID-19 from those with hepatitis (Chabrol et al., 2019). Healthcare professionals received training on infection management and personal protective equipment (PPE) to reduce the danger of co-infection. Training in infection prevention and control was provided to community health workers so they could provide patients with community education and assistance. Hepatitis services were effectively maintained during the epidemic via community-based hepatitis care approaches. Community health professionals were essential in the identification of hepatitis cases, support for treatment adherence, and provision of health education. The community's hepatitis cases were identified and managed by contact tracing and door-to-door screening. To increase knowledge of hepatitis symptoms and the significance of receiving treatment as soon as possible, community involvement and education were essential. Hepatitis and COVID-19 services were integrated to improve patient outcomes and increase the effectiveness of healthcare delivery. It was possible to diagnose COVID-19 and hepatitis simultaneously and treat co-infections appropriately thanks to dual screening and testing. Upgrades to health information systems allowed for the collection of data on both diseases, which made coordinated response operations easier. Healthcare professionals were guaranteed to be well-prepared to handle co-infections through collaborative training programs. To control hepatitis and other infectious diseases, the health system needs to be strengthened, as the COVID-19 pandemic brought to light. Investments in healthcare infrastructure, training of healthcare workers, and improving supply chain management were essential. Strengthening laboratory capacity for hepatitis and COVID-19 testing enhanced diagnostic accuracy and disease surveillance. Health information systems were upgraded to facilitate data collection, analysis, and reporting.

The pandemic spurred research and innovation in hepatitis management. Studies on the impact of COVID-19 on hepatitis transmission and outcomes provided valuable insights for policy and programmatic adjustments. Innovations in diagnostic tools, such as combined rapid tests for hepatitis and COVID-19, improved diagnostic efficiency. Digital health technologies and data analytics enhanced disease surveillance and response strategies. The experience of managing hepatitis during the COVID-19 pandemic underscores the importance of building resilient health systems capable of responding to multiple public health threats. Sustained investments in hepatitis control programs, including prevention, diagnosis, and treatment, are essential. Strengthening community health systems and integrating hepatitis services with other health programs can improve overall health outcomes. Digital technology supported enhanced monitoring systems that furnish up-to-the-minute information for educated decision-making. Continuity in the fight against hepatitis and attaining elimination targets will rely heavily on joint initiatives at the national, regional, and global levels (Ghaffari et al., 2021). A coordinated approach was required as Northern Ghana's COVID-19 pandemic called for adaptive strategies. Disrupting hepatitis services, presenting diagnostic challenges, and putting pressure on healthcare providers were some of the things that this epidemic caused. Nevertheless, creative means of disease prevention, treatment delivery systems, including community collaboration, as well as strengthening health systems have been able to maintain hepatitis service provision. The lesson from such an experience is that there is a need for robust health systems and continued investments in hepatitis control to preserve vulnerable populations and maintain progress toward elimination.

e. **HIV**

The COVID-19 pandemic complicated HIV management, emphasizing the importance of integrated approaches and robust health systems for efficiently addressing co-infections. The COVID-19 pandemic hampered HIV services, causing delays in diagnosis, treatment disruptions, and limited access to healthcare facilities. Patients were discouraged from obtaining care due to movement restrictions, lockdowns, and concerns about COVID-19 transmission. COVID-19 cases overloaded healthcare facilities, diverting resources and focus away from HIV services. The pandemic also impacted supply chains, resulting in stockouts of key HIV drugs and diagnostic supplies.

HIV and COVID-19 share some common symptoms, such as fatigue and fever, complicating the diagnostic process. Differentiating between the two diseases required efficient diagnostic tools and trained healthcare personnel. The pandemic led to a surge in cases presenting with immune-related symptoms, overwhelming diagnostic facilities, and complicating HIV case detection. Integration of HIV and COVID-19 testing was essential to ensure timely and accurate diagnosis. Maintaining continuity of HIV treatment was critical during the pandemic to prevent treatment interruptions and AIDS-related complications. Public health authorities implemented strategies to ensure the availability of HIV medications, including decentralized distribution points and community-based treatment initiatives. Multi-month dispensing of HIV drugs and home-based care models were adopted to reduce the need for frequent health facility visits. Telehealth services and community health workers provided remote consultations and support to HIV patients. Infection control measures were crucial to prevent the transmission of HIV and COVID-19 in healthcare settings. Health facilities implemented protocols to separate HIV and COVID-19 patients, ensuring appropriate isolation and treatment. Personal protective equipment (PPE) and infection control training were provided to healthcare workers to minimize the risk of co-infection. Community health workers were trained in infection prevention and control to educate and support patients at the community level (Waston et al., 2022).

Community-based HIV care models were effective in maintaining HIV services during the pandemic. Community health workers play a vital role in HIV case detection, treatment adherence support, and health education. Door-to-door screening and contact tracing activities were conducted to identify and manage HIV cases at the community level. Community engagement and education were crucial in raising awareness about HIV symptoms and the importance of seeking timely care. Integrating HIV and COVID-19 services enhanced the efficiency of healthcare delivery and improved patient outcomes. Dual screening and testing for HIV and COVID-19 allowed for timely diagnosis and appropriate management of co-infections. Health information systems were upgraded to capture data on both diseases, facilitating coordinated response efforts. Joint training programs for healthcare workers ensured that they were equipped to manage co-infections effectively. The COVID-19 pandemic highlighted the need for strengthening the health system to manage HIV and other infectious diseases (Udoakang et al., 2023). Investments in healthcare infrastructure, training of healthcare workers, and improving supply chain management were essential. Strengthening laboratory capacity for HIV and COVID-19 testing enhanced diagnostic accuracy and disease surveillance. Health information systems were upgraded to facilitate data collection, analysis, and reporting.

Research and innovation in HIV management were sparked by the pandemic. Research on the effects of COVID-19 on HIV outcomes and transmission has yielded important information for programmatic and policy changes. Diagnostic efficiency was increased by advancements in diagnostic techniques, such as integrated fast tests for COVID-19 and HIV. Data analytics and digital health technologies improved illness surveillance and response plans. The COVID-19 pandemic management experience with HIV highlights the significance of developing robust health systems that can address various public health risks. Sustained investments in HIV control programs, including prevention, diagnosis, and treatment, are essential. Strengthening community health systems and integrating HIV services with other health programs can improve overall health outcomes (Ghana AIDS Commission, 2020). Collaborative efforts at the national, regional, and global levels are crucial to sustain progress in HIV control and achieve elimination goals. The COVID-19 epidemic in Northern Ghana requires the implementation of adaptive methods and a coordinated response to HIV. The epidemic produced severe interruptions in HIV services, posed diagnostic hurdles, and put a burden on healthcare resources. Nonetheless, HIV services were maintained through novel approaches to prevention, treatment, community participation, and health-system strengthening. This experience emphasizes the significance of strong health systems and ongoing HIV control efforts to protect vulnerable groups and preserve progress toward elimination (Ghana AIDS Commission, 2020).

4.5 Contribution of COVID-19 to the Neglect of Co-infections

What has happened is that the worldwide health systems in a significant way were affected by the COVID-19 pandemic, leading to severe consequences on the management of other communicable diseases like TB, Malaria, HIV, and Hepatitis B co-infections. It has caused pressure on healthcare facilities, diverted focus from these diseases and funding meant for them, and altered normal healthcare services thus neglecting their acute public health problems (Chanda-Kapata et al., 2022).

4.5.1 Diversion of Healthcare Resources

i. *Resource Allocation*

The COVID-19 pandemic led to health professionals, hospital beds, and other medical supplies being moved from their usual positions to the treatment and care of COVID-19-positive individuals (Heuschen et al., 2023; Nkansah et al., 2015). As a result, there are not enough resources for diagnostics, management, or treatment of co-infections such as hepatitis B, HIV, malaria, and tuberculosis (Obeng et al., 2022). Hospitals that are overwhelmed with COVID-19 patients have converted wards exclusively for such cases reducing the availability of beds for other infectious diseases (Obeng et al., 2022).

ii. *Impact on Routine Healthcare Services*

Routine healthcare services, including immunization programs, routine check-ups, and chronic disease management, have been considerably disrupted (Chanda-Kapata et al., 2022). This disturbance has caused delays in the detection and treatment of co-infections, worsening morbidity, and fatality rates (Heuschen et al., 2023). Preventive services, such as screening and early detection programs for diseases like Hepatitis B and tuberculosis, have been severely impeded, resulting in missed diagnoses and delayed treatment initiation, allowing diseases to develop uncontrolled (Abesig et al., 2020).

4.5.2 Reduced Access to Healthcare

i. *Healthcare Access Barriers*

As lockdowns, limitations on movement, and fear of getting COVID-19 have been enforced, the availability of health services has lessened for individuals considerably. Several people stayed away from seeking medical care for co-infection signs resulting in low healthcare accessibility (Adusi-Poku et al., 2023). Additionally, transportation interruptions prevented patients from getting to their healthcare centers, specifically in rural areas where transportation means are scarce (Owusu-Dabo et al., 2018).

ii. *Impact on Vulnerable Populations*

Vulnerable groups, such as those living with HIV, tuberculosis, and chronic Hepatitis B, have encountered increased barriers to getting critical medical care. The pandemic has worsened existing disparities in healthcare access, disproportionately harming vulnerable populations (Udoakang et al., 2023). Furthermore, the economic impact of the pandemic affected people's capacity to purchase healthcare services, medications, and transportation, limiting their access to care (Obeng et al., 2022).

4.5.3 *Interruption of Public Health Programs*

i. *Impact on Disease Control Programs*

Public health measures focused on managing co-infections have been halted, including Hepatitis B vaccination initiatives, malaria net distribution, and TB screening and treatment initiatives (Owusu-Dabo et al., 2018). These changes have enhanced the spread and burden of these diseases (Nkansah et al., 2015). HIV prevention and treatment programs have also suffered substantial setbacks, with limited access to antiretroviral medication (ART) and prevention services, resulting in treatment interruptions and an increased risk of HIV transmission (Udoakang et al., 2023).

ii. *Challenges in Public Health Messaging*

The emphasis on COVID-19 has overwhelmed other public health messages, lowering awareness and education regarding co-infections (Chanda-Kapata et al., 2022). Public health initiatives for diseases such as malaria and tuberculosis have fallen behind, resulting in lower public knowledge and involvement (Abesig et al., 2020). The focus on COVID-19 preventative efforts has occasionally clashed with current health interventions, such as using health facilities for routine immunizations and screenings (Heuschen et al., 2023).

4.5.4 *Impact on Healthcare Workers*

i. *Healthcare Worker Shortages*

An insufficient number of healthcare workers has impacted the delivery of essential services for co-infections, as fewer personnel are available to manage these diseases (Nkansah et al., 2015). Training and capacity-building initiatives for healthcare workers have been delayed or put on hold which has affected their ability to effectively manage and treat co-infections (Heuschen et al., 2023). The pandemic has put immense pressure on healthcare workers, resulting in exhaustion, ailments, and loss.

ii. *Risk of Co-Infections Among Healthcare Workers*

Healthcare workers are at increased risk of contracting co-infections due to their exposure to patients with infectious diseases. The added risk of COVID-19 has further complicated their work environment, making it challenging to manage multiple health threats simultaneously (Adusi-Poku et al., 2023).

4.5.5 *Impact on Research and Funding*

i. *Shift in Research Priorities*

The global focus on COVID-19 has shifted research priorities and funding toward understanding and combating the pandemic. This shift has led to reduced funding and attention for research on co-infections and other infectious diseases (Udoakang et al., 2023). Clinical trials and studies related to co-infections have been delayed or canceled, further hindering advancements in treatment and prevention (Chanda-Kapata et al., 2022).

4.6 The Impact of Nutrition in Infectious Diseases

Apart from the impacts of co-infections, the nutrition plays a crucial role in infectious diseases outcome in several ways including:

1. Immune system support: Adequate nutrition is essential for a healthy immune system, which helps fight off infections.
2. Pathogen growth and virulence: Nutrient availability can affect the growth and virulence of pathogens, such as bacteria and viruses.
3. Inflammation and oxidative stress: Nutrition influences inflammation and oxidative stress, which can impact disease severity and outcomes.
4. Gastrointestinal health: Nutrition affects the gut microbiome, which plays a critical role in immune function and infection susceptibility.
5. Vaccine efficacy: Nutrition can impact vaccine efficacy, with deficiencies in nutrients like vitamin D and zinc potentially reducing vaccine effectiveness.
6. Disease severity and outcomes: Nutrition can influence disease severity, duration, and outcomes, with malnutrition often worsening prognosis.
7. Antimicrobial resistance: Nutrition may impact antimicrobial resistance, with excessive antibiotic use in agriculture contributing to resistance development.
8. Host–pathogen interactions: Nutrition can affect host–pathogen interactions, influencing disease susceptibility and severity.

Key nutrients are play a role in infectious disease prevention and treatment such as:

1. Vitamin D: Essential for immune system regulation and pathogen clearance.
2. Zinc: Crucial for immune cell function, wound healing, and protein synthesis.
3. Iron: Important for immune cell function, but excessive iron can promote pathogen growth.
4. Omega-3 fatty acids: Anti-inflammatory effects may help reduce disease severity.
5. Probiotics: Beneficial bacteria supporting gut health and immune function.
6. Antioxidants: Vitamins C and E, polyphenols, and other antioxidants help reduce oxidative stress and inflammation.

a balanced diet is crucial in providing essential nutrients vital for maintaining immune function hence reducing the risk of infectious diseases.

4.7 Conclusion

In conclusion, this chapter has outlined the public health implications that arose during the upsurge of COVID-19 infection, when a lot of attention was shifted away from other common infections of public health interest such as malaria, hepatitis B, TB, HIV, etc. Our level of preparedness was a cause for concern, which affected attitudes and practices resulting in many people engaging in self-medication among others with these common conditions (malaria, hepatitis B, TB, HIV, etc.) who did not go to the hospital. Thus, low prevalences of these infections were recorded at the hospitals during the COVID-19 restrictions. Nutrition also plays a crucial role in combating infectious diseases and must, thus, be taken seriously by all. Based on the information outlined here, it recommended that the knowledge of the populace as well as the health workers on diseases outbreak be improved with education while pragmatic steps are embarked upon to improve on the infrastructure in the health sector. It is also recommended that proper data generation and usage be encouraged to improve our preparedness as a nation to address any pandemic that may confront us in the near future. Finally, enough resources are committed into research and development (R & D) from the government to minimize the over reliance on foreign donors, which affected our level of preparedness in harnessing data in real-time and providing vaccines etc., in managing the cases.

References

Abesig, J., Chen, Y., Wang, H., et al. (2020). Prevalence of viral hepatitis B in Ghana between 2015 and 2019: A systematic review and meta-analysis. *PLoS ONE, 15*, Article e0234348.

Afum, T., Asare, P., Asante-Poku, A., et al. (2021). Diagnosis of tuberculosis among COVID-19 suspected cases in Ghana. *PLoS ONE, 16*(12), Article e0261849. https://doi.org/10.1371/journal.pone.0261849

Alene, K. A., Wangdi, K., & Clements, A. C. A. (2020). Impact of the COVID-19 pandemic on tuberculosis control: An overview. *Tropical Medicine & Infectious Disease, 5*(3), 123. https://doi.org/10.3390/tropicalmed5030123

Alhassan, R. K., Nutor, J. J., & Arhinful, D. K. (2020). Reducing health inequities in tuberculosis control: The role of community-based interventions in Ghana. *BMC Public Health, 20*(1), 110. https://doi.org/10.1186/s12889020091110w

Alipanah N., Jarlsberg L., Miller C., Linh N., Falzon D., Jaramillo E., & Nahid P. (2018). Adherence interventions and outcomes of tuberculosis treatment: A systematic review and meta-analysis of trials and observational studies. *PLoS Medicine, 15*(7). https://doi.org/10.1371/journal.pmed.1002595

Asamoah, C. K., Asamoah, B. O., & Agardh, A. (2017). A generation at risk: A cross-sectional study on HIV/AIDS knowledge and stigmatizing behaviors among young women in Ghana. *Global Health Action, 10*(1), 1331538. https://doi.org/10.1080/16549716.2017.1331538

Asante, K. P., Owusu-Agyei, S., & Cairns, M. (2018). Malaria prevention and control in Ghana: Progress and challenges. *Journal of Tropical Medicine, 2018*, 1–8. https://doi.org/10.1155/2018/8454732

Boah, M., Yeboah, D., Kpordoxah, M. R., & Adokiya, M. N. (2023). Temporal trend analysis of the HIV/AIDS burden before and after ART implementation in Ghana. *BMC Public Health, 23*, 1399. https://doi.org/10.1186/s12889023163213

Chanda-Kapata, P., Ntoumi, F., Kapata, N., et al. (2022). Tuberculosis, HIV/AIDS, and malaria health services in sub-Saharan Africa: A situation analysis of the disruptions and impact of the COVID-19 pandemic. *International Journal of Infectious Diseases, 124*(Suppl 1), S41-46.

Chang M. H., Chen C. J., Lai M. S., Hsu H. M., Wu T. C., Kong M. S., Liang D. C., Shau W. Y., & Chen D. S. (1997). Universal hepatitis B vaccination in Taiwan and the incidence of hepatocellular carcinoma in children. *New England Journal of Medicine, 336*, 1855–1859. https://doi.org/10.1056/NEJM199706263362602

Croxford, S., Kitching, A., Desai, S., et al. (2017). Mortality and causes of death in people with HIV in the ART era. *The Lancet Public Health, 2*(1), e35–e46. https://doi.org/10.1016/S24682667(16)300202

Friedland, G., Churchyard, G., & Nardell, E. (2020). Tuberculosis and HIV co-infection: Current state of knowledge and research priorities. *The Lancet Infectious Diseases, 20*(1), e22–e31. https://doi.org/10.1016/S14733099(19)304773

Ghana AIDS Commission. (2020). National HIV and AIDS strategic plan 2021–2025.

Ghana Health Service (GHS). (2022a). National malaria control programme annual report.

Ghana Health Service (GHS). (2022b). National tuberculosis control programme annual report. https://www.tbghana.gov.gh/

Ghana Malaria Indicator Survey (GMIS). (2022). Ghana malaria indicator survey report. *Ghana Statistical Service.*

Ghebreyesus, T. A., Jakab Z., Ryan M. J., Mahjour J., Dalil S., Chungong S., Schmets G., Mcdarby G., Mcdarby R. M. S., & Saikat S. (2022). *Bulletin of the World Health Organization, 100*, 240–240A, https://doi.org/10.2471/BLT.22.287843

Heuschen, A. K., Abdul-Mumin, A., Abubakari, A., et al. (2023). Effects of the COVID-19 pandemic on general health and malaria control in Ghana: A qualitative study with mothers and healthcare professionals. *Malaria Journal, 22*, 78. https://doi.org/10.1186/s12936-023-04513-6

Inusah, A. W, Collins, G., Dzomeku, P., Head, M., & Ziblim, S. D. (2023). Knowledge, attitudes and practice towards yellow fever among nomadic populations: A cross-sectional study in yellow fever outbreak communities in Ghana. *PLOS Global Public Health, 3*(3), e0000733. https://doi.org/10.1371/journal.pgph.0000733

Loembé, M. M., & Nkengasong, J. N. (2021). COVID-19 vaccine access in Africa: Global distribution, vaccine platforms, and challenges ahead. *Immunity, 54*(7), 1353–1362. https://doi.org/10.1016/j.immuni.2021.06.017

Martinson, F. E., Weigle, K. A., Mushahwar, I. K., Weber, D. J., Royce, R., & Lemon, S. M. (1996). Seroepidemiological survey of hepatitis B in Ghanaian children. *Journal of Medical Virology, 48*, 278–283.

Mills, E. J., Bakanda, C., Birungi, J., et al. (2011). Life expectancy of persons receiving combination ART in low-income countries. *Annals of Internal Medicine, 155*(4), 209–216. https://doi.org/10.7326/000348191554201108160000358

National Malaria Control Programme (NMCP). (2022). Annual malaria report. *Ghana Health Service.*

National Tuberculosis Control Programme (NTCP). (2022). Annual report on TB in Ghana.

Nketiah-Amponsah, E., Afful-Mensah, G., & Ampaw, S. (2020). HIV-related stigma and access to healthcare in Ghana. *AIDS Research and Therapy, 17*(1), 1–10. https://doi.org/10.1186/s12981020002901

Nwaiwu A. U., Musekiwa A., Tamuzi A. L., Sambala E., & Nyasulu P. S. (2021). The incidence and mortality of yellow fever in Africa: A systematic review and metaanalysis. *BMC Infectious Diseases, 21*(1), https://doi.org/10.1186/s12879-021-06728-x.

Obeng, A. F., Attipoe, L., & Asare, D. (2022). The state of HIV care in Ghana: Achievements and future prospects. *Global Health Action, 15*(1), 199–211.

Ofori-Asenso, R., & Agyeman, A. A. (2016). Hepatitis B in Ghana: A systematic review and meta-analysis. *BMC Infectious Diseases, 16*, 130. https://doi.org/10.1186/s1287901614665

Owusu-Dabo, E., Adjei, G., Meyer, C. G., & Browne, E. (2018). Tuberculosis epidemiology and control in Ghana. *Infectious Diseases, 50*(8), 601–610. https://doi.org/10.1080/23744235.2018.1486855

Schweitzer, A., Horn, J., Mikolajczyk, R. T., Krause, G., & Ott, J. J. (2015). Estimations of worldwide prevalence of chronic hepatitis B virus infection: A systematic review of data published between 1965 and 2013. *The Lancet, 386*(10003), 1546–1555.

Udoakang, A. J., Djomkam Zune, A. L., Tapela, K., Nganyewo, N. N., Olisaka, F. N., Anyigba, C. A., Tawiah-Eshun, S., Owusu, I. A., Paemka, L., Awandare, G. A., & Quashie, P. K. (2023). The COVID-19, tuberculosis, and HIV/AIDS: Ménage à trois. *Frontiers in Immunology, 14*, 1104828. https://doi.org/10.3389/fimmu.2023.1104828

UNAIDS. (2023a). *Country factsheets: Ghana.* https://aidsinfo.unaids.org, https://www.unaids.org/en/resources/presscentre/featurestories/2025/june/20250605_ghana#:~:text=Ghana%20has%20an%20estimated%20330,monitoring%2C%20and%20human%20rights%20work

UNAIDS. (2023b). *Ghana country fact sheet: HIV and AIDS statistics.* https://www.unaids.org/en/regionscountries/countries/ghana

UNAIDS. (2023c). *Global AIDS monitoring report*. UNAIDS.

Watson, O. J., Barnsley, G., Toor, J., Hogan, A. B., Winskill, P., & Ghani, A. C. (2022). Global impact of the first year of COVID-19 vaccination: A mathematical modeling study. *The Lancet Infectious Diseases, 22*(9), 1293–1302. https://doi.org/10.1016/S1473-3099(22)00320-6

World Health Organization (WHO). (2023a). *Global tuberculosis report 2023.* WHO.

World Health Organization. (2023b). *World malaria report*. WHO.

Zaidi, J., Grapsa, E., Tanser, F., et al. (2013). Dramatic increase in HIV prevalence after ART scale-up. *AIDS, 27*(14), 2301–2305. https://doi.org/10.1097/QAD.0b013e328362e832

Okeke, A. A., Ohihoin, [illegible] & Anzaku [illegible] (2022). [illegible] of HIV [illegible] among pregnant women [illegible]. [illegible], 12(2), 129–211.
Opio-Asiimwe, K., S., Agyemang, A. A. [illegible] 2016). Hepatitis B in [illegible] Analysis [illegible]. BMC [illegible] [illegible] [illegible].
Oumu, Pinto, E., Anjo, G., Meyer [illegible] & Brower, F. (2016). [illegible] in [illegible] and [illegible]. [illegible] [illegible]. https://doi.org/10.[illegible]
14/0455
Schweitzer, A., Horn, J., Mikolajczyk, R. T., Krause, G., & Ott, J. J. (2015). Estimations of worldwide prevalence of chronic hepatitis B virus infection: A systematic review of data published between 1965 and 2013. [illegible] (10003), 1546–1555.
Oduwole [illegible], [illegible] Nyanga [illegible] [illegible]
A., [illegible], S., [illegible], L., Awodeji, [illegible]
The [illegible] HIV [illegible] Medicine [illegible]
1064 [illegible] https://doi.org/10.[illegible]
UNAIDS. (2023a). [illegible] https://www.unaids.org/[illegible]
[illegible]
[illegible]
UNAIDS. (2023). [illegible] HIV and AIDS [illegible]
[illegible]
UNAIDS. (2023). Global [illegible] [illegible] HIV [illegible]
Watson, G. J., Daniels, B., [illegible] A. [illegible] (2021). Global [illegible] of [illegible] [illegible] [illegible]
[illegible] (2021). [illegible] https://doi.org/10.[illegible]
World Health Organization. (2021). Global [illegible] report 2021 [illegible]
World Health Organization. (2017). [illegible] WHO.
Zou, [illegible], Ghosh, [illegible] [illegible] [illegible]. Antimicrob. [illegible] 2005, 47(14), 230 [illegible] https://doi.org/10.[illegible]

Part III
Disease Management

Chapter 5
Rolling out COVID-19 Rapid Detection Test Point of Care Diagnoses in Managing and Curbing COVID-19 in Ghana

Gideon Kofi Helegbe, Julius T. Dongdem, Peter Suwirakwenda Nyasulu, and Paul Armah Aryee

Abstract Since March 2020 when COVID-19 was declared a pandemic by WHO, the world has been hit with several strains of the virus. Currently, there are six clusters of COVID-19 based on a group of symptoms, which indicate how unwell a patient could become. A new normal has developed and everyone's life has changed including huge losses to businesses.

With the daily increase in COVID-19 cases amidst inadequate vaccine and indefinite treatment, early detection is recommended for quick/immediate decisions to ensure effective control of the virus. Meanwhile, even though the COVID-19 results by standard PCR have been more accessible than in the early days of the COVID-19 pandemic, the cost still limits many people to patronize it, thus, making a case for a rapid diagnostic test kit.

In this brief, we shall explore the situation on COVID-19, the management and the available tests for the detection of COVID-19 cases, and why the RDT test kit is seen as an obvious choice for point-of-care. The merits and demerits of the RDT test kits for COVID-19 will also be discussed.

Keywords COVID-19 · MERS-CoV · SARS Cov-2 · Ghana · COVID-19 variants

---

G. K. Helegbe (✉) · J. T. Dongdem
Department of Biochemistry and Molecular Medicine, School of Medicine, University for Development Studies, Tamale, Ghana
e-mail: ghelegbe@uds.edu.gh

P. S. Nyasulu
Division of Epidemiology and Biostatistics, Faculty of Medicine and Health Sciences, Stellenbosch University, Cape Town, South Africa

P. A. Aryee
Department of Nutritional Sciences, School of Allied Health Sciences, University for Development Studies, Tamale, Ghana

P. S. Nyasulu
Division of Epidemiology and Biostatistics, School of Public Health, Faculty of Health Sciences, University of the Witwatersrand, Johannesburg, South Africa

F. Mphande and P. Nyasulu (eds.), *Evaluating Outbreak Potential of Infections in Tropical Climates*, https://doi.org/10.1007/978-981-95-0618-7_5

Abbreviation

COVID-19	Corona Virus Disease -2019 (SARS CoV-2)
RDT	Rapid detection kit
MERS-CoV	Middle East Respiratory Virus -Corona virus
SARS-CoV-2	severe acute respiratory syndrome coronavirus 2
WHO	World Health Organization

5.1 Introduction

Coronaviruses are common pathogens that infect the human respiratory system. Within the past two decades, SARS-CoV in 2003, Middle East Respiratory Virus (MERS-CoV)in 2012, and SARS-CoV-2 (COVID-19) in 2019 have contributed to three major outbreaks, with the latter leading to the COVID-19 pandemic. The world witnessed the first reported cases of SARS-CoV-2 in December 2019, which was identified in Wuhan, Hubei Province, China, in December 2019. The whole-genome sequencing was used to identify the virus (Liu et al., 2020), and initial symptoms included cough, fever, and dyspnoea. On 11 February 2020, the World Health Organization (WHO) officially named the disease COVID-19 and was declared a pandemic on 11 March 2020 (Harapan et al., 2020).

SARS-CoV-2 is an enveloped single-stranded RNA virus that belongs to the Beta coronavirus genus. It can mutate and undergo several re-combinations of genes giving rise to new variants. Vaccines were rolled out to manage the spread. Even though several concerns were observed about resistance to the vaccine, the available vaccines can still prevent hospitalization, severe disease, and deaths. Meanwhile, booster vaccines have been developed to improve immune response against new variants. The spike protein, required for virus attachment and entry into host cells, is the primary cause of SARS-CoV-2's global spread. A lot of variants have been discovered, highlighting the importance of continued research and monitoring, including the use of a testing system such as the point-of-care RDTs in a low-resource setting like Ghana.

5.2 COVID-19 in Ghana

The COVID-19 pandemic has had a profound impact on Ghana, as it has on the rest of the world. The first case of COVID-19 in Ghana was confirmed on 12 March 2020 (Ofori-Adjei et al., 2020). In Ghana, a total of 172, 075 individuals were diagnosed with COVID-19 (COVID-19 Updates | Ghana), as of 7 April 2024, according to the Ghana Health Service (GHS, 2020). Out of the infected individuals, 170, 592 recovered, while the number of deaths stood at 1462. With the first reported and increasing cases, the country has been working tirelessly to combat the spread of the virus. A vulnerable group that was severely affected by COVID-19 were pregnant women. COVID-19 in pregnancy was associated with consistent and substantial increases in severe maternal morbidity and mortality and neonatal complications in the pregnant women with the disease (Villar et al. 2021). This data should alert clinicians, other health workers, and pregnant individuals to enforce strictly all the recommended COVID-19 preventive measures.

5.2.1 COVID-19 Variants in Ghana

Several COVID-19 variants have been detected in Ghana, including the Alpha, Beta, Gamma, Delta variants, and Omicron (Asante et al., 2024; Adu, 2023), which characterized the early (Ngoi 2020) and the subsequent transmission (Morang'a et al., 2022). The Ghana Health Service (GHS) and the Noguchi Memorial Institute for Medical Research (NMIMR) together with West Africa Center for Cell and Infectious Pathogens (WACCBIP) have been conducting genomic sequencing to identify and track the variants. These variants of SARS-CoV-2 with a higher transmission and immune evasion characteristics certainly are of great public health concern since it can cause outbreaks and sustain the transmission in the population. Thus, there is a need for regular surveillance to identify these early enough for immediate and targeted response and policy decisions. A study by Asante et al. (2022), was enough for the Ghana government to decide on the reopening of land borders and ease travel restrictions related to the pandemic. From this study, it emphasized the point that data is needed for policy decisions through a collaborative approach to addressing public health crises. Furthermore, effective communication with transparency, and enhancing the preparedness of a country's health systems will determine how a policy decision may ensure how nations, including Ghana, can succeed in the fight against COVID-19, especially in bringing economies to normality by lifting lockdowns or other restrictions (Assan et al., 2022).

The WHO has shown that with current data there are some new variants (JN.1, KP2, LP.8.1, among others) of COVID-19 circulating (WHO dashboard, 2025), for which it is recommended that there should be continuous surveillance and monitoring at the genomic level.

5.3 Vaccine Acquisition and Distribution

5.3.1 Vaccine Efforts in Ghana

Vaccination was employed as one of the intervention strategies in managing the disease. COVID-19 vaccination among the people of Ghana was observed to be gradually increasing, even though it remains a challenge. It was in February 2021, through the initiative of COVAX Facility (a global initiative, which ensured equitable access to COVID-19 vaccines) that Ghana received the first batch of COVID-19 vaccines. The country has since received additional vaccine doses from various sources. The main types of vaccines used in Ghana are AstraZeneca (developed in Oxford, UK), Sputnik-V (from Moscow, Russia), Moderna (developed in Cambridge, Massachusetts, USA), Pfizer-BioNTech (developed by German and USA), and Janssen (by Johnson & Johnson, USA) (Table 5.1). Other sources that have donated these vaccines included the African Union's African Vaccine Acquisition Trust (AVAT) and bilateral donations. Table 5.1 shows the vaccine types, and the number of COVID-19 vaccine doses administered per 100 people as of 3 March 2023.

Meanwhile, there have been different reactions to the vaccine acceptance and promotion. While women were more prone to accept the vaccine, their male counterparts did not (Adjaottor et al., 2022). Furthermore, education about COVID-19 vaccines, the desire to protect oneself, vaccines being cost-free, family against COVID-19, and seeing others receive the COVID-19 vaccine influenced the vaccine acceptance rate (Afrifa-Anane et al., 2022). On the other hand, contamination fears, the danger in believing COVID-19 information, were significant predictors of COVID-19 vaccination acceptance. Additionally, long queues at the vaccination centres, fear of side effects, misconceptions about the vaccines, and shortage of vaccines were the main barriers against COVID-19 vaccination (Afrifa-Anane et al., 2022). What this means is that individual, institutional, and vaccine-related factors influence or hinder COVID-19 vaccination among the populace, while Fig. 5.1 shows the distribution of those fully vaccinated.

Source Ghana Health Service (2024a).

Since the development of COVID-19 vaccines, Ghana has 14,867,012 individuals at least who have taken one dose (46.3% of the total population). The number of fully vaccinated individuals was 11,782,2609 (36.7% of the population), while 6,991,825 individuals have received a booster (GHS dashboard, accessed 19 December 2024).

Table 5.1 Vaccine types and the number of dosages in the Ghanaian population as of 3 March 2023

Vaccine Type	Dosage(mL)
AstraZeneca	10,545,038
Sputnik-V	18,368
Moderna	1,065,357
Pfizer-BioNTech COVID-19 vaccine	7,903,938
COVID-19 vaccine Janssen	8,983,153

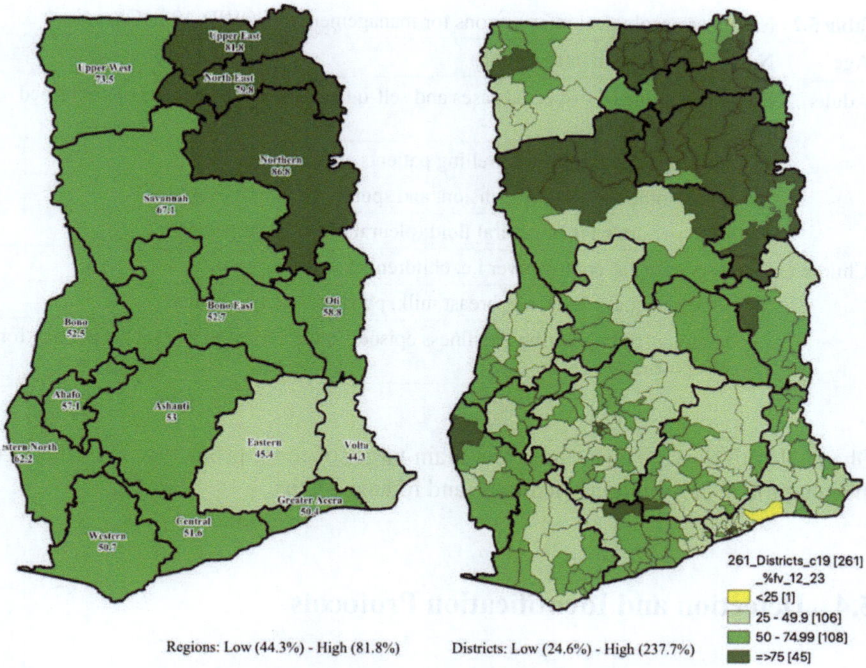

Fig. 5.1 Proportion (%) of persons fully vaccinated by region and districts in Ghana *Source* Ghana Health Service (2024a)

Fig. 5.1 shows the percentage of fully vaccinated individuals in the various regions of Ghana as of 31 December 2023 (GHS, 2023).

5.3.2 Management of COVID-19 in Ghana

COVID-19 treatment modules in Ghana were based on the severity of the symptoms of the COVID-19 infections. Efficient management of the COVID-19 cases was based on the protocols established by the GHS. These protocols include isolation and treatment of confirmed cases, contact tracing, and quarantine of suspected cases. COVID-19 treatment centres were also established across the length and breadth of the, making this very accessible and timely. Also, treatment can be classified into pharmacologic and non-pharmacologic interventions (Table 5.2).

(i) Pharmacological Treatment.

This treatment method involves the admission of antiviral medications and other supportive therapies. The administration and treatment protocols are created and developed by the WHO (Table 5.3), which are the most prominent methods that the

Table 5.2 Non-pharmacological interventions for management of COVID-19 in Ghana

Age	Non-pharmacologic interventions
Adults	Early quarantine of suspected cases and self-quarantine of all contacts of confirmed cases with follow-up.
	Psycho-social support by counselling patients and contacts.
	Chest physiotherapy, lung expansion, and sputum clearance exercises.
	Aspiration or drainage of pleural fluid (pleural effusion), if present.
Children	Tepid sponging to control fever i.e. children <5 years
	Providing adequate fluids e.g. breast milk, porridge, coconut water.
	Encouraging feeding during the illness episode and offering an extra meal per day for 2 weeks post-recovery.

Ghana Health Service agent use. The main target of these protocols was to reduce the symptoms, prevent complications, and reduce deaths.

5.4 Detection and Identification Protocols

To ensure a systematic and scientific approach in the detection and management of COVID-19 cases, Ghana established protocols in the detection and identification of these COVID-19 variants. The NMIMR and the Kumasi Centre for Collaborative Research (KCCR) are the primary institutions responsible for genomic sequencing. The GHS and the Ministry of Health (MOH) have also established a network of laboratories across the country for COVID-19 testing. The objective of these various centres across the country was to reduce the turn-around time in getting the results from the laboratory.

5.4.1 Detection Kits

There are currently 2 types of diagnostic tests available for COVID-19. They are antigen-based, which include enzyme-linked immunosorbent assays (ELISA) and molecular-based methods, such as polymerase chain reaction (PCR), loop-mediated isothermal amplification (LAMP), and CRISPR. The ELISA method is used to detect viral protein markers on the surface of the virus, while molecular-based tests amplify the viral genetic material present in the sample. Similarly, in Ghana, several COVID-19 detection kits are available, including PCR-based tests and rapid diagnostic tests (RDTs). However, the availability of RDTs is limited, particularly in rural areas.

Table 5.3 Symptoms and treatment guidelines for COVID-19

Severity	Treatment
Asymptomatic	**First line—evidence rating (C) hydroxychloroquine (Oral)** *adults:* 200 mg 8-hourly for 10 days *children:* 3 mg/kg 8-hourly (max 200 mg/dose) for 10 days **second line—evidence rating (C) chloroquine phosphate (Oral)** *adults:* 500 mg (300 mg base) 12-hourly for 5 days *children:* <60 kg: 5 mg base/kg 12-hourly for 5 days >60 kg: 500 mg (300 mg base) 12-hourly for 5 days
Mild/moderate illness or pneumonia	**First line—evidence rating (C) hydroxychloroquine (Oral)** (same as asymptomatic) **PLUS azithromycin (Oral)** *adults:* 500 mg day 1, then 250 mg once daily from day 2 to day 5 *children:* 10 mg/kg daily for 3 days (not recommended for children below 6 months) **OR doxycycline (Oral)** *adults:* 100 mg once daily for 5 days (contraindicated for children and pregnant women) **second line—evidence rating (C) chloroquine phosphate (Oral)** (same as asymptomatic) **PLUS** azithromycin or doxycycline as per above dosages
Severe illness (without ARDS, CRS, or DIC/ coagulopathy)	**Hydroxychloroquine, chloroquine, azithromycin, or doxycycline** (as per mild illness dosages) **AND (if available) convalescence plasma (evidence rating C)** 200–250 ml plasma from a COVID-19 recovered patient with significant levels of anti SARS-CoV-2 antibodies (IgG and IgM) **AND methyl prednisolone, IV (evidence rating C)** *adults:* 80 mg–120 mg or 1–2 mg/kg daily for 3–5 days *children:* Initial dose: 0.5–1.6 mg/kg/day in 3–4 divided doses (based on severity and patient response) **OR Remdesivir** *adults:* 200 mg IV load, then 100 mg IV 24-hourly for 2–10 days *children:* <40 kg: 5 mg/kg IV load then 2.5 mg/kg 12-hourly >40 kg: 200 mg IV load then 100 mg IV 24-hourly for 2–10 days
Severe illness (with ARDS, CRS, or DIC/ coagulopathy)	**Same as severe illness without ARDS, CRS, or DIC AND tocilizumab, IV (single dose) (evidence rating C)** *adults:* 400 mg or 8 mg/kg (max: 800 mg) single dose *children:* <30 kg: 12 mg/kg single dose >30 kg: Same as adults **AND (if available)** Remdesivir (same as above)

Source MOH, 2020 (COVID-19 Guidelines for Ghana) and Ismaila et al., 2021

5.4.2 Importance of Point-of-Care RDTs

Point-of-care RDTs are essential for Ghana, as they enable rapid testing and diagnosis of COVID-19 in remote and resource-limited areas. This can help reduce the spread of the virus and improve patient outcomes. Many countries around the world have already adopted point-of-care RDTs, and Ghana can benefit from their experience. Studies have been done to show the effectiveness and reliability of the point-of-care RDTs. While other studies have indicated its dependability in Ghana (Bani et al., 2024), others being specific for a certain variant, the Omicron (Aboagye et al., 2024), some were of the opinion that in as much it is useful, one needs to be cautious in its usage, and more data needed form further studies (Abdul-Mumin et al., 2021). These authors observe that SARS-CoV-2 Ag-RDTs appear to have a rather low sensitivity and particularly a low specificity under real-life conditions in Africa (Abdul-Mumin et al., 2021). Thus, the role of existing Ag-RDTs in countries with high-temperature climates and limited resources needs to be discussed further. Nevertheless, all these studies indicate that point-of-care RDTs are useful tools to use in limited resource settings for early detection and management of COVID-19 cases.

5.4.3 *Features of COVID-19 Rapid Diagnostic Tests (RDTS)*

RDTs are based on host antibody detection on a nitrocellulose membrane. Easy to operate and portable, these tests are suited for Point-of-Care testing (POCT) analyses of fingerpick blood, saliva, or nasal swab fluids. Samples are dropped on a loading pad and transferred via capillary motion. During this flow, antibodies in the sample bind to nanoparticles, and the whole complex is captured downstream at designated spots on the membrane by anti-human antibodies (Lee & Song, 2024). The results are usually displayed as coloured lines for the naked eye detection, a control line confirming test reliability, and test line (s) indicating the presence of target antibodies. Most assays use gold nanoparticles for signal generation, whereas carbon or coloured latex nanoparticles are alternative labelling candidates. The kit contains a sample pad, conjugate pad, IgM line, IgG line, control line, and an absorption pad. It uses the lateral flow mechanism to work effectively (Lee & Song, 2024).

5.4.4 *The Need for a Rapid Diagnostic Test for the COVID-19 Disease*

From the statistics of the cases of COVID-19, it is obvious that the cases are increasing at an alarming rate and are of great public health interest. Meanwhile, the needed treatment was not definitive, and the reported low acceptability of the vaccine usage as well as the inadequate amount to reach those ready to be vaccinated made a case for early detection and treatment. This will have an adverse effect on the pragmatic steps taken to control the spread of the virus and mitigate the impact of the different strains due to the mutation of the virus. Thus, efforts to control will depend on early detection, isolation and quarantine, contact tracing, care, and management (Nyazika et al., 2020; Wang, 2020). Therefore, it is imperative to institute diagnostic strategies with high analytical sensitivity and specificity to enable large-scale testing and rapid detection of SARS-CoV-2 (Marcel, 2020). As a result of this development, the need for COVID-19 tests should be point-of-care, widely available, and implemented outside of hospital settings to prevent overwhelming situation of the health care system as well as the risk of nosocomial transmission to other patients and healthcare workers (Castro et al., 2021).

5.4.5 Benefits of and Concerns in the Use of COVID-19 RDTs

The lack of RDTs in Ghana can lead to delayed diagnosis and treatment of COVID-19, particularly in rural areas. This can result in increased transmission of the virus, poor patient outcomes, and strain on the healthcare system. With the few studies conducted in a low-resource setting like Ghana indicating its reliability when compared to the molecular-based detection (Bani et al., 2024, Aboagye et al., 2024; Abdul-Mumin et al., 2021), it goes without saying that the benefits of using the point-of-care RDTs far outweigh the disadvantages.

There are several benefits of the COVID-19 RDTs which include, its being easy to use (Mallari et al., (2023), used in low-resource setting with results ready within 15–30 mins and able to identify past infections (Winter and Hegde 2020). It is also relatively far cheaper, and does not need high technical know-how or training, does not need electricity, and is easily performed outside the hospital setting and laboratory environment. Since it is difficult to use clinical characteristics to distinguish between patients with COVID-19 having malaria-like symptoms, the use of point-of-care RDTs in the detection of IgM is useful in predicting CT values for SARS-CoV-2 real-time PCR and therefore transmission (Dadzie et al., 2024).

Despite the benefits in the use, some claim it is too early and should be used for research purposes (Chtioui et al., 2020), while others claim there have been few research work on their validation. Those who propose for their use suggests that the RDTs have the potential to fill at least a portion of the 'testing gap' (WHO, 25 November, 2020) as well as offer the possibility of rapid case detection (Mallari et al., 2023), especially of the most infectious patients, at or near the point of care and for the fact that it will be readily available in low-resource settings in low—and middle—income countries (LMICs) due to their relatively cheaper cost.

The challenges in the use of these COVID-19 RDTs are that they require extensive design and troubleshooting of test antibodies that will react to viral proteins in the sample and deep knowledge of viral proteins produced in various tissue environments. In addition, the test may yield false negatives if the viral protein production is low or if there is not enough virus replication in the sampled area. Additional challenges noted with the RDTs usage are the likelihood of cross-reactivity, which may result in false positives, thus, creating panic, unnecessary quarantine, and contact tracing. This will call for regulatory policies, an effective health education plans (Mallari et al., 2023) by and through the media, press conferences by scientists, researchers, Ghana Health Service, etc. The other challenge with the introduction of RDTs leads to the potential influx of numerous COVID-19 RDTs, which calls for research in testing and evaluating them.

5.5 Recommendations

Based on the review made here, the following are recommended.

1. In as much as the response to the pandemic has been favourable, there is a need to appreciate the role of the RDTs in picking up cases early during surveillance without much capital investment for immediate targeted intervention and policy directives.
2. There is a need to validate more RDTs to boost confidence as the RDTs can be used to complement the SAR-CoV-2 RT-PCR as a surveillance tool.
3. The government of Ghana must provide funding for research and be committed, and not be involved in knee-jerk reaction.
4. The Ministry of Health (MoH), Ghana must improve on the healthcare services to boost public confidence to increase patronage.
5. The Ghana Government Must Implement Strategies to Enhance Positive Attitudes towards Vaccines.

5.6 Conclusion

Ghana has made significant progress in combating the COVID-19 pandemic, but there is still a need to improve detection and diagnosis, particularly in rural areas. Different strains of COVID-19 due to the high mutation rate have generated a lot of public health interest. Thus, the need for early detection and treatment has been discussed and resolutions made especially in the low—and middle-income countries (LMICs). The adoption of point-of-care RDTs can play a critical role in achieving this goal. Therefore, effective control of the SAR-CoV-2 pandemic, like any other infectious disease outbreak, relies on early detection, isolation, care, and management of almost all cases. Due to the likelihood of influx of RDTs from potential unreliable sources, there is a need to validate more RDTs to boost confidence as the RDTs can be used to complement the SAR-CoV-2 RT-PCR as a surveillance tool, which will allow for large-scale testing and rapid detection of SARS-CoV-2 cases. The RDTs will also be useful to address the logistical challenges associated with using the SAR-CoV-2 RT-PCR as a sole surveillance tool and improve timely detection of the true spread and tempo of the SAR-CoV-2, especially in resource-limited settings.

References

Abdul-Mumin, A., Abubakari, A., Agbozo, F., Abdul-Karim, A., Nuertey, B. D., Mumuni, K., Anna-Katharina, H., Lisa, H., Claudia, M. D., Olaf, M., & Albrecht, J. (2021). Field evaluation of specificity and sensitivity of a standard SARS-CoV-2 antigen rapid diagnostic test: A prospective study at a teaching hospital in northern Ghana. *PLOS Glob Public Health, 1*(12), e0000040. https://doi.org/10.1371/journal.pgph.0000040

Aboagye, F.T., Annison, L., Hackman, H. K., Acquah, M. E., Ashong, Y., Owusu-Frimpong, I., Egyam, B. C, Annison, S., Osei-Adjei, G., & Antwi-Baffour, S. (2024). Comparative evaluation of RT-PCR and antigen-based rapid diagnostic tests (ag-RDTs) for SARS-CoV-2 detection: Performance, variant specificity, and clinical implications. *Microbiology Spectrum Virology, 12*(6). https://doi.org/10.1128/spectrum.00073-24.

Abu-Faraj, Zia (2020).

Adjaottor, E. S., Addo, F.-M., Ahorsu, F. A., Chen, H.-P., & Ahorsu, D. K. (2022). Predictors of COVID-19 stress and COVID-19 vaccination acceptance among adolescents in Ghana. *International Journal of Environmental Research and Public Health, 19*, 7871. https://doi.org/10.3390/ijerph19137871

Adu et al., 2023.

Afrifa-Anane, G. F., Larbi, R. T., Addo, B., Agyekum, M. W., Kyei-Arthur, F., Appiah, M., et al. (2022). Facilitators and barriers to COVID-19 vaccine uptake among women in two regions of Ghana: A qualitative study. *PLoS One, 17*(8), e0272876. https://doi.org/10.1371/journal.pone.0272876

Asante, D., Twumasi, M. A., Sakyi, A. S. K. et al. (2022). A socio-geographic perspective of health and economic impacts of COVID-19 on poor households in ghana. *GeoJournal, 87*, 4113–4125. https://doi.org/10.1007/s10708-021-10487-2

Asante, I. A., Lwanga, C. N., Takyi, C., Sekyi-Yorke, A. N., Quarcoo, J. A., Odikro, M. A., Kploanyi, E. E., Donkor, I. O., Addo–Lartey, A., Duah, N.A., Odumang, D.A., Lomotey, E. S., Boatemaa, L., Kwasah, L., Nyarko, S. O., Affram, Y., Asiedu-Bekoe, F., & Kenu, E. (2024). Detection of SARS-CoV-2 variants imported through land Borders at the height of the COVID-19 pandemic in Ghana, 2022. *Cureus, 16*(8), e68220. https://doi.org/10.7759/cureus.68220.

Assan, A., Hussein, H., & Agyeman-Duah, D. N. (2022). COVID-19 lockdown implementation in Ghana: Lessons learned and hurdles to overcome. *Journal of Public Health Policy., 43*, 129–139. https://doi.org/10.1057/s41271-021-00330-w

Bani, S., Amakye, E. K., Akomea, S., Nyarko, E. N., Dodoo, D., Aidoo, C., Fynn-Buadu, M., Adom, M., Bani, F., & Christian, O. C. (2024). An evaluation of the sensitivity and specificity of three COVID-19 rapid Immunochromatographic test kits compared to real-time reverse transcriptase-polymerase chain reaction (rRT-PCR) among clinical samples. *Cureus, 16*(6), e63294. https://doi.org/10.7759/cureus.63294

Castro, M. C., Gurzenda, S., & Turra, C.M. et al. (2021). Reduction in life expectancy in Brazil after COVID-19. *Nature Medicine, 27*, 1629–1635. https://doi.org/10.1038/s41591-021-01437-z

Chtioui, M. J., Grati, H., Harzallah, N., Christine, M., Jebali, O., Trabelsi, A., Ahmed, M. B., Thabet, L., Mhalla, S., Moussa, M. B., Messaoud, T., Romdhane, H. B., Toumi, A., & Hamouda, C. (2020). Rapid diagnostic tests: Pros, cons and potential use in the COVID-19 management in Tunisia. *La Tunisie Médicale, 98*(8–9), 639–642.

COVID-19 Updates. Ghana.; https://ghs.gov.gh/covid19/. Accessed 7th April, 204.

Dadzie, A., Kuffour, A. S., & Turkson, A., et al. (2024). COVID-19 in patients presenting with malaria-like symptoms at a primary healthcare facility in Accra. *Ghana. PLoS ONE, 19*(2), e0298088. https://doi.org/10.1371/journal.pone.0298088

Freitas, A. R. R., Beckedorff, O. A., Cavalcanti, L. P. G., Siqueira, A. M., Castro, D. B., Costa, C. F. D., Lemos, D. R. Q., & Barros, E. N. C. (2021). The emergence of novel SARS-CoV-2 variant P.1 in Amazonas (Brazil) was temporally associated with a change in the age and sex profile of COVID-19 mortality: A population based ecological study. *Lancet regional health. The Americas, 1*, 100021. https://doi.org/10.1016/j.lana.2021.100021

Ghana Health Service. (2024a). Dashboard accessed 19th December, 2024.

Ghana Health Service. (2024b). Dashboard accessed 19th December, 2023.

Harapan, H., Itoh, N., Yufika, A., Winardi, W., Keam, S., Te, H., & Mudatsir, M. (2020). Corona virus disease 2019 (COVID-19): A literature review. *Journal of Infection and Public Health, 13*(5), 667–673. https://doi.org/10.1016/j.pulmoe.2020.10.013

Ismaila, H., Asamani, J. A., Lokossou, V. K., Oduro-Mensah, E., Nabyonga-Orem, J., & Akoriyea, S. K. (2021). The cost of clinical management of SARS-COV-2 (COVID-19) infection by level of disease severity in Ghana: A protocol-based cost of illness analysis. *BMC Health Services Research, 21*(1), 1–10.

Lee, Y. K., & Song, H. S. (2024). Recent advances in electrochemical and Nanophotonic biosensors for SARS-Cov-2 detection. *BioChip Journal, 18*, 171–185. https://doi.org/10.1007/s13206-024-00138-2

Liu, Y. C., Kuo, R. L., & Shih, S. R. (2020). COVID-19: The first documented Corona virus pandemic in history. *Biomedical journal, 43*(4), 328–333.

Mallari, E. U., Keller, S., Febre, J. F., Timbol, J., Powers, R., Peregrino, R. R., Slyzkii, A., Mulder, C., Magno, M. V., & Spruijt, I. (2023). Feasibility and acceptability of COVID-19 self-testing in the Philippines. *PHA, 13*(4), 119–122. e-ISSN 2220–8372.

Marcel et al., 2020.

MOH, 2020 (Covid-19 guidelines for Ghana).

Morang'a, C. M., Ngoi, J. M., Gyamfi, J., Amuzu, D. S. Y., Nuertey, B., Soglo, P., Appiah, V., Asante, I. A., Owusu-Oduro, P., Armoo, S., Adu-Gyasi, D., Amoako, N., Oliver-Commey, J., Owusu, M., Sylverken, A., Fenteng, E. D., M'cormack, V. V., Ei-Maya, F. T., Quansah, E. B., Ayivor-Djanie, R., Amoako, E. K., Ogbe, I. T., Yemi, B. K., Osei-Wusu, I., DNA, M., Saiid, S., Tapela, K., Dzabeng, F., Magnussen, V., Quaye, J., Opurum, P. C., Carr, R. A., Ababio, P. T., Abass, A.-K., Akoriyea, S. K., Amoako, E., Kumi-Ansah, F., Boakye, O. D., Mibut, D. K., Odoom, T., Ofori-Boadu, L., Allegye-Cudjoe, E., Dassah, S., Asoala, V., Asante, K. P., Phillips, R. O., Osei-Atweneboana, M. Y., Gyapong, J. O., Kuma-Aboagye, P., Ampofo, W. K., Duedu, K. O., Ndam, N. T., Bediako, Y., Quashie, P. K., Amenga-Etego, L. N., & Awandare, G. A. (2022). Genetic diversity of SARS-CoV-2 infections in Ghana from 2020-2021*, 13*, 2494. https://doi.org/10.1038/s41467-022-30219-5. www.nature.com/naturecommunications

Ngoi, J.M., Quashie, P. K, & Morang'a, C. M., et al. (2020). Genomic analysis of SARS-CoV-2 reveals local viral evolution in Ghana. *Experimental Biology and Medicine, 246*(8), 960–970. https://doi.org/10.1177/1535370220975351

Nyazika, T. K., Kaela, R., Mugoni, M., Musomekwa, K., Kyei-Baafour, E., Chiwanda, S., Mapondera, P. T., Makawa, T. S., Sithole, E. M., Mavunganidze, G., Manasa, J., Jambo, K. C., & Musarurwa, C. (2020). Implementation of antibody rapid diagnostic testing versus real-time reverse transcription-PCR sample pooling in the screening of COVID-19: A case of different testing strategies in Africa. *mSphere, 5*, e00524-20. https://doi.org/10.1128/mSphere%2000524-20

Ofori-Adjei, D., Lartey, M., & Koram, K. A. (2020). Ghana and the COVID-19 pandemic. *Ghana Medical Journal, 54(4) supplement*, 1–2. https://doi.org/10.4314/gmj.v54i4s.1

Torres-Castro, R., Vasconcello-Castilloa, L., Alsina-Restoy, X., Solis-Navarroa, L., Burgos, F., Puppo, H., & Vilaró, J. (2021). Respiratory function in patients post-infection by COVID-19: A systematic review and meta-analysis. *Pulmonology, 27*, 328–337.

Villar, J., Ariff, S., Gunier, R. B., Thiruvengadam, R., Rauch, S., Kholin, A., Roggero, P., Prefumo, F., Silva do Vale, M., Arturo Cardona-Perez, J., Maiz, N., Cetin, I., Savasi, V., Deruelle, P., Easter, S. R., Sichitiu, J., CPS, C., Ernawati, E., Mhatre, M., Teji, J. S., Liu, B., Capelli, C., Oberto, M., Salazar, L., Gravett, M. G., Cavoretto, P. I., Nachinab, V. B., Galadanci, H., Oros, D., Ayede, A. I., Sentilhes, L., Bako, B., Savorani, M., Cena, H., Garcia-May, P. K., Etuk, S., Casale, R., Abd-Elsalam, S., Ikenoue, S., Aminu, M. B., Vecciarelli, C., Duro, E. A., Usman, M. A., John-Akinola, Y., Nieto, R., Ferrazzi, E., Bhutta, Z. A., Langer, A., Kennedy, S. H., & Papageorghiou, A. T. (2021). Maternal and neonatal morbidity and mortality among pregnant women with and without COVID-19 infection. *JAMA Pediatrics, 175*(8).

Wang, C., et al. (2020). A novel coronavirus outbreak of global health concern. *The Lancet, 395*, 470–473. https://doi.org/10.1016/S0140-6736(20)30185-9

WHO dashboard (2025); Accessed 28th February 2025.

Winter, A. K., & Hegde, S. T. (2020). The important role of serology for COVID-19 control. *The Lancet Infectious Diseases, 20*, 758–759. https://doi.org/10.1016/S1473-3099(20)30322-4

Chapter 6
COVID-19 Pandemic's Negative Effect on the Lives of People Living with HIV

Regis Rugira Marie Modeste and Furaha Akimanimpaye

Abstract Four decades on, HIV has transformed into a chronic condition. Similar to chronic illnesses' management, the success of HIV management and well-being of patients living with HIV depend on the support that the patients receive, as well as their engagement in self-management activities. With the advent of COVID-19, there was a considerable disruption in the provision of care, and that had a negative effect on the well-being of people living with HIV (PLWH). As a result of regulations, access to health services was reduced. In institutions where patients had the opportunity to support each other in support groups, such gatherings were discontinued in an effort to ensure social distancing. The healthcare system diverted all the effort towards COVID-19, and as a result, the risk of loss to follow-up was increased, and access to medication needed was impacted. The isolation and social distancing required to reduce the risk of COVID-19 transmission caused the isolation of patients from their own social networks. Not only did they lose support from healthcare providers, but they also lost connection and support from their own social networks. Mental well-being is an important aspect of the overall well-being of PLWH, and isolation is one of the aspects that would negatively affect their well-being. Similarly, the regulations related to the hard lockdown where people were limited in their movements also brought an additional risk for PLWH as an active lifestyle is important in maintaining well-being. COVID-19 also brought a huge financial challenge to the communities. Opportunities for employment were reduced, a number of people lost their jobs, and those involved in small businesses and other informal activities were not able to earn an income through their businesses. Lack of financial means has a great impact on people living with HIV as they need to be able to provide food for themselves and their families.

Keywords People living with HIV · COVID-19 · HIV management · HIV patient care · HIV self-management

---

R. R. M. Modeste (✉)
Department of Nursing and Midwifery, Stellenbosch University, Cape Town, South Africa
e-mail: rmodeste@sun.ac.za

F. Akimanimpaye
School of Nursing, University of the Western Cape, Cape Town, South Africa

F. Mphande and P. Nyasulu (eds.), *Evaluating Outbreak Potential of Infections in Tropical Climates*, https://doi.org/10.1007/978-981-95-0618-7_6

Abbreviations

HIV	Human Immunodeficiency syndrome
PLWH	People living with HIV
PMTCT	Prevention of Mother-to-Child Transmission
COVID-19	Corona Virus Disease 2019 (SARS CoV -2)
ART	Anti-retroviral treatment
NNRTIs	Non-nucleoside reverse transcriptase inhibitors

6.1 Introduction—HIV Management in Endemic Countries

It has been more than four decades now that the world is battling with the HIV epidemic. The burden of HIV remains high at a global level and more concerning in many of the sub-Saharan countries where it remains endemic, with noted concerns about increased number of new infections in about 28 countries (UNAIDS, 2024: 7). The impact of HIV epidemic extends from individual to a societal negative impact. At an individual level, people living with HIV (PLWH) encounter a number of challenges that need a comprehensive approach to ensure better health outcomes to those infected as well as those affected.

The advent of the COVID-19 pandemic was accompanied with multiple regulations that had a negative impact on the process and progress of HIV management and subsequently resulted in a number of negative consequences for those living with HIV. This chapter will present the burden of HIV and how HIV is managed in endemic countries, then the negative impact COVID-19 had on people living with HIV in the various aspects of their lives will be presented.

Despite the enormous number of lives lost since the start of the HIV epidemic, there have been extraordinary advances that have changed the course of epidemic. Such advances include the advent of antiretroviral medication, more comprehensive approaches in the management of HIV, empowerment of people living with HIV in their own HIV self-management, more support systems in the community and health care system, as well as task shifting approaches for the care of those living with HIV. The fight against HIV includes efforts towards the prevention of new HIV infections, as well as the management of HIV infections for those who are already infected. This has resulted in a reduced HIV incidence and mortality, while at the same time it has contributed to an increased number of people living with HIV worldwide, with a good understanding that HIV can be successfully managed as a chronic condition.

The goal of HIV management is to improve patients' health outcomes, and that is mainly done through the provision of antiretroviral therapy for the suppression of HIV viral load and supplemented by the active involvement in HIV self-management by those living with HIV. In addition, the HIV management contributes to the reduction of HIV transmission to the population through the PMTCT programmes, the uptake of PrEP, as well as the provision of post-exposure prophylaxis when needed.

6.2 Health Challenges of People Living with HIV

The HIV infection affects the people living with the infection in a variety of ways, and as noted by Shaw and Matin (2022), HIV is a multisystem disease. The people living with HIV (PLWH) are affected at physical and social level. HIV infection affects the PLWH physically by weakening the immune system, leading to the development of a number of opportunistic infections. Oral candidiasis, cytomegalovirus (CMV), and diarrhoea are some of the main gastrointestinal-related complaints noted among PLWH (Shaw & Matin, 2022; Woldegeorgis et al., 2023). For the respiratory system, Tuberculosis and Pneumocystis pneumonia (PCP) remains a major concern in PLWH (Woldegeorgis et al., 2023). With advent of COVID-19, data from literature suggest due to the immune deficiency, there was an increased risk of poor health outcomes for PLWH who have COVID-19 infection (BHIVA, DAIG, EACS, GESIDA, & Polish Scientific AIDS Society, 2021; Hoffmann et al., 2021). The PLWH also experience dermatological problem, with Herpes zoster and kaposis sarcoma being part of the commonly reported opportunistic infections (Woldegeorgis et al., 2023). The central nervous system is equally affected, with cryptococcal meningitis and toxoplasmosis featuring as part of the common opportunistic infections even in those on HIV treatment (Shaw & Matin, 2022; Woldegeorgis et al., 2023).

On the social level, PLWH continue to be affected by the rampant stigma, despite HIV having transitioned from being a deadly disease to a chronic manageable condition (Friedland et al., 2020; Lo Hog Tian et al., 2021). The continued HIV-related stigma is linked to limited access to healthcare services, social support, and access to treatment, and contributes to the worsening of health outcomes for PLWH. HIV stigma remains and has been noted even in healthcare institutions, and at times, it presents with delayed care provision and negative experiences when engaging with healthcare professionals (Friedland et al., 2020; Yuvaraj et al., 2020). Experiences of HIV stigma are linked to poor health outcomes. PLWH who experience high levels of HIV-related stigma have been reported to have higher viral loads, lower social support, poor quality of life, their mental health status is negatively affected, and their risk of misusing alcohol and drugs increases (Kemp et al., 2019). Furthermore, due to limited social support and the added stress from the experienced stigma, adherence to treatment is also reduced (Friedland et al., 2020; Kemp et al., 2019; Lo Hog Tian et al., 2021). Adherence to HIV treatment is crucial to achieve effective HIV management and viral suppression, which ensures better health outcomes, as undetectable viral load leads to a positive outcome where HIV is no longer transmissible (U=U) (Eisinger et al., 2019).

6.2.1 HIV Patient Care

The management of HIV requires a multidisciplinary approach to ensure maximum success. The main components of HIV management are early diagnosis and early initiation of antiretroviral treatment for PLWH. Once treatment has been initiated, regular follow up and monitoring as well as adherence to treatment are crucial. With the current advances in HIV treatment, treatment guidelines recommend universal access to ART for all PLWH, and the initiation is recommended as soon as the person is diagnosed (Gandhi et al., 2023). The adoption of universal HIV treatment guidelines has increased in the low-and middle-income countries (Brazier et al., 2024). As part of the HIV patient care, annual viral load monitoring is required; however, the implementation remains unacceptably low, as Brazier et al. (2024) reported that, in 25 countries, more than 25% of patients had no record of annual viral load testing. Regular monitoring is crucial to improve the continuity of care and assess the effectiveness and efficiency of the ART programmes (Pham et al., 2022).

The ART treatment includes different classes of medication, and they all function by blocking the HIV cycle at different points. To increase the effectiveness of the treatment, it is necessary to combine different classes. The first class is made of Nucleoside reverse transcriptase inhibitors (NRTIs), and nucleotide reverse transcriptase inhibitors (NtRTIs). Medication in this class of reverse transcriptase inhibitors target reverse transcriptase enzyme, blocking the conversion of viral RNA into DNA hence stops HIV replication (Moranguinho et al., 2023). The second class of ART is the Non-nucleoside reverse transcriptase inhibitors (NNRTIs), that binds itself to the reverse transcriptase enzyme, blocking the transcription process. Integrase inhibitors are another class of ART that block the virus from inserting itself into the human DNA (Moranguinho et al., 2023). Dolutegravir is one of the integrase inhibitors that has been successful in ensuring viral suppression in people on ART (Schramm et al., 2022), and is part of the recommended first line ART (McCluskey et al., 2021). Protease inhibitors (PI) are another class of ART; they block the HIV cycle by blocking the protease enzyme, which interferes with partition of the polyproteins into small pieces needed to create new viral particles (Moranguinho et al., 2023). The advances in HIV treatment have produced a combination of different classes into one tablet, reducing the pill burden for the PLWH and enhancing adherence (Simon et al., 2024). The success of ART relies on adherence, and poor adherence can lead to resistance to ART (McCluskey et al., 2021).

In addition to ART, it is crucial to identify factors that could interfere with HIV treatment and engage a multidisciplinary team to address the barriers. In low-and middle-income countries, the common barriers are often linked to lack of financial means, infrastructure, and support services (McCluskey et al., 2021). The lack of financial means is related to the transport challenges, where PLWH miss the opportunity to access health care services as they do not have money for transport, or in some cases, where there is financial cost associated with accessing health care services (Bouabida et al., 2023). Additionally, lack of financial means is related to unemployment, food insecurity, living in an overcrowded home, or even homelessness. In such situations, the PLWH are not able to access healthcare services, and take the prescribed treatment.

Infrastructure challenges are other factors that can interfere with patient care, when the healthcare institutions are not fully equipped to provide comprehensive care, or experience stockout of ART treatment (Ijumba, 2002; UNAIDS, 2024). The availability of the healthcare services with regard to the opening hours can also lead to reduced accessibility to HIV care services, especially when there is lack of flexibility to accommodate the PLWH that have work responsibilities (Dandachi et al., 2020; Lazarus et al., 2023). The low healthy literacy levels are also part of challenges in accessing HIV care, as they result in poor understanding of the illness and its management and have a negative impact on the patients' engagement into care as well as adherence to treatment (Areri et al., 2020; Bouabida et al., 2023). Regardless of the various advances in HIV treatment, the success of the treatment depends on the patients' active involvement in their own care, as such involvement in the form of HIV self-management enhances their ability to navigate the various challenges they encounter.

6.2.2 *HIV Patient Self-Management*

Patients' active involvement in HIV care and management is important as it enhances treatment outcomes, mitigates the impact of HIV in those living with the infection, and improves health-related quality of life (Lazarus et al., 2023). As noted by Dadi et al. (2024), HIV self-management is beneficial in the management of minor symptoms, and the reduction in hospitalization. HIV self-management involves the active management of the HIV in terms of taking medication and attending to daily physical health, as well as accessing the needed social support as required for better health outcomes while living with HIV infection (Areri et al., 2020). Some of the strategies implemented as part of HIV self-management include engaging in physical exercises, adherence to treatment, managing symptoms, reducing stress, using their social networks for effective HIV self-management, as well as dealing with stigma (Areri et al., 2020). There is a myriad of factors that interfere with HIV self-management, and such factors have a potential to reduce not only the participants' efforts in HIV self-management, but also their quality of life (Areri et al., 2020). One of the main factors is the HIV-related stigma, that is associated with poor self-efficacy. Accepting the HIV diagnosis and being able to disclose the serostatus is often hindered by the fear of stigma and discrimination that could lead to losing their partners (Areri et al., 2020; Dadi et al., 2024; John & Chipwaza, 2022). Up to a fifth of participants in a study conducted in Tanzania did not disclose their HIV status, and in cases where disclosure happened, it was delayed by six (6) months (John & Chipwaza, 2022).

6.3 Burden of Disease and Gaps

The HIV epidemic continues to be a heavy burden globally, and more so in the African region that carried over 65% of the total number of people living with HIV by the end of the year 2023 (UNAIDS, 2024). Despite the decrease in new infections globally, there is an unacceptable increase in some of the low-and middle-income countries such as the Philippines (Gangcuangco & Eustaquio, 2023), and an increase in new cases of 0.18 per 1000 uninfected people in the European region (World Health Organization, 2024). Furthermore, there are reports that HIV incidence is increasing in 28 countries (UNAIDS, 2024). There were 39.9 million people living with HIV in the year 2023, and this burden is heavily carried by women and girls, as they account for 53% of people living with HIV (UNAIDS, 2024). Despite the various interventions and investment geared at the prevention and management of HIV, by the end of the year 2023, there were still about 9.3 million people who were not receiving antiretroviral therapy, and about five million people who remained unaware of their HIV status (UNAIDS, 2024). This highlights the need to accelerate and strengthen the existing structures, as there is a high risk of not achieving the 2030 target of ending AIDS. The focus of HIV programmes needs to affirm a comprehensive and inclusive approach by striving to include the key populations that are at an increased risk of infection and transmission of HIV.

Although the PMTCT programme has been implemented and is evaluated as a successful intervention, there are still about 1.4 million children younger than 15 years who are living with HIV, and 86% of those are in sub-Saharan Africa (UNAIDS, 2024). This highlights the heavy burden in sub-Saharan Africa, and further interventions are needed to eliminate perinatal HIV infection. Girls and young women are also highly affected, as there is high incidence among those aged 15–24 years, with records of up to 4000 new infections among young women aged 15–24 years (Payagala & Pozniak, 2024). The advances in ART have brought success in the fight against the HIV epidemic and turned HIV into a manageable chronic condition; however, the goal to eliminate HIV remains unachieved. Furthermore, treatment access has not been ensured for all PLWH, and in Sub-Saharan Africa, there are about 4.7 million PLWH who have not accessed treatment, and up to 9.3 million globally (UNAIDS, 2024). The complexities related to the management of HIV include the regular non-adherence reported in various studies, with a related myriad of factors that lead to non-adherence. Factors such as stigma, lack of social support, and depression have been noted to inhibit adherence to ART, and such non-adherence can lead to PLWH progressing into advance HIV disease, resistance to ART as well as developing opportunistic infections that can lead to hospitalization or diminished quality of life (Paramesha & Chacko, 2019; Stelzle et al., 2025).

6.3.1 Morbidity

The treatment advances have provided potential for PLWH to live longer. Remaining in care by adhering to ART regiment and being actively engaged in HIV self-management are necessary for the improved quality of life for PLWH. However, as a result of the various factors that interfere with the management of HIV, some PLWH progress to advanced HIV disease. Literature has noted that PLWH who disengage from care and those who are not virally suppressed are more likely to have advanced HIV disease (Stelzle et al., 2025). Hence, despite the advances in treatments, HIV-related illnesses have been reported as the main causes of hospitalization, up to 42% of all admissions (Burke et al., 2025). The HIV-related hospitalizations were documented in adults and children, and in most of the WHO regions, and were mainly related to tuberculosis, *Pneumocystis jirovecii* pneumonia, and cryptococcal disease (Burke et al., 2025). The continued reports of advanced HIV diseases and hospitalization due to HIV-related illnesses highlight that HIV remains a concern and the provision of comprehensive HIV care needs to be strengthened and include monitoring, prevention, diagnosis, and treatment (Burke et al., 2025; Stelzle et al., 2025). This is crucial as weaknesses in HIV management lead to the development of opportunistic infections and increased in morbidity among PLWH, while at the same time it puts a burden to the health care system and often threatens the financial stability of individuals and their families (Payagala & Pozniak, 2024; UNAIDS, 2024). Furthermore, the consequence of being admitted in hospital include increased risk of mortality, with in-hospital mortality being reported at 17%, and reports that 20% of PLWH who were admitted in hospital died (Burke et al., 2025).

6.3.2 *Mortality*

With the continued heavy burden of HIV, for those who progress to advanced HIV disease and those who develop opportunistic infections, the risk of dying is higher (Burke et al., 2025). There has been meaningful improvement as the number of people dying from AIDS-related complications has been reduced by 51%, with reports of about 630,000 AIDS-related deaths in the year 2023, compared to 1.3 million AIDS-related deaths reported in 2010 (Payagala & Pozniak, 2024; UNAIDS, 2024). However, this is still way below the target of less than 250,000 deaths by the year 2025 (UNAIDS, 2024). Tuberculosis and cryptococcal meningitis are the main causes of death among PLWH (UNAIDS, 2024). HIV-related mortality remains a health concern, and children are heavily affected. Children account for 3% of PLWH, however, they constitute 12% of all AIDS-related deaths.

Improving HIV management to ensure adherence and active involvement in HIV self-management are necessary to reduce HIV-related mortality (Kemp et al., 2019; UNAIDS, 2024). Early initiation of ART is a valuable strategy to reduce the mortality rate (UNAIDS, 2024). It is also crucial to ensure that PLWH remain in care, hence adherence to ART and active involvement in HIV self-management will improve the health outcomes of PLWH. However, due to various challenges, this is not always the case. COVID-19 was one of such challenges as it interrupted the usual functioning of the population and the health care institutions (Sukmaningrum et al., 2024).

6.4 Impact of COVID-19 on HIV Management in LMIC

The emergence of the severe acute respiratory syndrome coronavirus-2 (SARS-CoV-2) in December 2019 heralded a global crisis, now acknowledged as the COVID-19 pandemic (Salinas-Escudero et al., 2021). This unprecedented health emergency has strained healthcare systems worldwide, impacting both the general public and vulnerable groups, notably people living with HIV (PLWH) (Waterfield et al., 2021). PLWH face unique challenges due to their compromised immune systems and underlying health conditions, rendering them susceptible to severe COVID-19 illness (Waterfield et al., 2021). Diagnosis of COVID-19 in PLWH is complicated by symptom overlap with HIV-related pulmonary complications, posing diagnostic challenges. Furthermore, a significant increase in severe COVID-19 cases might have placed immense pressure on healthcare systems, potentially causing disruptions to the continuity of HIV treatment and care (Haileamlak, 2021; Waterfield et al., 2021).

Studies conducted across LMIC have explained the impact of COVID-19 on PLWH (Jones et al., 2021; Madzima et al., 2022; Poteat et al., 2020; Santos et al., 2021). While initial data suggested a relatively low mortality rate among PLWH with COVID-19, recent findings from South Africa and Zimbabwe indicate a heightened mortality risk, primarily associated with comorbidities like diabetes and hypertension (Lee et al., 2021; Madzima et al., 2022). Hospitalization rates among affected PLWH, particularly older individuals with comorbidities, underscore the severity of cases.

Global efforts to control COVID-19 included various containment measures, inadvertently disrupting HIV services reliant on face-to-face interactions. Despite global vaccination campaigns, delayed distribution of vaccinations in African countries hindered efforts, exacerbating challenges in HIV/AIDS management (Madzima et al., 2022). These disruptions, along with strains on healthcare infrastructure and medication supply chains, have affected PLWH's mental and social health, with potential disruptions in HIV prevention programmes like pre-exposure prophylaxis (PrEP) and interruptions in antiretroviral therapy (ART) supply chains (Jewell et al., 2020a, 2020b; Hogan et al., 2020).

The COVID-19 pandemic poses significant challenges for PLWH globally, necessitating comprehensive strategies to ensure their well-being and care continuity amid this crisis. Policymakers must comprehend the impact of these disruptions to formulate strategies for maintaining uninterrupted service delivery during the pandemic (Walker et al., 2020).

6.4.1 Mental Well-Being and Social Network Support

Both HIV and COVID-19, despite their differing modes of transmission, bring profound fear and anxiety regarding contagion (Waterfield et al., 2021). Similar to the early stages of the HIV epidemic, apprehension about contracting COVID-19 persists due to the absence of established vaccines or proven therapeutic remedies to mitigate symptoms and prevent fatalities. This apprehension not only fosters mental health concerns but also perpetuates the stigma surrounding both diseases. While extensive research has been conducted on HIV-related stigma and effective stigma-reduction interventions, emerging evidence underscores the mental health burden and stigma associated with COVID-19 (Stangl et al., 2013; Ho et al., 2020; Armitage & Nellums, 2020; World Health Organization, 2020a; Sukmaningrum et al., 2024).

Among people living with HIV (PLWH), mental health challenges such as anxiety, depression, and substance abuse are prevalent and are both influenced by and contribute to their condition (Waterfield et al., 2021). Similarly, pandemic-related fear can exacerbate existing mental health conditions and potentially trigger new ones, particularly among the elderly who may face heightened social isolation. Recognizing these mental health ramifications, the World Health Organization (2020b) has issued recommendations for addressing psychosocial concerns amidst the COVID-19 outbreak.

While much remains to be understood about the interplay between HIV and the evolving COVID-19 pandemic, existing evidence suggests a profound impact on the emotional and social health of PLWH. Previous studies have documented anxiety and depressive disorders among PLWH, and it is anticipated that the COVID-19 outbreak may exacerbate these symptoms due to widespread fear, including misinformation on social media (Brandt et al., 2017; Tasnim et al., 2020).

A study conducted in the United States revealed various psychosocial challenges faced by individuals living with HIV, including difficulties with sleeping and eating, increased alcohol or substance use, and exacerbation of existing chronic conditions due to worry and stress over the coronavirus (Madzima et al., 2022; Panchal et al., 2020). These challenges were further compounded by the limited physical and psychosocial support available as a result of COVID-19 containment measures.

Similar findings emerge from research conducted in African countries like Zimbabwe and India, where the psychological effects of the pandemic range from disruptions in sleep and eating habits to increased levels of stress and impaired cognitive abilities (Chenneville et al., 2020; Marbaniang et al., 2020).

Social distancing measures and lockdowns have had a profound effect on the mental well-being of individuals living with HIV during the COVID-19 pandemic. These stringent measures unintentionally severed crucial social connections vital for their mental health. Traditional face-to-face interactions in support groups, which provided essential emotional support and a sense of belonging, became inaccessible due to the pandemic. Consequently, PLWH faced distressing social isolation and a disruption in their support networks, making it challenging to establish new virtual connections due to lingering fears of stigma. The resulting loneliness exacerbates levels of depression and anxiety, which in turn can have adverse effects on physical health and immune function. Moreover, the absence of in-person support limits effective communication and emotional expression, posing challenges for mental health interventions and comprehensive care.

6.4.2 Support from Healthcare Providers

Understanding the impact of the COVID-19 pandemic on healthcare monitoring and overall well-being of people living with HIV (PLWH) is essential yet challenging, given the evolving nature of the crisis and limited available data (Liu et al., 2020). Particularly in resource-limited settings with weak healthcare systems, there is insufficient information regarding the continuity of HIV care during the outbreak.

The enforced confinement measures implemented to mitigate the spread of COVID-19 have resulted in disruptions in the supply chain, potentially leading to poor adherence to antiretroviral therapy (ART) among PLWH (Kowalska et al., 2020). Concerns about increased exposure to the coronavirus in healthcare settings further discouraged PLWH from attending follow-up visits, exacerbating the challenges in healthcare monitoring. Recent reports from the South African National Laboratory Service indicate a concerning 10% decline in viral load testing in the public sector, highlighting a disruption in HIV care services.

The highly transmissible nature of COVID-19 has overwhelmed healthcare systems globally, impacting not only COVID-19 patients but also individuals requiring other medical services (Liu et al., 2020). With older adults and those with pre-existing conditions facing elevated risks of severe illness or mortality, healthcare facilities are under immense pressure to manage the influx of patients.

People living with HIV faced additional challenges during the pandemic, including disruptions in non-emergency medical appointments and limited access to resources for virtual care (Kowalska et al., 2020). The slow adoption of telehealth services aggravated the continuity of HIV care, further compounded by potential COVID-19 exposure during in-person appointments.

Moreover, the pandemic-induced isolation has heightened mental health issues among PLWH, particularly affecting marginalized communities overrepresented among those affected by HIV (Kowalska et al., 2020). Restrictions on movement and social interaction disproportionately impact people of colour and economically disadvantaged individuals, exacerbating existing health disparities.

In Eastern Europe, where HIV specialists were mobilized to attend to COVID-19 patients, shortages of medical staff have led to disruptions in routine medical services (Kowalska et al., 2020). Clinics were compelled to suspend in-person appointments, delay blood tests, and prioritize the distribution of ART, further straining healthcare resources.

Reports from South Africa, Zimbabwe, Kenya, and Nigeria underscore the challenges in accessing chronic medication during lockdown measures, with significant proportions of PLWH facing difficulties obtaining antiretroviral drugs (Hosken, 2020). Supply chain disruptions and delays in medication delivery contribute to the limited availability of ART stock, posing a threat to the continuity of HIV care in sub-Saharan Africa.

In summary, the COVID-19 pandemic placed unprecedented pressure on healthcare systems globally, exacerbating existing challenges in HIV care continuity and access to medication for PLWH and hindering the appropriate support from the healthcare providers. Addressing these challenges requires coordinated efforts to ensure the uninterrupted provision of healthcare services amidst the ongoing crisis.

6.4.3 *Financial Well-Being*

The financial implications of the COVID-19 pandemic have echoed globally, causing a surge in unemployment rates and exacerbating economic inequalities. While discussions on the broader implications have been abundant, attention has dropped towards specific subgroups, particularly older individuals living with HIV (PLHIV), who are deemed especially vulnerable to the economic repercussions (Brown & Weissman, 2020).

Extensive research has delved into the impact of COVID-19 on employment and income among PLHIV. Santos et al. (2021) revealed that 11.0% of surveyed PLHIV experienced a substantial loss of around 30.0% of their income due to the pandemic. Studies conducted in the United States have shed light on the significant hurdles faced by PLHIV, with one-third experiencing reduced work hours and nearly one in five losing their jobs directly attributable to COVID-19 (Cooley et al., 2021; Jones et al., 2021). Similar findings were reported by Sanchez et al. (2020) in a US-based study.

In New York, Gwadz et al. (2021) uncovered alarming statistics, with only 8.0% of participants employed and 43.0% lacking funds for basic necessities, signalling severe poverty among PLHIV. Furthermore, Poteat et al. (2020) demonstrated that transgender women living with HIV faced disproportionate challenges, including higher rates of unemployment, incomes below the federal poverty level, and heightened risks of violence compared to non-HIV-positive transgender women.

Comparative studies conducted by Jones et al. (2021) between PLHIV in the US and Argentina revealed contrasting coping mechanisms, with PLHIV in Argentina exhibiting more effective adaptations attributed to the country's enduring economic crisis. On the other hand, National lockdown measures, particularly in lower-income countries like Uganda, have posed significant hurdles for accessing healthcare services. Suspension of transportation systems has impeded access to distant clinics, while returning migrant workers to rural areas have lost access to HIV care available in urban centres. Even for those overcoming these barriers, financial strains resulting from income loss make it arduous to afford essential healthcare. This convergence of lockdown measures and financial hardships presents a critical challenge for PLHIV in accessing necessary medical care.

In summary, these studies underscore the multifaceted financial challenges faced by PLHIV during the COVID-19 pandemic and underscore the urgent need for targeted interventions to mitigate their adverse effects.

6.5 Integrated HIV Management

An interruption in antiretroviral therapy (ART) presents a critical threat to the management of HIV, potentially leading to a significant increase in HIV-related deaths. This risk persists even after the disruption ends, as individuals who experience interrupted ART may face a depletion in their CD4 cell count, leaving them vulnerable to mortality (Brown & Weissman, 2020). Countries with high HIV incidence rates, such as South Africa, experience substantial shifts in both HIV incidence and mortality due to interruptions in ART. South Africa's large population receiving ART, coupled with the temporary halt in new treatment initiations, exacerbates the situation, leading to additional deaths among those who experience delays in initiating ART (Brown & Weissman, 2020).

Amidst disruptions caused by the COVID-19 pandemic, ensuring uninterrupted access to ART remains a paramount goal for HIV programmes. A prolonged break in ART supply could result in additional deaths comparable in magnitude to those prevented by measures aimed at mitigating the COVID-19 epidemic itself (Brown & Weissman, 2020). Policy adjustments, such as implementing changes in ART delivery, issuing multi-month prescriptions, or providing medication outside healthcare facilities, can mitigate some adverse effects of service interruption in the long run. However, if interruptions occur, programmes may face challenges reverting to their previous state, leading to further detrimental effects among individuals facing prolonged disruptions in ART access (Brown & Weissman, 2020).

Integrated management of HIV entails a comprehensive approach to addressing various facets of HIV care and treatment. The emergence of COVID-19 has posed significant challenges globally, straining healthcare systems worldwide and impacting individuals requiring medical services beyond COVID-19 treatment (Liu et al., 2020). Physical distancing measures recommended by the World Health Organization (WHO) have exacerbated economic, psychosocial, and educational challenges, particularly affecting people living with HIV (PLWH) (WHO, 2020a). PLWH face additional challenges during the pandemic, including disruptions in HIV care continuity, slow adoption of telehealth services, potential COVID-19 exposure during in-person appointments, and exacerbated mental health issues due to isolation (Liu et al., 2020).

COVID-19 exacerbates disparities within the HIV epidemic, emphasizing the need for targeted interventions for marginalized communities, particularly PLWH. The pandemic has significantly impacted healthcare delivery for other diseases, leading to shifts in disease burden trends and necessitating longer-term antiretroviral dispensing to address irregular drug supply issues (Liu et al., 2020). PLWH face compounded challenges influenced by social determinants of health (SDoH), with heightened vulnerability due to weakened immune systems from HIV, systemic health disparities, limited healthcare access, and social factors like economic instability or inadequate living conditions (Liu et al., 2020).

Addressing these challenges for PLWH necessitates a comprehensive approach involving healthcare systems, policymakers, communities, and support networks.

Combatting stigma and discrimination, leveraging telemedicine, providing economic support programmes, and offering virtual community-based initiatives are essential strategies to enhance access to healthcare and maintain treatment continuity for PLWH during the COVID-19 pandemic (Liu et al., 2020; WHO, 2020b). Rebuilding and maintaining social support networks are critical to alleviating the adverse effects of social isolation and promoting the well-being of PLWH (Liu et al., 2020). Collaboration with communities can lead to innovative solutions to address the unique challenges faced by PLWH during the pandemic.

6.6 Way Forward

What has not been ascertained, and therefore points to a need for specific studies, is whether the people living with HIV who died during the COVID-19 era actually died of COVID-19 or other complications. In this regard, it is imperative that the COVID-19 response or any other pandemic be programmatically integrated with that of HIV to ensure that all relevant data is collected. To date, there has been strong infrastructure and principles applied in the fight against HIV epidemic, and as noted by Collins et al. (2023) such strengths can be relied on to support the response to any other epidemic, which would facilitate continuity of care for everyone.

References

Areri, H., Marshall, A., & Harvey, G. (2020). Factors influencing self-management of adults living with HIV on antiretroviral therapy in Northwest Ethiopia: A cross-sectional study. *BMC Infectious Diseases, 20*, 879. https://doi.org/10.1186/s12879-020-05618-y

Armitage, R., & Nellums, L. B. (2020). COVID-19 and the consequences of isolating the elderly. *The Lancet Public Health, 5*(5), e256.

BHIVA, DAIG, EACS, GESIDA & Polish Scientific AIDS Society. (2021). *Statement on risk of COVID-19 for people living with HIV (PLWH)*. Retrieved December 1, 2024, from https://www.bhiva.org/joint-statement-on-risk-of-COVID-19-for-PLWH-and-SARS-CoV-2-vaccine-advice

Bouabida, K., Chaves, B. G., & Anane, E. (2023). Challenges and barriers to HIV care engagement and care cascade. *Frontiers in reproductive health, 5*, 1201087.

Brandt, C., Zvolensky, M. J., Woods, S. P., Gonzalez, A., Safren, S. A., & O'Cleirigh, C. M. (2017). Anxiety symptoms and disorders among adults living with HIV and AIDS: A critical review and integrative synthesis of the empirical literature. *Clinical Psychology Review, 51*, 164–184.

Brazier, E., Tymejczyk, O., Wools-Kaloustian, K., Jiamsakul, A., Torres, M. T. L., Lee, J. S., et al. (2024). Long-term HIV care outcomes under universal HIV treatment guidelines: A retrospective cohort study in 25 countries. *PLoS Medicine, 21*(3), e1004367. https://doi.org/10.1371/journal.pmed.1004367

Brown, M. J., & Weissman, S. B. (2020). The impact of COVID-19 on older adults living with HIV: HIV care and psychosocial effects. *Journal of Gerontological Social Work, 63*(6–7), 602–606.

Burke, R. M., Sabet, N., Ellis, J., Rangaraj, A., Lawrence, D. S., Jarvis, J. N., Falconer, J., Tugume, L., Bidwell, G., Berhanu, R. H., & MacPherson, P. (2025). *Causes of hospitalisation among people living with HIV worldwide, 2014–23: A systematic review and meta-analysis*. The Lancet HIV.

Chenneville, T., Gabbidon, K., Hanson, P., & Holyfield, C. (2020). The impact of COVID-19 on HIV treatment and research: A call to action. *International Journal of Environmental Research and Public Health, 17*(12), 4548.

Collins, C., Isbell, M. T., Karim, Q. A., Sohn, A. H., Beyrer, C., & Maleche, A. (2023). Leveraging the HIV response to strengthen pandemic preparedness. *PLOS Global Public Health, 3*(1), e0001511.

Cooley, S. A., Nelson, B., Doyle, J., Rosenow, A., & Ances, B. M. (2021). Collateral damage: Impact of SARS-CoV-2 pandemic in people living with HIV. *Journal of Neurovirology, 27*, 168–170.

Dadi, T. L., Tegene, Y., Vollebregt, N., Medhin, G., & Spigt, M. (2024). The importance of self-management for better treatment outcomes for HIV patients in a low-income setting: Perspectives of HIV experts and service providers. *AIDS Research and Therapy, 21*, 28. https://doi.org/10.1186/s12981-024-00612-9

Dandachi, D., Dang, B. N., Lucari, B., Teti, M., & Giordano, T. P. (2020). Exploring the attitude of patients with HIV about using telehealth for HIV care. *AIDS Patient Care and STDs, 34*(4), 166–172.

Eisinger, R. W., Dieffenbach, C. W., & Fauci, A. S. (2019). HIV viral load and transmissibility of HIV infection: Undetectable equals untransmittable. *Jama, 321*(5), 451–452. https://doi.org/10.1001/jama.2018.21167

Friedland, B. A., Gottert, A., Hows, J., Baral, S. D., Sprague, L., Nyblade, L., McClair, T. L., Anam, F., Geibel, S., Kentutsi, S., & Tamoufe, U. (2020). The people living with HIV stigma indhex 2.0: Generating critical evidence for change worldwide. *AIDS, 34*, S5–S18.

Gandhi, R. T., Bedimo, R., Hoy, J. F., Landovitz, R. J., Smith, D. M., Eaton, E. F., Lehmann, C., Springer, S. A., Sax, P. E., Thompson, M. A., & Benson, C. A. (2023). Antiretroviral drugs for treatment and prevention of HIV infection in adults: 2022 recommendations of the international antiviral society–USA panel. *JAMA, 329*(1), 63–84.

Gangcuangco, L. M. A., & Eustaquio, P. C. (2023). The state of the HIV epidemic in The Philippines: Progress and challenges in 2023. *Tropical Medicine and Infectious Disease, 8*(5), 258.

Gwadz, M., Campos, S., Freeman, R., Cleland, C. M., Wilton, L., Sherpa, D., Ritchie, A. S., Hawkins, R. L., Allen, J. Y., Martinez, B. Y., Dorsen, C., Collins, L. M., Hroncich, T., Cluesman, S. R., & Leonard, N. R. (2021). Black and Latino persons living with HIV evidence risk and resilience in the context of COVID-19: A mixed-methods study of the early phase of the pandemic. *AIDS and Behavior, 25*, 1340–1360.

Haileamlak, A. (2021). The impact of COVID-19 on health and health systems. *Ethiopian Journal of Health Sciences, 31*(6), 1073. https://doi.org/10.4314/ejhs.v31i6.1

Ho, C. S., Chee, C. Y., & Ho, R. C. (2020). Mental health strategies to combat the psychological impact of COVID-19 beyond paranoia and panic. *Annals of the Academy of Medicine, Singapore, 49*(1), 1–3.

Hoffmann, C., Casado, J. L., Härter, G., Vizcarra, P., Moreno, A., Cattaneo, D., Meraviglia, P., Spinner, C. D., Schabaz, F., Grunwald, S., & Gervasoni, C. (2021). Immune deficiency is a risk factor for severe COVID-19 in people living with HIV. *HIV Medicine, 22*(5), 372–378.

Hogan, A. B., Jewell, B. L., Sherrard-Smith, E., Vesga, J. F., Watson, O. J., Whittaker, C., Hamlet, A., Smith, J. A., Winskill, P., Verity, R., Baguelin, M., Lees, J. A., Whittles, L. K., KEC, A., Bhatt, S., Boonyasiri, A., Brazeau, N. F., et al. (2020). Potential impact of the COVID-19 pandemic on HIV, tuberculosis, and malaria in low-income and middle-income countries: A modelling study. *The Lancet Global Health, 8*(9), e1132–e1141.

Hosken, G. (2020). *Coronavirus fears keep HIV, TB patients from medication. Sunday Times, Johannesburg (May 17, 2020)*. Retrieved February 25, 2024, from https://www.timeslive.co.za/sunday-times/news/2020-05-17-coronavirus-fears-keep-hiv-tb-patients-from-medication/

Ijumba, P. (2002). 'Voices' of primary health care facility workers: Human resources. *South African health review, 2002*(1), 181–200.

Jewell, B. L., Mudimu, E., Stover, J., Ten Brink, D., Phillips, A. N., Smith, J. A., Martin-Hughes, R., Teng, Y., Glaubius, R., Mahiane, S. G., Bansi-Matharu, L., Taramusi, I., Chagoma, N., Morrison, M., Doherty, M., Marsh, K., Bershteyn, A., et al. (2020a). Potential effects of disruption to HIV programmes in sub-Saharan Africa caused by COVID-19: Results from multiple mathematical models. *The lancet HIV, 7*(9), e629–e640.

Jewell, B. L., Smith, J. A., & Hallett, T. B. (2020b). Understanding the impact of interruptions to HIV services during the COVID-19 pandemic: A modelling study. *EClinicalMedicine, 26*.

John, M. E., & Chipwaza, B. (2022). HIV status disclosure among adults attending care and treatment clinic in Kilombero district, south-eastern Tanzania. *International Journal of Africa Nursing Sciences, 17*, 100434. https://doi.org/10.1016/j.ijans.2022.100434

Jones, D. L., Ballivian, J., Rodriguez, V. J., Uribe, C., Cecchini, D., Salazar, A. S., Cassetti, I., & Alcaide, M. L. (2021). Mental health, coping, and social support among people living with HIV in the Americas: A comparative study between Argentina and the USA during the SARS-CoV-2 pandemic. *AIDS and Behavior, 25*, 2391–2399.

Kemp, C. G., Lipira, L., Huh, D., Nevin, P. E., Turan, J. M., Simoni, J. M., Cohn, S. E., Bahk, M., Berzins, B., Andrasik, M., & Mugavero, M. J. (2019). HIV stigma and viral load among African-American women receiving treatment for HIV. *AIDS, 33*(9), 1511–1519.

Kowalska, J. D., Skrzat-Klapaczyńska, A., Bursa, D., Balayan, T., Begovac, J., Chkhartishvili, N., Gokengin, D., Harxhi, A., Jilich, D., Jevtovic, D., Kase, K., Lakatos, B., Matulionyte, R., Mulabdic, V., Nagit, A., Papadopoulos, A., Stefanovic, M., et al. (2020). HIV care in times of the COVID-19 crisis—Where are we now in central and Eastern Europe? *International Journal of Infectious Diseases, 96*, 311–314.

Lazarus, J. V., Wohl, D. A., Cascio, M., Guaraldi, G., Rockstroh, J., Hodson, M., Richman, B., Brown, G., Anderson, J., & Fuster-RuizdeApodaca, M. J. (2023). Long-term success for people living with HIV: A framework to guide practice. *HIV Medicine, 24*, 8–19.

Lee, K. W., Yap, S. F., Ngeow, Y. F., & Lye, M. S. (2021). COVID-19 in people living with HIV: A systematic review and meta-analysis. *International Journal of Environmental Research and Public Health, 18*(7), 3554.

Liu, Y., Gayle, A. A., Wilder-Smith, A., & Rocklöv, J. (2020). The reproductive number of COVID-19 is higher compared to SARS coronavirus. *Journal of Travel Medicine.*

Lo Hog Tian, J. M., Watson, J. R., Ibáñez-Carrasco, F., Tran, B., Parsons, J. A., Maunder, R. G., Card, K. G., Baral, S., Hui, C., Boni, A. R., & Ajiboye, M. (2021). Impact of experienced HIV stigma on health is mediated by internalized stigma and depression: Results from the people living with HIV stigma index in Ontario. *BMC Public Health, 21*, 1–10.

Madzima, B., Makoni, T., Mugurungi, O., Mudariki, G., Mpofu, A., Dube, F., Munangaidzwa, L., & Taramusi, I. (2022). The impact of the COVID-19 pandemic on people living with HIV in Zimbabwe. *African Journal of AIDS Research, 21*(2), 194–200.

Marbaniang, I., Sangle, S., Nimkar, S., Zarekar, K., Salvi, S., Chavan, A., Gupta, A., Suryavanshi, N., & Mave, V. (2020). The burden of anxiety during the COVID-19 pandemic among people living with HIV (PLHIV) in Pune, India. *Research Square, 3.*

McCluskey, S. M., Pepperrell, T., Hill, A., Venter, W. D., Gupta, R. K., & Siedner, M. J. (2021). Adherence, resistance, and viral suppression on dolutegravir in sub-Saharan Africa: Implications for the TLD era. *AIDS, 35*(Supplement 2), S127–S135.

Moranguinho, I., Taveira, N., & Bártolo, I. (2023). Antiretroviral treatment of HIV-2 infection: Available drugs, resistance pathways, and promising new compounds. *International Journal of Molecular Sciences, 24*(6), 5905.

Panchal, N., Kamal, R., Orgera, K., Cox, C., Garfield, R., Hamel, L., & Chidambaram, P. (2020). The implications of COVID-19 for mental health and substance use. *Kaiser Family Foundation, 21*, 1–16. https://www.kff.org/coronavirus-covid-19/issue-brief/the-implications-of-covid-19-for-mental-health-and-substance-use/

Paramesha, A. E., & Chacko, L. K. (2019). Predictors of adherence to antiretroviral therapy among PLHIV. *Indian Journal of Public Health, 63*(4), 367–376.

Payagala, S., & Pozniak, A. (2024). The global burden of HIV. *Clinics in Dermatology, 42*(2), 119–127.

Pham, M. D., Nguyen, H. V., Anderson, D., Crowe, S., & Luchters, S. (2022). Viral load monitoring for people living with HIV in the era of test and treat: Progress made and challenges ahead–a systematic review. *BMC Public Health, 22*(1), 1203.

Poteat, T. C., Reisner, S. L., Miller, M., & Wirtz, A. L. (2020). In medRxiv (Ed.), *COVID-19 vulnerability of transgender women with and without HIV infection in the eastern and southern US*.

Salinas-Escudero, G., Toledano-Toledano, F., García-Peña, C., Parra-Rodríguez, L., Granados-García, V., & Carrillo-Vega, M. F. (2021). Disability-adjusted life years for the COVID-19 pandemic in the Mexican population. *Frontiers in Public Health, 9*, 686700.

Sanchez, T. H., Zlotorzynska, M., Rai, M., & Baral, S. D. (2020). Characterizing the impact of COVID-19 on men who have sex with men across the United States in April 2020. *AIDS and Behavior, 24*(7), 2024–2032.

Santos, G. M., Ackerman, B., Rao, A., Wallach, S., Ayala, G., Lamontage, E., et al. (2021). Economic, mental health, HIV prevention and HIV treatment impacts of COVID-19 and the COVID-19 response on a global sample of cisgender gay men and other men who have sex with men. *AIDS and Behavior, 25*, 311–321.

Schramm, B., Temfack, E., Descamps, D., Nicholas, S., Peytavin, G., Bitilinyu-Bangoh, J. E., Storto, A., Lê, M. P., Abdi, B., Ousley, J., & Kalua, T. (2022). Viral suppression and HIV-1 drug resistance 1 year after pragmatic transitioning to dolutegravir first-line therapy in Malawi: A prospective cohort study. *The Lancet HIV, 9*(8), e544–e553.

Shaw, J., & Matin, N. (2022). Opportunistic infections in HIV. *Medicine, 50*(5), 294–297.

Simon, M., Derrick, S., Kosanam, S., & Pasupula, R. (2024). Pill burden: A major barrier to HAART adherence and fixed dose combinations (FDCS) as its solution-a mini-review. *Current HIV Research, 22*(3), 143–152.

Stangl, A. L., Lloyd, J. K., Brady, L. M., Holland, C. E., & Baral, S. (2013). A systematic review of interventions to reduce HIV-related stigma and discrimination from 2002 to 2013: How far have we come? *Journal of the International AIDS Society, 16*, 18734.

Stelzle, D., Rangaraj, A., Jarvis, J. N., Razakasoa, N. H., Perrin, G., Low-Beer, D., Doherty, M., Ford, N., & Dalal, S. (2025). Prevalence of advanced HIV disease in sub-Saharan Africa: A multi-country analysis of nationally representative household surveys. *The Lancet Global Health, 13*(3). https://doi.org/10.1016/S2214-109X(24)00538-2

Sukmaningrum, E., Levy, J., Negara, M. D., Devika, D., Wardhani, B. D. K., Wulandari, L. P. L., & Januraga, P. P. (2024). Lived experience, social support, and challenges to health service use during the COVID-19 pandemic among HIV key populations in Indonesia. *BMC Health Services Research, 24*(1), 774.

Tasnim, S., Hossain, M. M., & Mazumder, H. (2020). Impact of rumors and misinformation on COVID-19 in social media. *Journal of Preventive Medicine and Public Health, 53*(3), 171–174.

UNAIDS (Joint United Nations Programme on HIV/AIDS). (2024). *The urgency of now: AIDS at a crossroads*. Geneva. Licence: CC BY-NC-SA 3.0 IGO [Online]. Retrieved November 10, 2024, from https://www.unaids.org/sites/default/files/media_asset/2024-unaids-global-aids-update_en.pdf

Walker, P. G., Whittaker, C., Watson, O. J., Baguelin, M., Winskill, P., Hamlet, A., et al. (2020). The impact of COVID-19 and strategies for mitigation and suppression in low-and middle-income countries. *Science, 369*(6502), 413–422.

Woldegeorgis, B. Z., Zekarias, Z., Adem, B. G., Obsa, M. S., & Kerbo, A. A. (2023). Prevalence and determinants of opportunistic infections among HIV-infected adults receiving antiretroviral therapy in Ethiopia: A systematic review and meta-analysis. *Frontiers in Medicine, 10*, 1087086.

World Health Organization (WHO). (2020a). *Mental health and psychosocial considerations during the COVID-19 outbreak*. Retrieved April 26, 2024, from https://www.who.int/docs/default-source/coronaviruse/mental-health-considerations

World Health Organization (WHO). (2020b). *Maintaining essential health services: operational guidance for the COVID-19 context interim guidance.* Retrieved March 19, 2023, from https://www.who.int/publications/i/item/WHO-2019-nCoV-essential_health_services-2020.2

World Health Organization (WHO). (2024). *HIV statistics, globally and by WHO region, 2024. Global HIV programme.* Retrieved December 20, 2024, from https://www.who.int/teams/global-hiv-hepatitis-and-stis-programmes/hiv/strategic-information/hiv-data-and-statistics

Waterfield, K. C., Shah, G. H., Etheredge, G. D., & Ikhile, O. (2021). Consequences of COVID-19 crisis for persons with HIV: The impact of social determinants of health. *BMC Public Health, 21*(1), 299. https://doi.org/10.1186/s12889-021-10296-9

Yuvaraj, A., Mahendra, V. S., Chakrapani, V., Yunihastuti, E., Santella, A. J., Ranauta, A., & Doughty, J. (2020). HIV and stigma in the healthcare setting. *Oral Diseases, 26*, 103–111.

Part IV
Preparedness and Response

Chapter 7
COVID-19 Response in Island Nations, Challenges, Lessons Learned, and Way Forward

Fingani Annie Mphande

Abstract Island nations are a unique ecosystem often isolated geographically. This isolation can be an advantage but also a limitation. While their remote locations provide a buffer against the initial spread of disease, this same isolation also creates logistical issues of access to medical supplies, healthcare support, and vaccines in times of emergencies. Heavy dependence on tourism created economic vulnerability for island nations and territories during border closures in response to the COVID-19 pandemic. The COVID-19 pandemic posed unique challenges for island nations, highlighting both their geographic advantages and systemic vulnerabilities. This chapter will explore the COVID-19 responses in island nations, evaluate some of the challenges encountered, and the unique responses to the pandemic. The lessons learned and response strategies as well as propose recommendations for future preparedness.

Keywords Carribean community · COVID-19 response · Indian ocean islands · Low and Middle-income countries · Pacific community · Small island developing states (SIDS)

List of Abbreviations

NCD	Non-communicable diseases
CARPHA	Caribbean Public Health Agency
CARICOM	Caribbean Community
DALYs	Disability adjusted life years
PAHO	American Health Organization
PICT	Pacific Island countries and territories
LMIC	Low and middle income countries

F. A. Mphande (✉)
Faculty of Medicine, King Mongkut's Institute of Technology Ladkrabang, Bangkok, Thailand
e-mail: yadoster@gmail.com

F. Mphande and P. Nyasulu (eds.), *Evaluating Outbreak Potential of Infections in Tropical Climates*, https://doi.org/10.1007/978-981-95-0618-7_7

ESKD	End stage kidney disease
SIDS	Small island developing states

7.1 Introduction

Island nations are ecosystems with unique plant and animal populations but also home to populations that have adaptations due to their geographic isolation and surroundings. Globally, island nations are located in the seven oceans with vast archipelagos spanning the oceans. From the pacific island nations encompassing Melanesia, Micronesia, and Polynesia to the Caribbean nations in the Atlantic and Indian Ocean island nations. Rich in culture and natural beauty, accessibility to these islands varies tremendously. The Caribbean islands comprise over 7000 islands with 30 territories and 13 independent island countries. Covering western and central pacific, the pacific islands are made up of over 25,00 islands and 14 countries and territories, and Indian ocean islands with approximately 2000 islands (Table 7.1). Population sizes vary between the islands and so do health systems and resource capabilities.

The uniqueness of island nations is the small populations and vast areas covering thousands of kilometres. The small populations often bring challenges in human resources while the vast areas bring challenges not only of human resources but also infrastructure. Fragile health communities in the Caribbean struggled during the pandemic; the tourism sector was greatly affected putting economies at risk and with small businesses especially those that depended on tourism were at a standstill. According to the global burden of disease report 2019, ischeamic heart disease, stroke, and diabetes were among the top 10 non-communicable diseases (NCD) in small island nations and territories (Vos et al., 2020).

7.2 Disease Burden and Co-morbidities

A high burden of disease in small island nations is attributed to NCD (Razzaghi et al., 2019; Rivera-Andrade & Luna, 2014; Yisahak et al., 2014). With the highest reported premature mortality rates in the Americas, over 60% of Caribbean adults are overweight with up to 80% prevalence in some of the countries (Caribbean Public Health Agency -CARPHA, 2017; Ordunez et al., 2015). The human and economic costs of NCD are high ranging from amputations that greatly affect the quality of life to financial costs both at family and national level (Hennis et al., 2004).

Table 7.1 Island nation countries and estimated populations as of 2023

Caribbean island nations (Population)	Indian ocean island nations	Pacific island nations
Antigua and Barbuda (96,696)	Comoros (850,397)	Australia
The Bahamas (401,283)	Madagascar (31,195,932)	Cook Islands (14,987)
Barbados (281,114)	Mauritius (1,261,040)	Federated States of Micronesia (112,630)
Cuba (11,347,169)	Seychelles (119,770)	Fiji (948,300)
Dominica (74,183)	Sri Lanka (22,037,000)	French Polynesia
Dominican Republic (11,424,748)	Maldives (525,994)	Kiribati, (132,530)
Grenada (120,809)	Mayotte (316,015)	Nauru (11,875)
Haiti (11,972,522)	La Reunion (874,883)	New Caledonia
Jamaica (2,839,175)		New Zealand
Saint Kitts and Nevis (53,120)		Niue (11,875)
Saint Lucia (187,211)		Palau (17,727)
Saint Vincent and the Grenadines (108,058)		Papua New Guinea (10,826,800)
Trinidad and Tobago (1,507,782)		Republic of Marshall Islands (38,827)
Guadeloupe (375,106)		Samoa (216,663)
		Solomon Islands (800,005)
		Tonga (106,017)
		Tuvalu (11,204)
		Vanuatu (319,137)

Source https://data.worldbank.org/indicator/SP.POP.TOTL

7.2.1 Caribbean Islands

According to the World Bank, non-communicable diseases account for 75% of deaths in the Caribbean countries. Cardiovascular disease, cancer, and diabetes are the leading cause of deaths in the region. The economic costs ranging from 1.36% to 8% as well as direct and indirect costs have a huge impact on the countries and the population (https://www.worldbank.org/en/country/caribbean/brief/the-economic-impact-of-non-communicable-diseases-in-the-caribbean). To mitigate these challenges, countries are working hard to reduce the burden. Some of the measures include policies to control alcohol and tobacco consumption. The declaration of Port of Spain (2007) by the member states of the Caribbean Community (CARICOM) emphasized on standardization of care and policies that encourage healthy living (https://www.worldbank.org/en/region/lac/publication/noncommunicable-diseases-care-in-the-eastern-caribbean).

7.2.2 *Indian Ocean Islands*

In the Indian Ocean islands, NCD are a concern. In Maldives, smoking, obesity, diabetes, hypertension, and hypercholesterolemia were reported as a challenge (Aboobakur et al., 2010). In Seychelles, stroke, hypertension, and diabetes have been reported for the past decades (Bovet, Viswanathan, Shamlaye, Romain, & Gedeon, 2010). In a 2023 report, WHO stated NCD as a major health problem in Seychelles with cardiovascular disease, chronic respiratory disease, cancer, and diabetes listed among the public health challenges (WHO, 2023). Similarly, neighbouring Mauritius has a high prevalence of NCD, which was a cause of concern during the COVID-19 pandemic (World Health Organization, 2020). For Sri Lanka, NCD account for approximately 80% of deaths and contribute to over 70% of disability adjusted life years (DALYs) (Kyu et al., 2018). Diabetes and hypertension are among the NCD affecting Sri Lanka with primary healthcare provisions to address the challenges (Nair et al., 2023).

7.2.3 *Pacific Islands*

Apart from diabetes, obesity and hypertension are another set of NCD affecting island states. A study from three pacific islands, Fiji, Kiribati, Vanuatu obesity was observed to be higher in urban than rural areas. Higher prevalence rates of diabetes, hypertension, and higher cholesterol levels were also reported (Foster et al., 2018; Taylor et al., 1992). Efforts to reduce the risk of obesity by setting up various regulations including dietary regulations were reported in both pacific (Fiji, Nauru, and Tonga) and Caribbean (Barbados, Dominica, and Jamaica) islands (Foster et al., 2018). The per cent deaths from all major NCDs was 83% and 79% for Barbados and Jamaica, respectively. While the prevalence of obesity was 33.2%, 26.8% and 25.9% for Barbados, Jamaica, and Dominica, respectively (Foster et al., 2018).

In the pacific islands, NCD remain a challenge with six of the top 10 countries globally with a high prevalence of diabetes using age adjusted comparative prevalence in adults coming from this region (International Diabetes Federation (IDF), 2025). French Polynesia, New Caledonia, Northern Mariana Islands, Marshal Islands, and Kiribati are among the top 10 countries. Between 2015 and 2017, Fiji reported the highest number of deaths from major NCDs (cardiovascular diseases, cancers, chronic respiratory diseases, and diabetes), with a prevalence of 93% and prevalence of obesity at 35.9%. The prevalence of obesity was highest in Nauru at 45.1% followed by Tonga at 41.1% (Foster et al., 2018).

7.3 COVID-19 and Response in Selected Small Island Nations

To understand the impact and response of COVID-19 in small island nations will be reviewed. Six island states were selected; Caribbean island states (Trinidad and Tobago and Haiti), Indian Ocean Islands (Mauritius and Sri-Lanka), and two pacific island states (Fiji and New Caledonia). The impact, preparedness, and response to COVID-19 in these countries are hereby reviewed.

7.3.1 COVID-19 and Caribbean Islands and Territories

As the pandemic was growing in other parts of the world, Caribbean governments were preparing even before registering cases of COVID-19. Border closures were initiated, curfews were put in place, gatherings were controlled, while stay at home orders were implemented on the ground (Murphy et al., 2020). Movement was controlled into and within the country. School closures, control of social events and gatherings as well as closure and or limited access to businesses and public places were implemented as within country non-pharmaceutical control measures (Murphy et al., 2020). By April 2020, curfews, partial and full lockdowns were implemented in The Bahamas, Barbados, while Trinidad and Tobago only implemented a full lockdown. Antigua and Barbuda implemented curfews and full lockdown while Jamaica implemented curfews and partial lockdown. Belize and Jamaica only implemented partial lockdowns. These measures were associated with reduction of human movement (Murphy et al., 2020). During the pandemic, preparedness and response to the pandemic followed cooperation with regional organizations including CARPHA (https://caribbean.eclac.org/information-resources/website/caribbean-public-health-agency-carpha-coronavirus-disease-2019-covid), Pan American Health Organization (PAHO) (https://paho-covid19-response-who.hub.arcgis.com/), and the Caribbean Association of Medical Councils (CAMC) (https://www.camcouncils.org/). These organizations provided information through situational reports, provided statistical analysis, and developed guidelines for use in the region (Umakanthan et al., 2022). Effects of the pandemic included loss of livelihood as some people lost their jobs resulting in economic impact on families. Similarly, the economic impact was felt on countries in the region as tourism took a plunge due to border closures affecting economies in the region. The number of COVID-19 cases and deaths varied between countries (Table 7.2).

The number of deaths per 100,000 population for Caribbean island territories as of January 2022, were estimated above the global rate (71.07 deaths per 100,000 population) except for Haiti (6.93 deaths per 100,000 population), Dominica (65.5 deaths per 100,000 population), Dominican Republic (39.62 deaths per 100,000 population), and St Kits and Nevis (53 deaths per 100,000 population) (Schwalb et al., 2022).

Table 7.2 Cumulative COVID-19 cases as of 2023 in selected Caribbean Island Countries and territories

Country/Territory	Cumulative COVID-19 Cases	Cumulative deaths	Population	Percent Cumulative cases/ total population
Antigua and Barbuda	6,607	146	96,696	6.83
Barbados	108,525	593	281,114	38.61
Cuba	1,113,662	8,530	11,347,169	9.81
Dominica	16,047	74	74,183	21.63
Dominican Republic	661,103	4,384	11,424,748	5.79
Grenada	19,693	238	120,809	16.30
Guyana	74,439	1,302	826,350	9.01
Haiti	34,298	860	11,972,522	0.29
Jamaica	157,165	3,611	2,839,175	5.54
Saint Kitts and Nevis	6,607	46	53,120	12.44
Saint Lucia	30,271	410	187,211	16.17
Saint Vincent and the Grenadines	9,674	124	108,058	8.95
Suriname	82,501	1,406	628,890	13.12
The Bahamas	39,127	593	401,283	9.75
Trinidad and Tobago	191,496	4,390	1,507,782	12.70

7.3.1.1 Trinidad and Tobago and COVID-19

Trinidad and Tobago, an island with a population of 1,365,805 was not spared from COVID-19. Despite control measures in place, 191,496 COVID-19 cases and 4,390 cases were reported. Waves of Gamma and Omicron strains were reported between 2020 and 2023 (Dookeeram et al., 2023).

Counter Measures

Lockdowns and social distancing were implemented to prevent community spread. Financial boost was obtained for support of emergency response including health personnel managing COVID-19 patients (Dookeeram et al., 2023). Despite hurdles to obtain the COVID-19 vaccines, vaccination was rolled out and 53% of the population was vaccinated with Astrazeneca as well as Sinopharm by the year 2021 (Maharaj et al., 2021).

Lessons Learned

Trinidad and Tobago was able to adapt their healthcare system by creating a "Parallel healthcare system" isolating routine healthcare service from COVID-19 patients. Trinidad and Tobago ranked number one by a report by Oxford University assessing response to COVID-19 based on 4 of the six WHO criteria for rolling back lockdown measures (Hale et al., 2020). The country demonstrated political will, collaborative actions, evidence-based and informed decision-making as well as timely coordination and respect for science. These attributes contributed to the successful management of COVID-19 irrespective of the health system and or resource capabilities (Hunte et al., 2020).

Strengthening of the healthcare workforce through training during the pandemic as well as provision of PPE, quarantine facilities as well as psychological support for frontline workers was one of the strategies used to support the health workforce in the country. Open communication and bolstering local manufacturing of needed supplies such as face masks, face shields, as well as sanitisers assisted with the control efforts. Maintenance of health information systems, including surveillance, contact tracing, as well as treatment (Hunte et al., 2020).

7.3.1.2 Haiti and COVID-19

Since the earthquake in 2010, Haiti has suffered wave upon wave of catastrophic natural disasters as well as civil unrest. The natural disasters, cholera outbreak, coupled with civil unrest affected various sectors in the country including health systems, financial and agricultural sectors (Kianersi et al., 2021). In 2020, the onset of the COVID-19 pandemic added to the various hurdles Haiti was going through. COVID-19 cases in Haiti were recorded with a cumulative total of 34,785 cases. The Haitian population has gone through a lot of natural disasters and experiences that could have assisted with coping with the pandemic (Blanc et al., 2020).

The benefits and harms of lockdown were evaluated and adherence remained a challenge for most of the population, with the need to meet everyday needs and limited trust in the health system attributing to some of the contributing factors (Bardosh et al., 2023). Still lower numbers of COVID-19 cases were reported in the country where hand hygiene, mask wearing with persons exhibit symptoms would go to hospital proved successful (Fujita & Sabogal, 2021).

Counter Measures

When the pandemic hit, a state of emergency was declared in Haiti, followed by stay home orders. Borders were closed and movement between certain regions was within the country were restricted (Bardosh et al., 2023).

Lessons Learned

COVID-19 was a crisis that added to the strain on Haiti which was already struggling to recover from the past crises. The resilience and coping strategies for the Haitian population are worth exploring.

7.3.2 *COVID-19 and Indian Ocean Island Countries and Territories*

Indian Ocean islands and territories are beautiful destinations for tourists from all over the world. COVID-19 had an impact not only at the population but also on tourism (Mayr et al., 2020). Lockdown restrictions were implemented in Madagascar, Mauritius, and Sri Lanka, including inter-island travel bans in the Maldives to control the spread of the virus (Singh & Goel, n.d.). The confirmed total number of cases and deaths varied between countries (Table 7.3).

7.3.2.1 Mauritius and COVID-19

The Indian Ocean island of Mauritius, home to approximately 1.26 million people, was not spared from COVID-19 (WHO- Mauritius Country Office, 2020).

Counter Measures

Strong public health measures including lockdown were implemented together with border closures to control the spread of COVID-19 and strict laws were put in place to

Table 7.3 Cumulative COVID-19 cases as of 2023 in selected Indian Ocean Island Countries and territories

Country/Territory	Cumulative COVID-19 Cases	Cumulative deaths	Population	Percent Cumulative cases/ total population
Comoros	9,109	160	850,397	1.07
La Reunion	494,595	540	874,883	56.53
Madagascar	68,669	1,426	31,195,932	0.2
Maldives	186,694	316	525,994	35.49
Mauritius	334,323	1,056	1,261,040	26.51
Mayotte	42,027	316,015	316,015	13.30
Sri Lanka	672,812		22,037,000	3.05
Seychelles	51,899	172	119,770	43.32

combat misinformation (Musango et al., 2021; Ramphul, 2022). Strong governance, adherence to public measures, and open communication were key in combating the pandemic (Musango et al., 2021). Mauritius employed further outbreak control measures including quarantine, contact tracing, isolation, and mass testing (Musango et al., 2021). Vaccinations were implemented in January 2021, with the elderly first followed by the general public (Ramphul, 2022).

Lessons Learned

Mauritius demonstrated strong governance through multisectoral collaboration between various sectors both government and private sector which allowed for informed decision making and continuity. Guidelines and standard operating procedures were elaborated, and daily activities and operational plans were monitored through the Ministry of Health and Wellness. WHO protocols were used including some that were adapted to the local setting and capacities in the country incorporating changes in resource, lessons learned, and epidemiological context (Musango et al., 2021).

Clear and consistent communication was another attribute that allowed for success in combating COVID-19 in Mauritius. Creation of a National Communications Committee, a central communication mechanism responsible for relaying decisions from a high-level COVID-19 committee to the general public assisted in relaying accurate information during daily briefings and fighting miscommunication (Musango et al., 2021). Feedback from the population was essential in understanding the status of the population during the pandemic.

7.3.2.2 Sri Lanka and COVID-19

With a population of 21,919,000 in 2020, Sri Lanka had survived natural disasters and unrest and was now faced with the emerging COVID-19 pandemic. Collaboration between government and private sectors was crucial in the success in combating the pandemic (Wickramasinghe & Fernando, 2022).

Counter Measures

Local preparedness was initiated using a three-tier approach. The first was to declare facilities for COVID-19 treatment, secondly was declaration of isolation hospitals followed by identification of ICU and High dependency units (HDU) in the country. Hospital-based surveillance as well as existing respiratory disease surveillance systems were also used for COVID-19 surveillance. The Ministry of Health published guidelines for clinical management of COVID-19 and quarantine was implemented. Immunizations and field clinics for pregnant women were halted during the first wave of the pandemic (Wickramasinghe & Fernando, 2022).

Curfews and subsequent lockdown were initiated and travel restrictions from outside the country were gradually introduced. Disease detection, isolation, and mobility controls were put in place. Information was disseminated to the public through TV, radio, including websites, social media to reach the masses.

Lesson Learned

Weakened social adhesion, as well as mental health issues associated with quarantine and isolation due to COVID-19 affected the population. The three-tier approach assisted in the management of COVID-19 in the country (Wickramasinghe & Fernando, 2022).

7.3.3 COVID-19 and Pacific Island Countries and Territories

Apart from differences in population, culture, and geographical location, pacific island countries and territories (PICT) share some common characteristics. Geographically isolated, logistical challenges are a common feature among island nations. A huge burden of infectious diseases and NCDs is one feature of the PICT populations. These comorbidities are a risk factor to COVID-19 as well as other infectious diseases. Another shared characteristic is access to health services as well as financial constraints which affect healthcare services. The impact of climate change and natural disasters is an existing threat for these nations. Rapid border closures and restricting movement with the countries were some of the first countermeasures in response to the pandemic. As the pandemic progressed, health systems were challenged as the number of cases increased especially during the Delta wave. French Polynesia, Palau, and New Caledonia reported the highest number of cases with community transmission reported in Commonwealth of Northern Marianas, Fiji, Guam, Papua New Guinea (PNG), and Wallis and Futuna (Bell et al., 2022).

According to the Secretariat of the Pacific Community Public Health Division (SPC Public Health division https://php.spc.int/covid-19#pc-update), COVID-19 cases have plateaued in 2024 (Table 7.4). New Caledonia, Fiji, French Polynesia and Guam reported a substantially high number of cases. The quick response of PICT averted increase in COVID-19 cases and possibility of mortalities.

7.3.3.1 Fiji and COVID-19

According to latest WHO data on COVID-19 for Fiji (2023 report), from an estimated total population of 924, 145, the number of reported COVID-19 cases was 69,047 (7.47%) with 885 confirmed deaths (Sharma et al., 2022). Fiji reported its first case of COVID-19 in March 2020 but the 2021-Delta wave of COVID-19 resulted in a major outbreak with lasting impact on Fiji and its population (Sharma et al., 2022). The

Table 7.4 Cumulative COVID-19 cases in selected PICT as of 2023

Pacific Island Countries and territories	Cumulative COVID-19 Cases	Cumulative deaths	Population	Percent Cumulative cases/total population
American Samoa	8,431	34	47,521	17.74
Cook Islands	7,326	2	14,987	48.88
Fiji	69,117	885	948,300	7.29
Micronesia (Federated States of)	31,764	62	112,630	28.20
Guam	64,253	419	168,801	38.06
Kiribati	5,085	24	132,530	3.84
Marshall Islands	16,247	17	38,827	41.84
Northern Mariana Islands	14,594	48	45,143	32.33
New Caledonia	80,421	314	289,870	27.74
Nauru	5,485	1	11,875	46.19
Niue	1,074	0	11,857	9.06
French Polynesia	79,630	652	281,118	28.33
Papua New Guinea	46,842	670	10,826,800	0.43
Pitcairn	4	0	35	11.43
Palau	6,372	10	17,727	35.95
Solomon Islands	25,945	199	800,005	3.24
Tokelau	242	0	2,608	9.28
Tonga	16,966	12	106,107	15.99
Tuvalu	3,234	0	11,204	28.86
Vanuatu	12,029	14	319,137	3.77
Wallis and Futuna	3,831	10	11,194	34.22
Samoa	17,006	31	216,663	7.85

health system was overwhelmed by the number of cases with daily cases peaking at 1200. Unvaccinated individuals were the most affected comprising 80% of the reported deaths (Reading & Strugnell, 2021). Age, ethnicity, and treatment-seeking behaviour were reported as contributing factors to COVID-19 deaths in the population (Sharma et al., 2022).

Counter Measures

The swift response from Fiji was key in management of COVID-19 and stabilizing the country. Various countermeasures were employed, including reduction of population movement, and vaccination campaigns (Reading & Strugnell, 2021). Border closures and quarantine helped keep the pandemic at bay. People entering Fiji were subjected to a 14-day hotel quarantine, thereby limiting contact between new arrivals and the local population.

Spreading through the peri-urban areas of Suva and Viti Levu, vaccination as well as systematic mitigation through the Ministry of Health and other government agencies helped bring down the case numbers. A two-dose vaccination coverage estimated at over 70% of the population was commendable with donations from countries including Australia, New Zealand, Japan, and the United States (Reading & Strugnell, 2021).

Lessons Learned

The pandemic led to new developments in management of emerging infectious diseases and outbreak response. Molecular diagnostics technologies are now widely applied in the country, a key preparedness strategy for future outbreaks of similar magnitude. These new capabilities could strengthen diagnostics for other infectious diseases both emerging and endemic to the country. Strict adherence to WHO guidelines, open, transparent, and sustained communication as well as strong partnerships and engagement between various stakeholders allowed for success in managing the pandemic (Madewell et al., 2021).

The pandemic also revealed technological gaps, including data as well as access to internet which affected some of the response strategies such as contact tracing using downloadable apps such as CareFiji (Chand et al., 2021).

7.3.3.2 New Caledonia and COVID-19

The impact of COVID-19 on New Caledonia, a country with an estimated population of 295,333 was substantial. The territory recorded the highest number of cases among PICT. Apart from COVID-19, New Caledonia carries a huge burden of end stage kidney disease (ESKD), with the highest prevalence in the world, 3000 cases per million population inhabitants (Baroux et al., 2024). One of the impacts of COVID-19 for New Caledonia was the disruption of the transplant program for ESKD patients affecting travel of both individuals who needed surgery but also the expert surgeons (Haidar et al., 2022).

Counter Measures

Several countermeasures were applied in New Caledonia including screening people entering the country. Fourteen day quarantine was mandatory for people travellers entering the country (Kerbaj et al., 2020). Later, a safe travel zone was later declared allowing people to freely travel between New Caledonia and Wallis and Futuna, both French territories (Moury et al., 2021). Lockdowns were used to control community spread of COVID-19 within the territory.

Lessons Learned

Despite the success in managing the alpha variant of COVID-19, the Delta- variant on the contrary resulted in a major outbreak. Vaccination campaigns successfully reduced the number of cases (Ochida et al., 2023). Timely lockdown also played a crucial role in reducing the number of COVID-19 cases. The movement between territories and their metropolitan powers had an effect in introducing COVID-19 cases between the territories and their associated countries (Mcclure, 2021).

7.4 Challenges

For territories, movement between metropolitan countries and their island territories was a challenge in keeping COVID-19 out of the island territories as the metropolitan countries were inundated with COVID-19 cases. While logistics remained a challenge in getting resources in the archipelagos due to travel restrictions imposed in various countries globally.

Existing social structures presented a challenge to adherence to some of the control measures. Depending on the socioeconomic structures of families, some individuals still needed to go out to work. Low-income households were greatly affected by lockdowns and many had to choose between keeping the public health measures and going out to fend for their families (Alicea-Planas et al., 2021).

Inequitable distribution of vaccines experienced in other parts of the world was also experienced in the Caribbean as well as other island countries and territories in the pacific and Indian Ocean which depended on donations for COVID-19 doses (Umakanthan et al., 2022). COVID-19 fatigue led to cautious opening of businesses and gatherings were allowed with precautions but carried the risk of spreading COVID-19 (Umakanthan et al., 2022). Investment in the healthcare system made a difference in the response capabilities of countries to COVID-19 (Kousi et al., 2022). According to OECD reports, COVID-19 brought financial strains that affected livelihoods in small island developing states (SIDS) (OECD, 2021). Strain on health systems due to the surge of cases, including need for ICU beds and trained healthcare personnel was a reality for most island states and territories (Maharaj et al., 2021). Severe healthcare shortages were a major challenge in LMIC globally including

SIDS. Despite these challenges, island states and territories accomplished significant milestones in management of COVID-19 with lessons for many countries. The role of non-communicable diseases on the impact on COVID-19 healthcare outcomes in island nations and territories should not be underestimated. One of the risk factors for COVID-19 infections was comorbidities including diabetes, hypertension, and obesity, most of which are prevalent in most of the small island nations.

7.5 Accomplishments and Way Forward

Trustworthy and open communication was essential in building community trust as well as ensuring accurate information flow between decision makers and the general public.

Island nations just like the rest of the world struggled to adjust to the impact of COVID-19. With limited human resources and infrastructure, COVID-19 brought people from all walks of lives, economies, and businesses to a standstill. The healthcare systems were overwhelmed and had to adjust to manage the increased number of cases and demands for ICU bed space and equipment to support critically ill patients. While some countries had free healthcare, others used both public and private health facilities to manage the pandemic.

Outbreaks from emerging infectious diseases have been on the rise in the past decades and the COVID-19 pandemic revealed a lot of gaps in the healthcare system including limited data. Limited surveillance as well as diagnostic infrastructure contributed to the lack of data on COVID-19 in some countries. In the Caribbean, genomic surveillance was strengthened during the pandemic by the implementation of the COVID-19: Infectious disease Molecular epidemiology for Pathogen Control & Tracking (COVID-19 IMPACT) project. The IMPACT project established rapid SARS-CoV2 whole genome sequencing at the University of West Indies in Trinidad and Tobago. This allowed sequencing and rapid identification of strains from the Caribbean countries (Sahadeo et al., 2023). From 17 Caribbean member states (CMS), over 80% of the samples were sequenced with 91 lineages identified. The identified variants included variants of concern (VOC), Alpha, Beta, Gamma, Delta, and Omicron; variants of interest (VOI) Epsilon, Iota, Lambda, and Mu; and others (Resiere et al., 2021).

According to the World Bank, in the Latin America and Caribbean countries adherence to wide-scale public health measures played a role in reducing the loss of lives in the region (https://doi.org/https://doi.org/10.1787/532b0e2d-en).

7.6 Conclusion

While all island nations faced common constraints, geographic isolation, dependence on tourism, and limited healthcare systems, their responses were shaped by regional partnerships, governance styles, and vaccine accessibility. Pacific nations emphasized prevention through isolation, Caribbean states balanced health and economic needs, while Indian Ocean nations pursued rapid reopening backed by vaccination campaigns. These differences offer critical lessons in balancing public health, economic recovery, and regional solidarity.

References

Aboobakur, M., Latheef, A., Mohamed, A. J., Moosa, S., Pandey, R. M., Krishnan, A., & Prabhakaran, D. (2010). Surveillance for non-communicable disease risk factors in Maldives: Results from the first STEPS survey in Male. *International Journal of Public Health, 55*(5), 489–496. https://doi.org/10.1007/s00038-009-0114-y

Alicea-Planas, J., Trudeau, J. M., & Vásquez Mazariegos, W. F. (2021). COVID-19 risk perceptions and social distancing practice in Latin America. *Hispanic Health Care International, 19*(4), 254–259. https://doi.org/10.1177/1540415320985141

Bardosh, K., Jean, L., Desir, L., Yoss, S., Poovey, B., Beau de Rochars, M. V., & Noland, G. S. (2023). Was lockdown worth it? community perspectives and experiences of the Covid-19 pandemic in remote southwestern Haiti. *Social Science & Medicine, 331*, Article 116076. https://doi.org/10.1016/J.SOCSCIMED.2023.116076

Baroux, N., Magnat, É., Cauchy, M., Cantin, J.-F., Cohen, R., & Domingue-Mena, P. (2024). Prévalence de la maladie rénale chronique stades 3–5 en Nouvelle-Calédonie. *Néphrologie & Thérapeutique, 20*(3), 1–9. https://doi.org/10.1684/ndt.2024.77

Bell, L., van Gemert, C., Merilles, O. E., Cash, H. L., Stoové, M., & Hellard, M. (2022). The impact of COVID-19 on public health systems in the Pacific Island Countries and Territories. *The Lancet Regional Health - Western Pacific, 25*, Article 100498. https://doi.org/10.1016/j.lanwpc.2022.100498

Blanc, J., Louis, E. F., Joseph, J., Castor, C., & Jean-Louis, G. (2020). What the world could learn from the Haitian resilience while managing COVID-19. *Psychological Trauma: Theory, Research, Practice, and Policy, 12*(6), 569–571. https://doi.org/10.1037/tra0000903

Bovet, P., Viswanathan, B., Shamlaye, C., Romain, S., & Gedeon, J. (2010). Addressing non-communicable diseases in the Seychelles: towards a comprehensive plan of action. *Global Health Promotion, 17*(2_suppl), 37–40. https://doi.org/10.1177/1757975910363930

Caribbean Public Health Agency (CARPHA). (2017). Promoting Healthy Diets, Food Security, and Sustainable Development in the Caribbean Through Joint Policy Action Caricom Technical Brief. *Report*, (High Level Meeting to Develop a Roadmap on Multi-Sectoral Action in Countries to Prevent Childhood Obesity through Improved Food and Nutrition Security Barbados, 9–10 February 2017), 1.

Chand, S. S., Chand, A. A., & Chand, K. K. (2021). The use of careFiji app for contact tracing during the COVID-19 pandemic: Digital gap and challenges faced in Fiji. *International Journal of Surgery, 92*, Article 106023. https://doi.org/10.1016/j.ijsu.2021.106023

Dookeeram, D., Hariharan, S., Hambleton, I., Ali, K., Teelucksingh, S., Ramsewak, S., Dookeeram, D., & Maharaj, S. B. (2023). Experiences with SARS-CoV-2 (Covid-19) in Trinidad and Tobago, a small island developing state: Realities and opportunities. *The Lancet Regional Health - Americas, 26*, Article 100589. https://doi.org/10.1016/j.lana.2023.100589

Foster, N., Thow, A. M., Unwin, N., Alvarado, M., & Samuels, T. A. (2018). Regulatory measures to fight obesity in Small Island Developing States of the Caribbean and Pacific, 2015 – 2017. *Revista Panamericana de Salud Pública, 42*, 1–7. https://doi.org/10.26633/RPSP.2018.191

Fujita, Y., & Sabogal, A. (2021). *Perspective of localization of aid during COVID-19 Reflecting on the tensions between the top-down and bottom-up responses to the health emergency in Haiti.* www.iss.nl/en/library

Haidar, F., Issa, N., Gourinat, A. C., Savalle, M., Elodie, C., & Wyburn, K. (2022). The "New Caledonia COVID-19 Paradox": Dramatic indirect impact of the pandemic on organ donation and transplantation in a non-prevalence country. *Néphrologie & Thérapeutique, 18*(5), 472. https://doi.org/10.1016/j.nephro.2022.07.034

Hale, T., Phillips, T., Petherick, A., Kira, B., Angrist, N., Aymar, K., & Webster, S. (2020). *Lockdown rollback checklist: Do countries meet WHO recommendations for rolling back lockdown?*

Hennis, A. J. M., Fraser, H. S., Jonnalagadda, R., Fuller, J., & Chaturvedi, N. (2004). Explanations for the high risk of diabetes-related amputation in a Caribbean population of Black African descent and potential for prevention. *Diabetes Care, 27*(11), 2636–2641. https://doi.org/10.2337/diacare.27.11.2636

Hunte, S.-A., Pierre, K., St. Rose, R., & Simeon, D. T. (2020). Health systems' resilience: COVID-19 response in Trinidad and Tobago. *The American Journal of Tropical Medicine and Hygiene, 103*(2), 590–592. https://doi.org/10.4269/ajtmh.20-0561

International Diabetes Federation (IDF). (2025). *IDF Diabetes Atlas 2025*. https://diabetesatlas.org/resources/idf-diabetes-atlas-2025/

Kerbaj, J., Cazorla, C., De Greslan, T., Serie, M., Gourinat, A.-C., & Marot, B. (2020). COVID-19: The New Caledonia experience. *Clinical Infectious Diseases, 71*(16), 2279–2281. https://doi.org/10.1093/cid/ciaa600

Kianersi, S., Jules, R., Zhang, Y., Luetke, M., & Rosenberg, M. (2021). Associations between hurricane exposure, food insecurity, and microfinance; a cross-sectional study in Haiti. *World Development, 145*, Article 105530. https://doi.org/10.1016/J.WORLDDEV.2021.105530

Kousi, T., Vivacqua, D., Dalal, J., James, A., Câmara, D. C. P., Botero Mesa, S., & Hofer, C. B. (2022). COVID-19 pandemic in Africa's island nations during the first 9 months: A descriptive study of variation in patterns of infection, severe disease, and response measures. *BMJ Global Health, 7*(3), Article e006821. https://doi.org/10.1136/bmjgh-2021-006821

Kyu, H. H., Abate, D., Abate, K. H., Abay, S. M., Abbafati, C., Abbasi, N., & Murray, C. J. L. (2018). Global, regional, and national disability-adjusted life-years (DALYs) for 359 diseases and injuries and healthy life expectancy (HALE) for 195 countries and territories, 1990–2017: A systematic analysis for the Global Burden of Disease Study 2017. *The Lancet, 392*(10159), 1859–1922. https://doi.org/10.1016/S0140-6736(18)32335-3

Madewell, Z. J., Yang, Y., Longini, I. M., Halloran, M. E., & Dean, N. E. (2021). Factors Associated With Household Transmission of SARS-CoV-2. *JAMA Network Open, 4*(8), Article e2122240. https://doi.org/10.1001/jamanetworkopen.2021.22240

Maharaj, S. B., Ramsewak, S. S., Dookeram, D., & Franco, D. (2021). Did vaccine inequity lead to the second wave of COVID-19 infections in Trinidad and Tobago? *BMJ Global Health, 6*(8), Article e007096. https://doi.org/10.1136/bmjgh-2021-007096

Mayr, V., Nußbaumer-Streit, B., & Gartlehner, G. (2020). [Quarantine Alone or in Combination with Other Public Health Measures to Control COVID-19: A Rapid Review (Review)]. *Gesundheitswesen (Bundesverband der Arzte des Offentlichen Gesundheitsdienstes (Germany)), 82*(6), 501–506. https://doi.org/10.1055/a-1164-6611

Mcclure, H. (2021). *Surviving the pandemic: COVID-19 in the Pacific and health security*. https://pacificsecurity.net/resource/development-bulletin-82/

Moury, P.-H., Gourinat, A.-C., Riou, O., Laumond, S., Dupont-Rouzeyrol, M., Cazorla, C., & Mangeas, M. (2021). Successful COVID-19 elimination after an alpha variant outbreak in a "safe travel zone." *Travel Medicine and Infectious Disease, 44*, Article 102202. https://doi.org/10.1016/j.tmaid.2021.102202

Murphy, M. M., Jeyaseelan, S. M., Howitt, C., Greaves, N., Harewood, H., Quimby, K. R., & Hambleton, I. R. (2020). COVID-19 containment in the Caribbean: The experience of small island developing states. *Research in Globalization, 2*, Article 100019. https://doi.org/10.1016/j.resglo.2020.100019

Musango, L., Veerapa-Mangroo, L., Joomaye, Z., Ghurbhurrun, A., Vythelingam, V., & Paul, E. (2021). Key success factors of Mauritius in the fight against COVID-19. *BMJ Global Health, 6*(3), Article e005372. https://doi.org/10.1136/bmjgh-2021-005372

Nair, D., Thekkur, P., Fernando, M., Kumar, A. M. V., Satyanarayana, S., Chandraratne, N., & Harries, A. D. (2023). Outcomes and challenges in noncommunicable disease care provision in health facilities supported by primary health care system strengthening project in Sri Lanka: A mixed-methods study. *Healthcare, 11*(2), 202. https://doi.org/10.3390/healthcare11020202

Ochida, N., Dupont-Rouzeyrol, M., Moury, P.-H., Demaneuf, T., Gourinat, A.-C., Mabon, S., & Mangeas, M. (2023). Evaluating the strategies to control SARS-CoV-2 Delta variant spread in New Caledonia, a zero-COVID country until September 2021. *IJID Regions, 8*, 64–70. https://doi.org/10.1016/j.ijregi.2023.06.004

OECD. (2021). *COVID-19 pandemic Towards a blue recovery in small island developing states.*

Ordunez, P., Prieto-Lara, E., Pinheiro Gawryszewski, V., Hennis, A. J. M., & Cooper, R. S. (2015). Premature mortality from cardiovascular disease in the Americas – Will the goal of a decline of "25% by 2025" be met? *PLoS ONE, 10*(10), Article e0141685. https://doi.org/10.1371/journal.pone.0141685

Ramphul, K. (2022). The fight against COVID-19 in the small island of Mauritius. *Acta Bio-Medica : Atenei Parmensis, 92*(6), e2021452. https://doi.org/10.23750/abm.v92i6.12199

Razzaghi, H., Martin, D. N., Quesnel-Crooks, S., Hong, Y., Gregg, E., Andall-Brereton, G., Gawryszweski, V., Saraiya, M. (2019). 10-year trends in noncommunicable disease mortality in the Caribbean region. *Revista Panamericana de Salud Pública*, 1–11. https://doi.org/10.26633/RPSP.2019.37

Reading, P. C., & Strugnell, R. A. (2021). COVID-19 in Fiji. *Microbiology Australia, 42*(4), 192–195. https://doi.org/10.1071/MA21053

Resiere, D., Mehdaoui, H., Dyer, H., Chabartier, C., Cabié, A., Inamo, J., & Kallel, H. (2021). Covid-19 in the Caribbean: Lessons learned from the ongoing international medical and scientific cooperation. *Globalization and Health, 17*(1), 55. https://doi.org/10.1186/s12992-021-00706-3

Rivera-Andrade, A., & Luna, M. A. (2014). Trends and heterogeneity of cardiovascular disease and risk factors across Latin American and Caribbean Countries. *Progress in Cardiovascular Diseases, 57*(3), 276–285. https://doi.org/10.1016/j.pcad.2014.09.004

Sahadeo, N. S. D., Nicholls, S., Moreira, F. R. R., O'Toole, Á., Ramkissoon, V., Whittaker, C., Hill, V., McCrone, J. T., Mohammed, N., Ramjag, A., Brown Jordan, A., & Carrington, C. V. F. (2023). Implementation of genomic surveillance of SARS-CoV-2 in the Caribbean: Lessons learned for sustainability in resource-limited settings. *PLOS Global Public Health, 3*(2), Article e0001455. https://doi.org/10.1371/journal.pgph.0001455

Schwalb, A., Armyra, E., Méndez-Aranda, M., & Ugarte-Gil, C. (2022). COVID-19 in Latin America and the Caribbean: Two years of the pandemic. *Journal of Internal Medicine, 292*(3), 409–427. https://doi.org/10.1111/joim.13499

Sharma, N., Balak, D., Prakash, S., & Maguire, J. (2022). Descriptive analysis of deaths associated with COVID-19 in Fiji, 15 April to 14 November 2021. *Western Pacific Surveillance and Response Journal, 13*(4), 64–71. https://doi.org/10.5365/wpsar.2022.13.4.964

Singh, S., & Goel, D. (n.d.). *On the countries of Indian Ocean Region.*

Taylor, R., Badcock, J., King, H., Pargeter, K., Zimmet, P., Fred, T., Lund, M., Ringrose, H., Bach, F., & Wang, R. L. (1992). Dietary intake, exercise, obesity and noncommunicable disease in rural and urban populations of three Pacific Island countries. *Journal of the American College of Nutrition, 11*(3), 283–293. https://doi.org/10.1080/07315724.1992.10718229

Umakanthan, S., Bukelo, M. M., & Gajula, S. S. (2022). The Commonwealth Caribbean COVID-19: Regions resilient pathway during pandemic. *Frontiers in Public Health, 10*. https://doi.org/10.3389/fpubh.2022.844333

Vos, T., Lim, S. S., Abbafati, C., Abbas, K. M., Abbasi, M., Abbasifard, M., Abbasi-Kangevari, M., Abbastabar, H., Abd-Allah, F., Abdelalim, A., Abdllahi, M., & Murray, C. J. L. (2020). Global burden of 369 diseases and injuries in 204 countries and territories, 1990–2019: A systematic analysis for the Global Burden of Disease Study 2019. *The Lancet, 396*(10258), 1204–1222. https://doi.org/10.1016/S0140-6736(20)30925-9

WHO- Mauritius Country Office. (2020). *Best practices and experience of Mauritius' preparedness and response to COVID-19 pandemic*. Retrieved from https://www.afro.who.int/sites/default/files/2021-01/Mauritius-Inter-Action-Review-1-COVID-19-Report.pdf

WHO. (2023). *Country Disease Outlook, Seychelles*. https://www.afro.who.int/sites/default/files/2023-08/Seychelles.pdf

Wickramasinghe, D., & Fernando, V. K. (2022). Sri Lanka's fight against COVID-19: A brief overview. In *Pandemic Risk, Response, and Resilience* (pp. 129–142). https://doi.org/10.1016/B978-0-323-99277-0.00031-0

World Health Organization. (2020). Older people, and people with pre-existing conditions (such as heart diseases, diabetes, respiratory conditions) appear to be more susceptible to becoming severely ill with the virus. Retrieved May 26, 2025, from https://www.who.int/publications-detail/clinical-management-of-severeacute- respiratory-. Acesso em: 12 Maio 2022. https://www.who.int/publications-detail/clinical-management-of-severe-acute-respiratory-

Yisahak, S. F., Beagley, J., Hambleton, I. R., & Narayan, K. M. V. (2014). Diabetes in North America and The Caribbean: An update. *Diabetes Research and Clinical Practice, 103*(2), 223–230. https://doi.org/10.1016/j.diabres.2013.11.009

World Health Organization (WHO) COVID-19 Dashboard

United Nations Development Programme (UNDP) Island Vulnerability Reports

Ministry of Health – Fiji, New Zealand, Maldives, etc.

Academic Journals on Public Health and Island Economies

https://www.worldbank.org/en/country/caribbean/brief/the-economic-impact-of-non-communicable-diseases-in-the-caribbean

https://data.worldbank.org/indicator/SP.POP.TOTL

(https://www.worldbank.org/en/region/lac/publication/noncommunicable-diseases-care-in-the-eastern-caribbean

https://caribbean.eclac.org/information-resources/website/caribbean-public-health-agency-carpha-coronavirus-disease-2019-covid

https://paho-covid19-response-who.hub.arcgis.com/

https://www.camcouncils.org/

https://doi.org/10.1787/532b0e2d-en

Chapter 8
Fungal Co-infections and COVID-19: A Global Overview of Regional Trends, Risk Factors and Response Strategies

Fingani Annie Mphande

Abstract Fungal infections are one of the important but often neglected infections in humans with distribution worldwide. Approximately 1 in 8 individuals globally are affected by fungal diseases. A global increase in fungal co-infections has been reported in several regions between 1990 and 2021. Fungal infections affect the health, livelihood and quality of life with approximately 66.7% disability adjusted life years (DALYs) with a standardized DALY of 7789.55 per 100,000 population. Apart from cutaneous infections, a more severe and often fatal form of fungal disease is invasive fungal infections (IFI). These IFIs affect various organs with the ability to spread to other parts of the body. *Aspergillus spp.*, *Mucor spp.*, *Rhizopus spp.* and *Candida spp.* were the most common species reported with increased morbidity and mortality observed in severely ill patients during the COVID-19 pandemic. Current diagnostic approaches remain a challenge especially in limited resource settings affecting accurate diagnosis and timely treatment. This chapter will focus on fungal infections reported during and after the COVID-19 pandemic in all the WHO regions. Associated underlying diseases, treatment and response will also be discussed. The chapter will also explore policies on fungal infection prevention and control and their implementation globally. Strategies including optimal diagnostic approaches, routine screening and timely initiation of antifungal therapy will be analyzed.

Keywords Fungal infections · COVID-19 · COVID-19 Associated Pulmonary Aspergillosis (CAPA) · COVID-19 Associated Mucormycosis (CAM) · COVID-19 Associated Candidiasis (CAC) · *Candida auris* · *Pneumocystis jirovecii*

List of Abbreviations

COVID-19	Corona virus disease -2019
CAPA	COVID-19 Associated Pulmonary Aspergillosis

F. A. Mphande (✉)
Faculty of Medicine, King Mongkut's Institute of Technology Ladkrabang, Bangkok, Thailand
e-mail: fingani.mp@kmitl.ac.th

F. Mphande and P. Nyasulu (eds.), *Evaluating Outbreak Potential of Infections in Tropical Climates*, https://doi.org/10.1007/978-981-95-0618-7_8

CAM	COVID-19 Associated Mucormycosis
CAC	COVID-19 Associated Candidiasis
HIV	Human immunodeficiency virus
PJP	*Pneumocystis jirovecci* Pneumonia
ICU	Intensive Care Unit

8.1 Epidemiology Invasive Fungal Infection

Fungal infections are one of the important but often neglected infections in humans with distribution worldwide. Their ability to grow and proliferate on dead material, ability to grow at different temperatures, as well as ability to survive as mould and yeast (in some species) makes fungi successful pathogens to humans, animals as well as plants.

In humans fungi successfully grow on dead skin, nails and hair resulting in what are known as cutaneous infections. While some can invade deep tissues to cause subcutaneous and systemic infections. Although human to human transmission occurs for cutaneous fungal infections, this is a rare occurrence in subcutaneous and systemic infections (Benedict & Park, 2014; Hoenigl et al., 2022; Neblett Fanfair et al., 2012).

Fungi that are responsible for cutaneous infections are known as dermatophytes. Dermatophyte infections are commonly caused by three fungal species *Epidermophyton sp.*, *Microsporum sp.* and *Trycophton sp.* While subcutaneous infections are often introduced into the body through cuts, abrasions and or puncture into the skin, systemic infections can be acquired through inhalation and the pathogen can spread to other organs resulting in serious and at times fatal infections. Various fungal species are responsible for subcutaneous and systemic fungal infections. In general, fungal diseases are difficult to manage and hard to diagnose with infections often being chronic and difficult to resolve. Increase in immune impairment due to underlying disease as well as prolonged exposure to therapies has allowed for an increase in proliferation of fungal infections with some resulting in severe and or fatal outcomes. While the HIV epidemic led to immunosuppression and increased incidence of cryptococcal meningitis in infected individuals in the twentieth century, the twenty-first century has seen further increased immunosuppression. Medical advancements such as transplants, cancer therapies, treatment of autoimmune diseases as well as invasive therapies that involve intravascular catheters and surgeries, could increase the risk of fungal infections in immunocompromised individuals; specifically due to impaired immunity rendered during such procedures (Brown et al., 2012; Casadevall et al., 2018). This chapter will focus on fungal infections reported during and after the COVID-19 pandemic in all the WHO regions as well as underlying diseases. Treatment and response. Policies on management of fungal infections globally will also be addressed.

8.1.1 Burden of Pathogenic Fungal Infections and Geographical Distribution

More than 2.5 million people die from invasive fungal infections annually (Denning, 2024). Despite these advancements, antifungal drug resistance is on the rise highlighting further concerns and the management of fungal infections. A study on the burden of fungal skin diseases in 204 countries revealed an increase in the incidence and prevalence of the disease between 1990 and 2021 (Qin et al., 2024, Wong et al., 2024). It is estimated that approximately 1 billion people are affected by cutaneous fungal infections (Bongomin et al., 2017). The impact of fungal skin disease not only affects the health of the affected individuals but also the quality of life and livelihoods. The social and economic impacts of these diseases affect the social and economic well-being of affected individuals with an approximate 66.77% disability adjusted years (DALYs) (Qin et al., 2024). The DALYs are crucial in estimating the impact of a disease on the life of affected individuals by measuring mortality and morbidity which are expressed as years of health lost. Estimates from 2021 have shown an age standardized DALY of 7789.55 per 100,000 population (95% UI: 7059.28–8583.54) and age standardized incidence of 21,668.40 per 100,000 population (Qin et al., 2024). Age standardized prevalence for fungal skin diseases were highest among children between the ages of 5 and 9 years in Ethiopia, Mali, Central African Republic and Nigeria among countries having the highest incidences of tinea capitis (Qin et al., 2024). Approximately 138 million children are affected in Africa, representing a prevalence of 23% (Bongomin et al., 2017; Urban et al., 2021a). Apart from dermatophytes such as tinea and candidiasis, invasive infections including chronic pulmonary aspergillosis (CPA), allergic bronchopulmonary aspergillosis (ABPA), histoplasmosis and cryptococcosis have been reported in populations in Sub-Saharan Africa and globally (Koffi et al., 2021). Approximately 134 million are affected by Candidiasis annually. Systemic fungal infections cumulatively affect millions of people worldwide (Bongomin et al., 2017). Mortality due to fungal infections is reported at over 1.6 million, three times more than malaria (Bongomin et al., 2017). The highest burden of fungal infection is reported on the African region, followed by South Asia, Southeast Asia, Oceania, Latin America and the Caribbean. High-income countries have the lowest DALYs (Urban et al., 2021a).

Denning reviewed publications between 2010 and 2023, reported an annual incidence of chronic pulmonary aspergillosis in approximately 1.8 million individuals with a mortality rate of 18.5% while invasive candidiasis had an annual incidence of approximately 1.5 million with 63.3% mortality (Denning, 2024).

8.1.2 Diagnostic Approaches

Invasive fungal infections are rarely communicable, with limited human to human transmission in comparison to bacterial and viral diseases. This together with the tendency to cause chronic rather than acute infections has led to reduced interest in fungal infections. Currently, there are no vaccines or immunotherapies to fungal infections although there are some vaccines in development e.g. NDV-3A for treatment of recurrent vulvovaginal candidiasis (Edwards et al., 2018). Advances in detection of fungal infections have also been reported including galactomannan and 1,3 B-D- glucan for diagnosis of invasive aspergillosis, mass spectrometry for diagnosis on invasive fungal metabolites in serum and nucleic acid detection methods for detection of fungal pathogens (Buitrago et al., 2013; Mery et al., 2016; Miceli & Maertens, 2015).

Several risk factors are reported which play a role in disease severity and outcomes. In Sub-Saharan Africa and globally, the HIV/AIDS pandemic, limited resources including limited diagnostic capacity, drug resistance and climate change are some of the contributing factors to the increase in disease burden (Bongomin et al., 2020; Chanyachailert et al., 2023; Pfavayi et al., 2021; Urban et al., 2021a).

8.1.2.1 Diagnostic Approaches and Setting

Setting is a crucial determining factor on the approaches to management of various mycoses. While guidelines are in place for the management of various fungal infections, implementation of the recommended guidelines remains a challenge especially in limited resource settings. While risk factors to mycoses may be similar in different settings, availability of evidence in the various settings including local epidemiology, and susceptibility of fungal pathogens are essential in determining management principles and protocols. Various guidelines to fungal disease management are available from the European Confederation of Medical Mycology (ECMM) in cooperation with the Mycoses Study Group Education and Research Consortium (MSGERC), as well as country-based guidelines (Cornely et al., 2019; Kung et al., 2018). In April 2025, WHO published for the first time reports on tests and treatments for fungal infections. This follows the publication of fungal priority pathogens list publishedin2022 (https://www.who.int/publications/i/item/9789240060241 Table 8.1).

Aspergillus fumigatus responsible for various forms of aspergillosis and Candida auris responsible for invasive candidiasis are among the pathogens in the critical priority groups (Table 8.1).

The publication of the priority pathogen list aims to promote research and development of fungal infections, therapeutics and diagnostics to improve disease outcomes. The reports will enhance global understanding of fungal pathogens and improve response to fungal infections and antifungal resistance. The information also provides awareness to policy makers and the public as well as information that can assist in the design and implementation of measures to combat fungal infections and antifungal resistance globally. The WHO priority list of diseases is divided into three phases, critical priority, high priority and medium priority (Table 8.1). The designation of

Table 8.1 Priority fungal pathogens and associated disease

Priority level	Pathogen	Associated disease
Critical priority group	*Cryptococcus neoformans*	Cryptococcal meningitis
	Aspergillus fumigatus	Invasive apspergillosis (AI), Allergic broncopulmonary aspergillosis (ABPA)
	Candida auris	Invasive candidiasis
	Candida albicans	Candidiasis (Oral thrush, vulvovaginal candidiasis), candidaemia (Blood stream/ systemic infections)
High priority group	*Nakaseomyces glabrata (Candida glabrata)*	Candidiasis (Oral thrush, vulvovaginal candidiasis), candidaemia (Blood stream/ systemic infections)
	Eumycetoma causative agents	Mycetoma
	Fusarium spp.	Onychomycosis, keratitis, Endophthalmitis, Systemic infections
	Candida parapsilosis	invasive candidiasis, Endocarditis, wound and tissue infection, Meningitis, associated with peritonitis and abscesses
	Histoplasma spp	Systemic infection, histoplasmosis
	Mucorales	Mucormycosis
	Candida tropicalis	Candidiasis (Oral thrush, vulvovaginal candidiasis), candidaemia (Blood stream/ systemic infections)
Medium priority group	*Scedosporium spp.*	Candidiasis (Oral thrush, vulvovaginal candidiasis), candidaemia (Blood stream/ systemic infections)
	Lomentospora prolificans	Emerging fungal pathogen that causes disseminated disease
	Coccidiodes spp.	Coccidioiodomycosis
	Pichia kudravzeveii (C. krusei)	Emerging fungal pathogen, Candidiasis including VVC
	Cryptococcus gattii	Cryptococcosis
	Talaromyces marnafeii	Penicilosis
	Pneumocystis jirovecii	Pneumocystis pneumonia
	Paracoccidiodes spp.	Paracoccidiosis

priority level was based on number of deaths, annual incidence, current global distribution, trends in the last decade, inpatient care, complications and sequelae, antifungal resistance as well as access to diagnostics (https://www.who.int/publications/i/item/9789240060241). Despite the knowledge, challenges remain in LMIC, home to over 6.6 billion which is 80% of the world population. Knowledge of fungal infections specifically invasive fungal infections remains scanty with limited knowledge including among healthcare practitioners (https://data.worldbank.org/indicator/SP.POP.TOTL?name_desc=false). The knowledge gap is a critical issue as this determines the ability to accurately identify and diagnose fungal infections. Limited access to diagnostic tools exacerbates the limited diagnosis further limiting knowledge of existing fungal pathogens and hampering surveillance efforts (Fig. 8.1). Failure in accurate diagnosis of fungal infections implies limited knowledge in circulating fungal pathogens in a particular setting, hence poor quality of surveillance data should any exist. Reporting of priority pathogens can only occur if there is ability to diagnose these pathogens. The limited data and evidence on the burden of fungal infections in LMIC affect research efforts as well as identification of priorities in these countries. As such, the global priorities may not completely align with the needs in these countries. It is therefore crucial for LMICs to boost research in fungal infections by setting priorities that could improve diagnosis and identification of fungal infections further informing surveillance. With this knowledge, appropriate guidelines in management of fungal infections could be set up tailor made for the countries individually and as a group (Chakrabarti et al., 2023).

Collaboration between stakeholders within a country as well as in neighbouring countries and or regions is essential in combating fungal infections. The interconnectedness between diagnosis, surveillance as well as knowledge of circulating fungal pathogens within the region would assist in understanding risks and inform policy

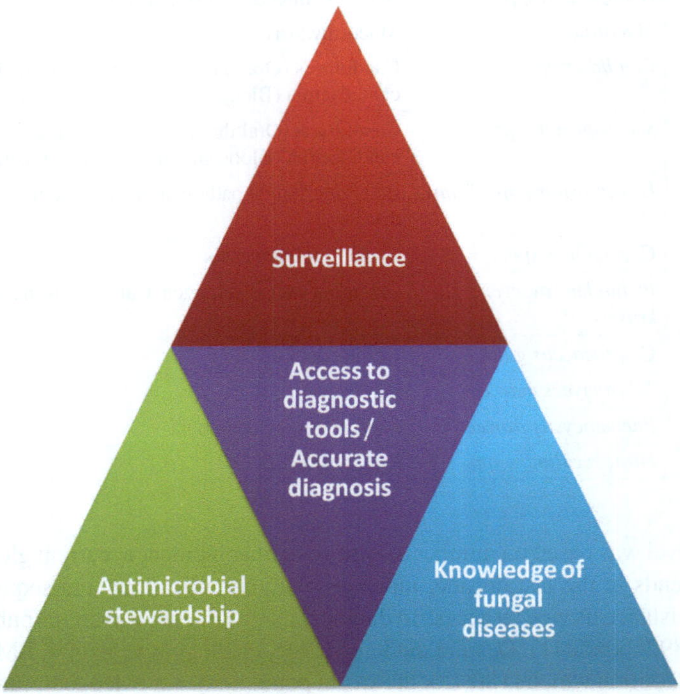

Fig. 8.1 Interconnectedness between surveillance, antimicrobial stewardship, access to diagnostic tools and knowledge of fungal diseases

for better preparedness. These include surveillance programmes, antimicrobial stewardship and access to diagnostic tools which would assist in accurate diagnosis (Fig. 8.1).

At the onset of COVID-19, complications arose in distinguishing co-infections of the viral disease with systemic fungal infections such as aspergillosis, mucormycosis and candidiasis. While guidelines were available for management of invasive fungal infections, challenges in accurate diagnosis with COVID-19 co-infections were observed (Fekkar et al., 2021). Radiological tests could not distinctively identify IFI and other supporting tests proved inaccessible specifically for LMIC (Hoenigl, 2022; Prattes et al., 2022). Lack of protective gear and limited infrastructure in LMIC meant a greater risk of nosocomial infections placing the already stretched healthcare workforce at risk of exposure.

Systemic infections including Covid Associated pulmonary Aspergillosis (CAPA), mucormycosis, candidemia, *Pneumocystis jirovecii* Pneumonia (PJP) and cryptococcosis are associated with high severity as they are common in critical cases often in ICU settings. In comparison, cutaneous infections such as oral candidiasis, dermatophytes and cutaneous mucormycosis present low to moderate severity. Systemic fungal infections involve the bloodstream and affect organs, hence are often severe and life-threatening. On the contrary, cutaneous infections affect the skin and mucuous membranes and are usually less severe (although they could result in high morbidity) but could become invasive should opportunity arise. Some examples include the progression of mucormycosis from skin cutaneous to systemic infection (Jeong et al., 2019; Prakash & Chakrabarti, 2019). Similarly, nosocomial infections with *C. auris*, that could start from the skin and may colonize the bloodstream through catheters and other invasive equipment have been reported in several countries in COVID-19 patients (Biran et al., 2023; Najeeb et al., 2022).

8.2 Fungal Infections and COVID-19 Co-infections

The COVID-19 pandemic disrupted infectious disease dynamics globally. COVID-19 infections often lead to prolonged hospital stays with increased susceptibility to secondary infections including fungal infections. Complications due to COVID-19 infections lead to immune dysregulation often attributed to corticosteroid use. These complications meant patients had to be treated in Intensive Care Units (ICU) where mechanical ventilation was often required, increasing the risk of secondary infections including fungal infections.

The prevalence of fungal infections has been a great concern since the onset of the COVID-19 pandemic with an increase in prevalence of some fungal infections in COVID-19 patients. Some of the most reported fungal infections associated with COVID-19 were CAPA with a prevalence of 5–30% reported in mechanically ventilated ICU patients and those on prolonged steroid therapy or with lung damage (Alanio et al., 2020; Dupont et al., 2021; Egger et al., 2022; Lamoth et al., 2020; Rutsaert et al., 2020; van Arkel et al., 2020). The mortality rate of CAPA was over

50% in some ICU settings, raising great concerns damage (Alanio et al., 2020; Dupont et al., 2021; Egger et al., 2022; Lamoth et al., 2020; Rutsaert et al., 2020; van Arkel et al., 2020). Another disease with high mortality if not treated early was COVID-19 Associated Mucormycosis (CAM). Widely reported in India, CAM registered a prevalence of 0.27%–0.5% in hospitalized patients with uncontrollable diabetes, corticosteroid use and use of oxygen therapy as risk factors (Chandley et al., 2022; Krishna et al., 2022; Pal et al., 2021; Pasquier, 2023). Candidemia was reported in COVID-19 patients with approximately 15% prevalence in ICU patients. *Candida albicans* and *C. auris* were the commonly reported pathogens (Chowdhary et al., 2017). Although less common, PJP was reported in immunocompromised or in individuals with severe COVID-related immunosuppression (Bhat et al., 2020; Mang et al., 2021).

During the pandemic, systemic and cutaneous fungal infections were encountered in both HICs and LICs (Tables 8.2 and 8.3). Cutaneous/mucosal fungal infections were reported to flare up in patients post-COVID-19 recovery (Table 8.2).

Table 8.2 Systemic fungal infections associated with COVID-19

Infection	Pathogen	Common regions	Prevalence	Risk factors
COVID-19 Associated Pulmonary Aspergillosis (CAPA)	*Aspergillus fumigatus*	HICs and ICU settings globally	10–30% (ICU)	Mechanical ventilation, Corticosteroids, lung damage
Mucormycosis (CAM)	*Rhizopus, Mucor spp.*	India, LMICs	0.3–0.5% in hospitalized COVID-19 patients (India)	Diabetes, steroid use, oxygen therapy
Candidemia (Invasive Candidiasis)	*Candida albicans, C. auris*	HICs and LMICs	5–15% (ICU)	Central lines, Immunosuppression
Pneumocystis jirovecii Pneumonia (PCP)	*Pneumocystis jirovecii*	Globally	Rare < 1%	Undiagnosed immunodeficiency, high steroid doses
Cryptococcosis	*Cryptococcus neoformans*	Sub-Saharan Africa, Southeast Asia	Very rare in COVID-19 patients	Profound immunosuppression, common in HIV positive patients

Table 8.3 Cutaneous fungal infections and COVID-19

Infection	Pathogen	Common regions	Risk populations	Risk factors
Cutaneous Mucormycosis	*Mucorales spp.*	India, Tropical LMICs	Rare, common in trauma or wound cases	Wound exposure, burns, poor hygiene
Candidiasis (oral, esophageal, cutaneous	*C. albicans*	Global	Common in hospitalized and ventilated patients and in COVID-19 and post-steroid patients	Immunosupression, prolonged antibiotic use
Dermatophyosis (Tinea)	*Trycophyton, Microsporum spp.*	Global	All ages, may flare post-COVID-19 infection	Poor hygiene, steroid misuse
Malassezia folliculitis	*Malassezia spp.*	Global	Young to middle-aged adult males, very rare in COVID-19	Humidity and steroid use

8.3 Transmission and Risk Factors Associated with Fungal Infections and COVID-19

Challenges in continuity of health promotion and disease prevention programmes due to the COVID-19 pandemic saw losses in progress in infectious disease prevention and control that were achieved in decades (Arisanti et al., 2024; Comella-del-Barrio et al., 2021; Facciolà et al., 2023; Mude et al., 2024). The increase in fungal infections during the pandemic was attributed to use of steroid/ corticosteroid treatment allowing opportunistic growth and spread of fungal infections (Li & Denning, 2023; Wilbourn et al., 2024). Use of mechanical devices including catheterization as well as long-term hospitalization and ICU has increased risks to fungal infections. Environmental conditions could lead to exposure to fungal spores. These include living conditions, as well as setting. Similarly, age is an important factor with children and the elderly being susceptible to certain fungal infections. Men have also been reported to be more affected with fungal infections compared to women (Qin et al., 2024; Urban et al., 2021b; Wang et al., 2025). Several risk factors have been reported in literature; these include host factors, environmental factors as well as social and economic factors (Fig. 8.2).

With COVID-19, a notable surge in mucormycosis was reported for example in India with immunosuppressive therapies as the main risk factor. Nosocomial infections of *C. auris* as well as challenges in diagnostics were reported due to overlapping symptoms between COVID-19 and respiratory fungal infections. The enormity of the COVID-19 pandemic resulted in limited diagnostic tools especially in overwhelmed healthcare systems and limited resource settings. Lack of diagnostic tools and therapies is an existing challenge in LMICs (Hoenigl et al., 2021).

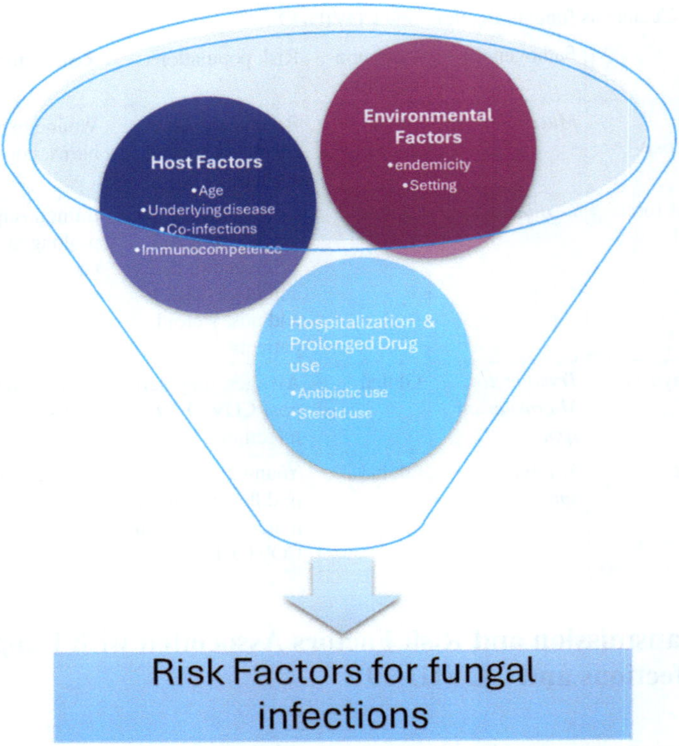

Fig. 8.2 An interplay of host, environmental as well as clinical factors plays a role in the risk to fungal infections in COVID-19 patients

8.3.1 Host Factors

Host factors play an important role in disease outcomes. In fungal infections, immune status, use of broad-spectrum antibiotics and steroids have been reported to influence fungal infections and outcomes (Arastehfar et al., 2020). Tolle et al., reported immune suppression, socio-economic status and living conditions as well as prolonged broad-spectrum antibiotic use has also been linked to increase in fungal infections Fungal immunology and pathogenesis in COVID-19 patients (Tolle & Standiford, 2013).

In populations with predisposing factors such as HIV, Diabetes and other underlying diseases, immunosuppression is a major challenge. Immunosuppression due to other infections and underlying diseases as well as medical conditions such as, tissue transplant, burns, prolonged treatment with antibiotics and or steroid treatment tend to exacerbate the risk to fungal infections (Dudoignon et al., 2024). Due to the chronic nature and slow development of fungal infections, misdiagnosis and lack of timely diagnosis especially in low resource settings has resulted in uncontrolled proliferation of disease resulting in further spread and complications. This was evident during the COVID-19 pandemic where complications from existing fungal infections increased the severity of COVID-19. During the pandemic, infections such as CAM, CAPA and COVID-19 associated candidiasis (CAC) were recognized (Kundu & Singla, 2022). Chavda et al., addressed some of the complications in COVID-19 patients with fungal co-infections (Chavda et al., 2023). The authors proposed a pathogenesis mechanism which involves immunocompromised states due to COVID-19 treatment which allows proliferation and growth of fungal pathogens within the host and exacerbates lung infections such as pneumonia. Intubation due to COVID-19 respiratory complications also provides opportunity for spread of systemic candidiasis. Thus, in trying to treat one disease, another pathogen takes opportunity and cause further poor outcomes in the host. Underlying infections can result in immune responses in the host which provide a favourable environment for growth of fungal pathogens. In Diabetic patients, increased glucose levels (hyperglycaemia) were related to COVID-19 complications. A systematic review conducted in India revealed that 80% of the patients with Mucormycosis and COVID-19 co-infections had diabetes mellitus (Singh et al., 2021). Hyperglycaemia provides opportunity for growth of filamentous fungi, including mucormycosis hence opportunities to invade cells, and play a role in ischemic necrosis in cases blockage of blood vessels occurs due to fungal filaments (Hernández & Buckley, 2025).

In the case of Candida infections, endogenous infections could pose a risk in immunocompromised individuals. Thus, individuals can easily be infected by existing yeast pathogens within the individual. This could possibly allow for systemic infections from superficial yeast infections and or equipment such as ventilators in patients in intensive care units (Arastehfar et al., 2020; Gangneux et al., 2022). As such, skin infections, open wounds and invasive therapies are risk factors for fungal co-infections.

Age is an important factor in disease outcomes and has been associated with severity of disease (Sanyaolu et al., 2020). During COVID-19 pandemic, six million fatalities were reported (Shishido et al., 2022). Similarities in presentation between COVID-19 and fungal respiratory co-infections were reported. Both diseases affect lungs; these include aspergillosis, pneumonia associated cryptococcus and pulmonary mucormycosis (Chavda et al., 2023). Hypersensitivity including stimulation of blood serum and allergic reactions affects disease outcomes (Chavda et al., 2023).

8.3.2 Environmental Factors and Underlying Social Determinants of Health

Settings play a critical role in exposure to fungal spores, especially endemic species. In areas where pathogenic fungal species are endemic, there is a higher likelihood of exposure to the population than those living in non-endemic areas (Shishido et al., 2022). For example, presence of *Coccidioides* in South Western United States, parts of Mexico and Central America; Aspergillus species worldwide, *fusarium spp.* and *mucorycosis*, as well as endemic mycoses such as penicilosis, histoplasmosis, coccidioidomycosis in certain localities are a risk to the population (Seagle et al., 2022). Living conditions could also contribute to exposure to fungal spores which could cause infections in susceptible individuals upon exposure. Rural communities often live in houses with dirt floors. This exposes these populations to fungal spores in the soil. Similarly, farmers are at high risk of exposure to fungal spores as they work in their farms. With climate change and search for fertile soils and farmlands, populations have encroached in areas which were inhabitable before exposing them to possible new fungal species in that novel environment.

8.3.3 Socioeconomic Factors

8.3.3.1 Management of COVID-19 and Fungal Infections, a Comparison Between HIC and LMIC

Social and economic factors play a major role in health outcomes. Economic disparities between HIC and LMIC determine not only access but also quality of healthcare. Socioeconomic factors played a great role in disparities in the COVID-19 response as well as management of fungal co-infections in the different settings.

Fungal infections in COVID-19 patients varied significantly between HIC and LMIC. While systemic infections such as aspergillosis and candidemia were prevalent in both settings, mucormycosis was highly detected in India. High-income countries with advanced healthcare systems had access to diagnostics and therapies which were barely accessible in differences in LMIC. Quality of patient care varied between HIC and MIC with patients in HIC having access to better ICU care, as well as access to vaccines, ventilators and immunosuppressants. Due to availability of diagnostic tools, HIC were able to detect, identify and report circulating COVID-19 strains faster giving them the opportunity to make informed decisions in management of the infection. On the contrary, LMIC struggled with detection and timely identification of circulating strains due to limited resources and diagnostic tools. Management of infections on the backdrop of comorbidities (Diabetes, hypertension and other chronic illnesses), malaria and HIV epidemic played a huge role on disease outcomes. Lack of diagnostic tools, personnel affected the ability to identify co-infections and allowed for poor infection prevention and control leading to nosocomial outbreaks (Cobb et al., 2021; Ngandu et al., 2022; Rosenthal et al., 2022).

Underreporting was a risk factor in LMIC due to limited diagnosis and infrastructure. The prevalence patterns for CAPA were estimated at 10–30%, while *C. auris* was estimated at 5–15% in ICU patients in HIC. On the contrary, it was difficult to estimate similar cases in LMIC leading to underestimation of the actual disease burden of fungal infections as well as estimate the morbidity and mortality due to COVID-19 and fungal co-infections (Table 8.4).

Table 8.4 Respiratory fungal infection and COVID-19, HIC vs LMIC

Factor	HIC	LMIC
Access to healthcare	Advanced healthcare system with ready access to diagnostic tools, vaccines and antifungal therapies	Limited access to healthcare infrastructure, diagnostic tools, vaccines and antifungal therapies
Prevalence	Higher detection rates due to availability of tools for identification, surveillance and record keeping which are essential for accurate estimation of prevalence	Poor detection and identification rates due to limited tools for identification, surveillance and poor record keeping which affect accurate estimation of prevalence
Diagnosis	Advanced diagnostic tools (PCR, bronchoscopy, galactomannan assays, advanced imaging tools)	Limited diagnostic tools and capacity due to resource constraints
Detection of CAPA	Higher detection due to availability of advanced diagnostic tools (10–30% detection in ICU patients with COVID-19) Prattes et al. (2022), Baddley (2011)	Underreported
Detection of candidiasis	5–15% detection of *C. auris* in ICU patients with severe COVID-19 as well as detection of hospital outbreaks Baddley (2011)	Underreported
Detection of mucormycosis	Rare (sporadic cases)	Underreported (0.3–0.5% reported in COVID-19 hospitalized patients in India) Rudramurthy et al. (2021)
Detection of PJP	Rare but potentially underdiagnosed in COVID-19 patients Baddley (2011)	Underreported

Rayens et al., elucidate that in the United States, evaluation of the risk of fungal infections requires increased evaluation by medical personnel and that this is associated demographic and socioeconomic factors (Rayens et al., 2022). Similarly, this applies to LMIC and highlights the need for trained health personnel and availability of tools to aptly detect and identify fungal infections. Limitations in diagnostic tools, underreporting, and underdiagnosis could be directly linked to overwhelmed healthcare systems with limited human and financial resources as well as infrastructure in place to manage the disease burden. There is need for specialized testing, availability and use of tools beyond light microscopy. Use of molecular, biochemical and proteomic techniques, such as PCR, sequencing as well as MALDI-TOF mass spectrometry, could assist in further identification as well as management of existing and emerging fungal infections.

8.3.4 Racial and Ethnic Identities and Risk for Fungal Infections

In some fungal infections, differences in susceptibility were reported in certain racial groups. Disparities in immunogenetic factors have been reported to exist between the Hmong and European population which contributes to their susceptibility to blastomycosis (Merkhofer et al., 2019). These observations are indicative of the possible role of immunogenetic factors in susceptibility to fungal infections. Similarly, inequities in distribution of fungal infections across races have been observed (Jenks et al., 2023).

The differences are often associated with various social factors, including setting, living environments, access to healthcare, occupation and age. Variations in the burden of comorbidities such as diabetes and hypertension have been reported among people of African and Hispanic descent in the United States (Cho et al., 2013). Overcrowding & Poor Housing among low resource populations is a challenge in urban settings. These include slum dwellers and homeless populations who often live in poorly ventilated quarters often overcrowded with minimal hygiene, often with dusty floors and damp walls increasing exposure to environmental fungi (e.g. *Aspergillus spp*). The health status of such populations also increases the risk of susceptibility specifically in immunocompromised individuals. Similarly, crowding posed high risk to exposure and acquisition to COVID-19 hence overlapping risks with respiratory fungal infections in these marginalized communities.

8.3.5 Rural Communities and Fungal Infections

Both rural and urban populations are also at risk of exposure to fungal infections due to underlying occupations. Farm workers are at risk of exposure from soil and animals. Similarly, construction workers are at risk of exposure to fungal spores in urban areas. Often ethnic minorities or undocumented immigrants, these workers could have limited access to healthcare. Underdiagnosis and misdiagnosis are a challenge in both rural and urban marginalized populations especially in LMIC where health insurance may not exist for many limiting these populations access to healthcare. Urban and rural settings pose varying threats in exposure to fungal infections (Table 8.5). While exposure to soil remains a common factor between both populations, rural farmers are at a greater risk of exposure due to frequent exposure to fungal spores. Similarly, construction workers in both settings face similar risks (Garber, 2001; Maertens et al., 2001; Sipsas & Kontoyiannis, 2008).

Table 8.5 Risk factors to fungal infections in Rural and Urban populations

Factor	Rural communities	Urban communities
Environmental exposure	High (soil, farming, construction)	Medium (mould in old/damp buildings), construction workers
Healthcare access	Limited access to health services (fewer clinics, longer distances)	Better access to health services, better access to financial resources and health insurance
Immunocompromised populations	Aging population often with (unattended/ undiagnosed) comorbidities	Populations living with (diagnosed/ undiagnosed/ misdiagnosed) comorbidities
Health literacy	Generally lower	Variable—higher in affluent areas, lower in underserved neighbourhoods

8.3.6 *Knowledge Levels and Health Seeking Behaviour for Fungal Infections*

During the COVID-19 pandemic, distrust for health systems grew in most populations leading to unfavourable public health outcomes (Gillibrand et al., 2024; Wong et al., 2024). The scare from the pandemic led to changes in health-seeking behaviour, with many afraid to seek treatment in the fear of contracting COVID-19 from the hospitals (Lopes et al., 2022). With fungal infections, delay in seeking treatment could result in poor prognosis for both cutaneous and systemic infections. While self-treatment with over the counter medication is likely to contribute to antimicrobial resistance (Choudhary et al., 2024). Use of traditional medicine for fungal infections has been reported with varying outcomes. These traditional remedies, however could be a window into future antimicrobial candidates although further research is essential (Aschale et al., 2021). Despite the availability of such remedies, information regarding fungal infections, risk factors and severity is limited among populations both in urban and rural settings as well as among health practitioners (Diongue et al., 2023; Oladele et al., 2020). This knowledge gap creates a greater risk of misdiagnosis among health personnel as well as risk of late diagnosis and health-seeking in populations. Lower literacy among populations and stigma that follows specifically cutaneous and or mucosal fungal infections has allowed for proliferation of infection as well as challenges in treatment and prognosis of disease outcomes. As such, there is a need for community awareness and public health campaigns on fungal infections in both urban and rural populations in LMICs and globally to ensure better management of these diseases (Chakrabarti et al., 2023; Loyse et al., 2019).

8.3.7 *Case Studies*

8.3.7.1 COVID-19 and Fungal Co-infections

Co-infections between COVID-19 and fungal infections specifically respiratory fungal infections were reported. COVID-19 associated Aspergillosis, CAC and CAM were reported in various countries around the world (Feys et al., 2021). In the Americas, CAPA was reported in the United States and Mexico, China, Pakistan and Iran for Asia, and in Europe, Austria, Belgium, France, Germany, Hungary, Greece, Italy, Spain, Netherlands, Switzerland and the UK reported incidence of CAPA (Feys et al., 2021). Among the factors reported, significant factors associated with CAPA were older age (Gangneux et al., 2022; Prattes et al., 2022; Z. Wang et al., 2025).

Various risk factors for co-infections were reported. These included host factors such as the severity of disease, as well as comorbidities and host immunity. Severely ill patients with comorbidities on admission were as a risk factor (Prattes et al., 2022). Similarly, solid organ transplant and malignancy were reported as a risk factor elsewhere (Gradoni et al., 2017; Muhammad Iqbal et al., 2012; Permpalung et al., 2023; White et al., 2019). Pulmonary and liver disease were another set of risk factors reported in patients with co-infections (Muhammad Iqbal et al., 2012; Permpalung et al., 2023; H. Wang et al., 2024). Prolonged use of corticosteroids including Tocilizumab was reported (Ergun et al., 2017; Fekkar et al., 2021; Gangneux et al., 2022; Permpalung et al., 2023; White et al., 2019). Negative pressure in ICU rooms was associated with proliferation of *Aspergillus fumigatus* (Ichai et al., 2020). COVID-19 associated aspergillosis was associated with increased mortality in affected patients (Prattes et al., 2022). Timely diagnosis could greatly impact disease outcomes, and it was reported as a risk factor, as failure to do so affected disease outcomes. The second wave of COVID-19 saw an increase in cases of mucormycosis, a life-threatening fungal infection globally. The development of the co-infections differed with CAPA reported to develop within the first month of infection (day 1–28) while CAM was observed from 10 to 15 days post diagnosis of COVID-19 (Huang et al., 2023). Timely diagnosis was essential for better patient outcomes for both co-infections. Risk factors for COVID-19 associated mucormycosis (CAM) included comorbidities such as diabetes and prolonged use of corticosteroids. Increased cases of invasive pulmonary aspergillosis in patients with severe COVID-19 with prevalence of CAPA estimated from less than 5% to greater than 30%. A multi-disciplinary approach was suggested for diagnosis and management of IPA and in patients with COVID-19. A study by Gangneux et al., showed that length of duration of mechanical ventilation was associated with proven/probable CAPA in ICU patients (Gangneux et al., 2022).

8.3.7.2 Mucormycosis and COVID-19

Mucormycosis (MM), also known as black fungus, is a lethal opportunistic disease with a yearly incidence of 1.7 cases per one million population. Mucormycetes are a group of mould, commonly found in the environment. The group consists of several species but of importance are the *Rhizopus* and *Mucor* species responsible for a serious and highly fatal infection known as mucormycosis (Richardson, 2009). Mucormycosis can be contracted through inhalation of spores (rhinocerebral and blood infections), introduction of spores through trauma and or breaks in the skin (cutaneous infections) and through ingestion of contaminated foods and products (Gastrointestinal mucormycosis) resulting in systemic infections that can spread to various organs in the body.

Five types of mucormycosis are reported globally. These include Rhinocerebral (sinus and brain) mucormycosis, Pulmonary (lung) mucormycosis, Cutaneous (skin) mucormycosis, Gastrointestinal mucormycosis, and disseminated mucormycosis. Each of these types presents differently often with specific indicative symptoms https://www.who.int/india/home/emergencies/coronavirus-disease-(covid-19)/mucormycosis#:~:text=The%20incidence%20rate%20of%20mucormycosis,to%201.7%20per%20million%20population). Rhinocerebral mucormycosis affects the sinuses and the brain, while pulmonary mucormycosis affects the lungs. Disseminated mucormycosis on the contrary can spread to various organs (Table 8.6).

8.3.7.3 Risk Factors of Mucormycosis

Risk factors for mucormycosis include uncontrolled diabetes, immunosuppression, stem cell and or organ transplant, hematologic malignancies and prolonged use of corticosteroids (Rammaert et al., 2012). Morbidity and mortality have been reported for mucormycosis with high costs of treatment as well as loss of lives (Kontoyiannis et al., 2014; Rammaert et al., 2012; Skiada et al., 2011). Several challenges have been reported in investigation of mucormycosis. Most cases of mucormycosis present with unique and often complicated histories making it difficult to pinpoint the source of mucormycosis in the healthcare and or within the environment. Though molecular methods exist, most are inaccessible in limited resource settings where diagnosis of the disease is often difficult. Diagnosis is also a challenge due to limited laboratory capacity and infrastructure for fungal species determination and research (Hartnett et al., 2019). During the COVID-19 pandemic, co-infections between COVID-19 and Mucormycosis were reported. A study by Arjmand et al., reported 58.1% COVID-19 associated with mucormycosis (CAM) in Iran. The study reported an increase in mucormycosis cases during the pandemic compared to pre-pandemic and with each successive wave of COVID-19. Risk factors identified in this study were diabetes mellitus, corticosteroid use and COVID-19 (Arjmand et al., 2022).

Estimating the global prevalence of mucormycosis remains a challenge due to limited data in most countries, despite this, mucormycosis has been reported in Africa

Table 8.6 Types of mucormycosis and their main features

Type of Mucormycosis	Site of infection	Symptoms/Presentation
Rhinocerebral mucormycosis	Sinuses, brain	Swelling on one side of the face
		Headache
		Nasal or sinus congestion
		Black lesions on nasal bridge or upper inside of mouth that quickly become more severe
		Fever
		Lethargy, seizures, slurred speech, partial paralysis
Cutaneous mucormycosis	Skin	Skin lesions,
		The infected area may turn black
		Pain
		Excessive redness or swelling around a wound
Pulmonary mucormycosis	Lungs	Fever
		Cough
		Chest pain
		Shortness of breath
		Hemoptysis
Gastrointestinal mucormycosis	GI tract	Abdominal pain
		Nausea and vomiting
		Gastrointestinal bleeding
Disseminated mucormycosis	Different organs/parts of the body	Usually occurs in immunocompromised individuals, or individuals with other underlying diseases as such it is not easy to pinpoint specific symptoms

(Cameroon, Kenya, Nigeria, Algeria and Malawi), Asia (Thailand, Pakistan, Philippines, Korea, Japan, India, Uzbekistan and Kazakhstan) Americas (Brazil, Chile, Colombia, United States, Canada, Dominican Republic, Mexico and Argentina), Australia as well as in the Eastern mediterranean (Qatar and Jordan) (Prakash & Chakrabarti, 2019). Incidences have been reported through the years in some countries with India reporting approximately 24% of invasive mycoses in the ICU patients being attributed to mucormycosis (Prakash & Chakrabarti, 2021). A notable increase in mucormycosis cases was observed in India during the COVID-19 pandemic (Prakash & Chakrabarti, 2021).

On the African continent, underreporting remains a major obstacle in estimating the burden of fungal infections including invasive fungal infections such as mucormycosis (Kalua et al., 2018; Osaigbovo et al., 2023). Studies report diabetes mellitus,

COVID-19, malignancies and neutropenia as risk factors for mucormycosis in African countries reporting the disease (Osaigbovo et al., 2023). Laboratory capacity remains a challenge and over 70% of the diagnosis was through histopathology. *Rhizopus oryzae/arrhizus* is the common species identified accounting for 71.1% of the cases (Osaigbovo et al., 2023). Despite limited access to therapeutic intervention, antifungal therapy was reported in 81.9% of the cases on the African continent with surgical intervention conducted on 59.8% of the cases. A survival rate of over 50% was also reported (Osaigbovo et al., 2023). Over 80% of the cases reported on the African continent are from North Africa, 15.4% in Southern Africa, 1.7% for East Africa, similarly 1.7% for West Africa and 0.2% for Central Africa (Osaigbovo et al., 2023). These estimates should be taken with consideration of considerable underreporting, underdiagnosis with limited capacity on knowledge of mucormycosis and its presentation in this setting.

Increased prevalence of mucormycosis during the pandemic could be due to interlinked risk factors such as diabetes mellitus, corticosteroid therapy and COVID-19. Increases in mucormycosis cases were reported with successive COVID-19 waves in Iran. According to Prakash et al., the global incidence of mucormycosis varies, with estimates ranging from 0.005 to 1.7 cases per million population with studies suggesting mucormycosis is more prevalent in developing countries like India and Mexico than in developed nations (Prakash & Chakrabarti, 2019). There has been a rise in mucormycosis cases globally, particularly in Asia and Europe. Many cases of mucormycosis may remain undiagnosed due to difficulties in collecting samples and low sensitivity of diagnostic tests.

A high burden of mucormycosis has been reported in India. India has a significantly higher burden of mucormycosis compared to other countries. A notable increase in mucormycosis cases in India, particularly during and after the COVID-19 pandemic. Diabetes mellitus, hematological malignancies, solid organ transplant and chronic kidney disease are common reported risk factors in India. Infections due to emerging pathogens including *Rhizopus microsporus, Rhizopus homothallicus* and *Apophysomyces* variabilis are on the rise in India. Some of the reported cases in India were nosocomial in origin, with contaminated medical equipment and procedures being potential sources of infection. Despite increased awareness, mucormycosis-associated morbidity and mortality remain high in India due to late diagnosis and treatment. Since 2021, mucormycosis has been a notifiable disease in India.

Apart from India, cases of mucormycosis have been reported from other WHO regions. In Europe, a multicentre study in Spain reported 0.43 cases per million population/year. While a population-based study in France reported an increase in prevalence from 0.7 to 1.2 cases per million between 1997 and 2006. In the United States, a survey from 2006 to 2014 identified 3,374 invasive fungal infections (IFIs), with Mucorales implicated in 1.1% of these infections. Similarly, in Canada the estimated incidence of mucormycosis is around 1.2 cases per million while in Australia the incidence is estimated at around 0.6 cases per million (Prakash et al., 2019). Consideration should be taken on these estimates as the numbers are prone to change with time and improved diagnostics as well as reporting. According to WHO, despite mucormycosis being not contagious and with no person to person spread yet reported, the surge in cases is on the increase. Diabetes is a predisposing factor and with the increase in diabetes in LMIC, and existence of fungal spores in the environment, this is a cause of concern with greater chances of mucormycosis in these regions.

8.3.7.4 Diagnosis

Early detection and commencement of treatment are crucial in mucormycosis infections, and it is advisable that treatment should commence without delay. Diagnosis remains a challenge in limited resource settings with biopsy and potassium hydroxide (KOH) often used in laboratories. Imaging, including CT scan of affected areas, can be used to support diagnosis.

8.3.7.5 Treatment

Detailed guidelines for management of mucormycosis are available, even though the disease is difficult to treat and often fatal. Intravenous antifungal therapy and surgical debridement have been used often in combination. Due to the complexity of the disease presentation, a multi-disciplinary approach is required to manage the disease.

8.3.8 Aspergillosis and COVID-19

Aspergillosis is a fungal infection caused by *Aspergillus species including A. fumigatus, A. flavus, A. tereus, and A. niger, A. lentulus, A. oryzae, A. nidulans, A. versicolor* and *A. sydowii* (Morgan et al., 2005, Steinbach et al., 2004, Lionakis et al., 2005, Khan et al., 2024). These fungal species are distributed worldwide with cases reported in Asia, Europe, Africa, the Americas as well as Oceania (Table 8.7).

Table 8.7 Aspergillus species associated with CAPA in COVID-19 Patients

Pathogen	Country Reported	Reference
Aspergillus spp.	China	Zhu et al. (2019)
Aspergillus fumigatus *A. flavus*	Belgium, France, Netherlands, Germany	Koehler et al. (2022) Rutsaert et al. (2020) Alanio et al. (2020) Van Arkel et al. (2020) Agrawal and Phulware (2021) (in pregnant women)
Aspergillus spp.	France Pandemic wave	Bretagne et al. (2021)
A. tereus *A. niger*	Iran	Abolghasemi et al. (2021)

There are different types of aspergilloses each with distinctive symptoms or presentation (Table 8.8). Invasive aspergillosis is described according to several criteria, including clinical and host factors (classical symptoms and radiological findings) (Donnelly et al., 2020). The host factors include hematologic malignancies, recent history of neutropenia, hematopoietic transplant or solid organ transplant. Use of corticosteroids and immunosuppressive therapies affects the host's immune system resulting in decreased immunity and giving chance to opportunistic infections (Baddley, 2011).

Chronic pulmonary aspergillosis (CPA) presents in different forms from aspergillomas to severe and often fatal conditions including subacute pulmonary aspergilosis (SAPA) formerly chronic necrotising pulmonary aspergillosis (CNPA) (Kosmidis & Denning, 2015).

According to Denning, invasive aspergillosis has been reported in approximately 2,113,000 cases with an annual mortality of 85.2% (1,801,000) in the context of chronic obstructive pulmonary disease, intensive care, lung cancer or haematological malignancy (Denning, 2024). On the contrary the mortality due to CPA was 18.5% with 340, 00 deaths from 1,83, 272 cases (Denning et al., 2024).

Aspergillosis is not a notifiable disease as such estimating the burden of aspergillosis is challenging. While literature reviews and modelling have been used to estimate the burden in some countries including Canada and Mexico, the challenge remains in estimating the burden in LMIC (Corzo-Leon et al., 2015). Hospital records are one option in estimating the burden of disease. Hospital databases as well as surveillance could provide trends in aspergillosis and fungal infections in general. The possibility of accurate data does not only rely on the availability of the database but also the diagnostic capabilities within the countries. In resource-limited settings, estimation of disease burden is compromised due to the limited capacity in fungal

Table 8.8 Types of Aspergilloses and their symptoms

Type	Main Feature	Who it Affects	Key Symptoms
Allergic Bronchopulmonary Aspergillosis (ABPA)	Allergic reaction to spores	Asthma, Cystic Fibrosis patients	Wheezing, coughing, mucus plugs
Chronic Pulmonary Aspergillosis (CPA)	Chronic lung infection	Lung disease patients (TB, COPD)	Weight loss, cough, fatigue
Aspergilloma ("Fungus Ball")	Mass of fungus in lung cavity	Old lung cavities (TB, abscess survivors)	Coughing blood, sometimes silent
Invasive Aspergillosis	Fungus invades tissues	Severely immunocompromised patients	Fever, chest pain, breathing issues
Cutaneous Aspergillosis	Skin infection	Immunocompromised or wound patients	Skin ulcers, lesions
Sinus Aspergillosis	Sinus infection	All patients, worse in immunocompromised	Facial pain, congestion, sinusitis

diagnostics. Poor estimation of disease burden and diagnostics contributes to willingness and commitment to surveillance. Database records in the United Statesshowed an increase in Aspergillosis by 57% from the year 2000 and 2013, these trends were possible to estimate due to availability of data (Vallabhaneni et al., 2017). Hence reliable data collection and management would assist in understanding the magnitude of effects of aspergillosis not only in the United States but also globally.

Limited true epidemiological studies contribute to difficulties in estimating the burden of disease. Aspergillus fumigatus is the main pathogen implicated in CPA. It is estimated that approximately 3 million people differ from CPA with Asia carrying the most burden (Bongomin et al., 2017).

8.3.8.1 Risk Factors

Risk factors for invasive aspergillosis include, pulmonary TB, complications from bronchopulmonary aspergillosis as well as complications from sarcoidosis, with evidence reports from Ghana, India and Vietnam (Denning et al., 2017, Bongomin and Denning, 2024).

Drug resistant strains of *A. fumigatus* have been reported leading to further complications in treatment of CPA. Khan et al. (2024) reported *A. fumigatus* as the prominent pathogen in Mainland China (75.14%) followed by *A. flavus* (12.25%), *A. niger* (6.14%) and *A. terreus* (3.33%). The study further reported underlying conditions including lung disease, previous TB episodes, organ transplant, organ failure as well as corticosteroid therapy (Khan et al., 2024).

During the COVID-19 pandemic, patients with COVID-19 presented a severely weakened immune system and were prone to fungal infections such as aspergillosis. COVID-19–Associated Pulmonary Aspergillosis (CAPA) was reported in critically ill COVID-19 patients, especially those in the ICU or on ventilators. Damage to the lungs caused by COVID-19 is believed to contribute to the ease of invasion and colonization of *Aspergillus spp.* resulting in disease. The risk was further increased by the use of corticosteroids (like dexamethasone) and immunosuppressive therapies which were used to treat severe COVID-19. Overlap of symptoms of CAPA and COVID-19 complicated the diagnosis which could have resulted in late diagnosis and treatment of CAPA. During the pandemic, CAPA was reported in Europe, Asia, as well as the Americas (Table 8.1).

8.3.9 Candidaemia and COVID-19

Candida albicans was isolated in COVID-19 patients with increased Candidaemia reported during the pandemic as well as poor disease outcomes (Denny et al., 2021; Liu et al., 2025; Seagle et al., 2022; Shin et al., 2024). Mechanical ventilation was used on the critically ill COVID-19 patients. A systematic review by Liu et al., showed associations between mechanical ventilation and candida infections with a prevalence ranging from 10- 56% of mechanically ventilated patients (Liu et al., 2025). Similar outcomes were reported in Croatia in mechanically ventilated surgical patients with a significantly higher mortality with 42% mortality observed in patients with isolated *Candida* than in the control group (19%, $p < 0.001$) (Glavaš Tahtler et al., 2024). A study by Gangneux revealed three significant factors, Age > 62 years, solid organ transplant and probable, and or possible CAPA infection as risk factors (Gangneux et al., 2022). Apart from *C. albicans*, *Candida auris* was reported during the COVID-19 pandemic with significant consequences on the healthcare system.

Candida auris remains a major threat globally due to increased healthcare settings as well as its ability to colonize and difficulty in decontamination (Schaefer et al., 2024). Often drug resistant, the identification of *C. auris* in a healthcare setting calls for a complete closure and careful decontamination of the premises, thereby affecting any healthcare operations in the affected setting (Dahiya et al., 2020; Du et al., 2020; Pristov & Ghannoum, 2019). During the COVID-19 pandemic, an increase in incidence of *C. auris* was observed globally. The increase was attributed to prolonged hospitalization, mechanical ventilation as well as antimicrobial use (Khojasteh et al., 2022). In the United States, the CDC reported a 95% increase in *C. auris* cases between 2020 and 2023 some of which were due to multidrug resistant strains. Multi-drug resistant strains were also observed in Israel. During a nationwide outbreak of *C. auris* between 2021 and 2022, cases of *C. auris* infections were reported in several hospitals in the country (Biran et al., 2023; Khojasteh et al., 2022). Association of *C. auris* and COVID-19 hospitalizations were observed and drug resistant strains were reported including in patients receiving mechanical ventilation (Biran et al., 2023). To manage *C.auris* cases in a hospital in Florida, various infection prevention measures were put in place. These included contact tracing, cleaning surfaces including floors and ultraviolet disinfection of rooms as part of room turnover procedures after patient discharge to mitigate the spread of *C. auris* in the hospital environment (Prestel et al., 2021).

8.4 Lessons Learned

8.4.1 Changing with Changing Times

Availability of resources allowed for flexibility in adapting to the needs during COVID-19 pandemic.

Management of invasive fungal infections, especially those with multi-drug resistant strains, requires specific protocols including isolation of infected individuals, as well as availability of therapeutic and personnel able to administer these therapies safely to the patient. Treatment of invasive fungal infections is often long and requires close monitoring as some of the medications could result in adverse effects taken long term. The emerging drug resistance could mean limited treatment options some of which are not available in certain settings. The burden of fungal infections including invasive fungal infections and prevalence of *C. auris* is yet to be established for example in LMIC which often lack the infrastructure and resources. Screening hospital settings could assist in reducing nosocomial infections through proper management of the known cases as well as implementation of preventive measures including hand hygiene and hospital hygiene.

8.4.2 The Threat of Underlying Diseases

While dealing with the risk of infectious diseases, it is the non-communicable diseases that are a major threat in disease outcomes. Diabetes, hypertension, malignancies, organ transplants as well as age, long-term treatment with antibiotics and corticosteroids were the major determinants to disease outcomes during COVID-19. These threats remain as an increase in non-communicable diseases is reported globally. India which reported a high number of mucormycosis cases recorded that diabetes mellitus was a major contributing factor to the increase in cases apart from corticosteroid use during the COVID-19 pandemic. Management of non-communicable diseases is thus essential in preparing for emerging infectious diseases. The COVID-19 pandemic showed gaps as well as interconnectedness between the burden of non-communicable diseases and infectious disease outcomes. Addressing these gaps is essential in preparing for the next pandemic.

8.4.3 When Life Support Becomes a Threat

During the COVID-19 pandemic, critically ill patients required support through treatment in ICU as well as mechanical ventilation and other invasive procedures to manage the infection. Unfortunately, the measure trying to save the life of the individual also puts the patient at risk of life-threatening diseases including invasive fungal infections. Guidelines are in place to assist in reduction of these risks but implementing these guidelines remains at the capability and availability of resources in individual countries. While the knowledge, infrastructure as well as resource gaps remain, tackling the next pandemic remains a major challenge especially in resource limited settings where the burden of fungal infections remains unclear and surveillance programmes and or records remain scarce. Without this information, underestimation of the disease burden remains and resources to manage these unknown and or underreported burdens will remain minimal and or non-existent.

8.4.4 Weighing the Risk

The lessons learned during the COVID-19 pandemic and the co-infections that were observed during the period could prove essential for better preparedness and response. Challenges in diagnosis between HIC and LMIC could influence adherence to guidelines as well as types of tests used for diagnosis of fungal co-infections (Kanj et al., 2024). Fungal infections increase the severity of disease. Use of catheters and ventilators increased the risk of exposure to fungal infections (Chavda et al., 2023). The risk of invasive fungal infections increased in severely ill COVID-19 patients requiring invasive treatment in the ICU treatment (Kanj et al., 2024).

8.5 Recommendations for Bridging the Gaps

8.5.1 Addressing the Gap of Knowledge

One thing that is clear is that knowledge gaps do exist at family, community, national, regional and global level. Addressing these gaps in a multi-sectoral manner would assist in achieving better outcomes. For instance, targeted family education on health benefits of nutrition and lifestyle in reducing non-communicable diseases could result in better understanding of risk factors associated with non-communicable diseases. Similarly, educating families on fungal infections, risks, sources of disease and underlying factors could encourage changes in treatment seeking behaviour. In the health sector, educating health personnel in presentation of various fungal infections and the risk factors presented in the healthcare system would assist in better diagnosis, management and treatment of fungal infections. Emphasis on hygiene and nosocomial infections is essential.

8.5.2 Bridging the Diagnosis Gap

Diagnosis remains a major challenge in limited resource settings. It is crucial to encourage research and innovation and develop tools that would assist diagnostics needs in LMIC as well as rural and vulnerable communities globally. Availability of healthcare facilities, diagnostic laboratories as well as diagnostic tools remains a challenge for many. Better diagnosis could assist in greater understanding of circulating fungal pathogens and targeted treatment for those pathogens.

8.5.3 Addressing the Resource Gaps

Availability of resources is key in addressing the gaps that currently exist globally. The knowledge gap, financial gap, as well as the challenges in access to various resources that could assist in reducing these existing gaps are a requirement. Equitable distribution of healthcare resources at family, community and national level is crucial in better health outcomes at both national and global level. Lack of diagnostic tools, treatment and other therapies including vaccines results in loss of lives, loss of productivity and most of all economic losses that will affect the development of the affected populations. Perpetual gaps in healthcare are a systematic process that have hindered growth and development of most LMICs creating an atmosphere of rampant diseases that go untreated due to limited resources, a struggling healthcare system and governments succumbing to loss of lives due to preventable diseases. Limited productivity, political uncertainties and struggling governance have all contributed to the growing gaps. Thus, setting up policies that are tailor made for the populations and are culturally appropriate is vital. Community engagement with local leaders is essential especially in working with rural and indigenous communities.

8.5.4 The Power of Surveillance and Data

Surveillance is key to data collection. Without appropriate data, it is difficult to estimate the burden of disease. As such accurate surveillance is crucial in creating databases and further avenues of data collection should be explored in LMIC. Currently, surveillance data in LMIC is limited; this affect decision making as the resolutions could be made on faulty data. Better surveillance will ensure optimal estimation of disease burden thus informing policy.

8.6 Conclusion

COVID-19 unearthed existing gaps in resources, knowledge as well as challenges brought about by co-infections. In trying to treat COVID-19, patients were exposed to even further risk of complications due to opportunistic fungal infections. Existing co-morbidities exacerbated the severity of COVID-19 co-infections. Despite existing management policies for fungal infections, and COVID-19 co-infections, implementation varied in different settings due to various disparities including availability of resources. The chapter has discussed various strategies through the case studies presented. The need to improve surveillance mechanisms, implement optimal diagnostic approaches, routine screening and timely initiation of antifungal therapy especially in limited resource settings could be the first step in addressing the existing gaps in identification, diagnosis, treatment and management of fungal infections.

References

Abolghasemi, S., Hakamifard, A., Sharifynia, S., Pourabdollah Toutkaboni, M., Azhdari Tehrani, H. (2021). Fatal invasive pulmonary aspergillosis in an immunocompetent patient with COVID-19 due to aspergillus terreus: A case study. *Clinical Case Reports, 9*, 2414–2418. https://doi.org/10.1002/ccr3.4051

Agrawal, S., & Phulware, R. H. (2021, August 20). COVID-19 associated pulmonary aspergillosis (CAPA) in a pregnant woman. *Autopsy and Case Reports 11*, e2021313. PMID: 34458181; PMCID: PMC8387078. https://doi.org/10.4322/acr.2021.313

Alanio, A., Dellière, S., Fodil, S., Bretagne, S., & Mégarbane, B. (2020). Prevalence of putative invasive pulmonary aspergillosis in critically ill patients with COVID-19. *The Lancet Respiratory Medicine, 8*(6), e48–e49. https://doi.org/10.1016/S2213-2600(20)30237-X

Arastehfar, A., Carvalho, A., van de Veerdonk, F. L., Jenks, J. D., Koehler, P., Krause, R., Cornely, O. A., S Perlin, D., Lass-Flörl, C., & Hoenigl, M. (2020). COVID-19 Associated Pulmonary Aspergillosis (CAPA)-from immunology to treatment. *Journal of Fungi (Basel, Switzerland), 6*(2). https://doi.org/10.3390/jof6020091

Arisanti, R. R., Saputri, G. N., Ahmad, R. A., & Utarini, A. (2024). Impacts of COVID-19 on malaria elimination strategies in Asia: A scoping review. *Narra J, 4*(3), e1492. https://doi.org/10.52225/narra.v4i3.1492

Arjmand, P., Bahrami, M., Mohammadie, Z. E., Taherynejad, M., Khorasani, N. Y., Mehrad-Majd, H., Roshanzamir, I., & Bakhshaee, M. (2022). Mucormycosis in pre <scp>-COVID</scp> -19 and <scp>COVID</scp> -19 era: A study of prevalence, risk factors and clinical features. *Laryngoscope Investigative Otolaryngology, 7*(5), 1343–1350. https://doi.org/10.1002/lio2.899

Aschale, Y., Wubetu, M., Abebaw, A., Yirga, T., Minwuyelet, A., & Toru, M. (2021). A systematic review on traditional medicinal plants used for the treatment of viral and fungal infections in Ethiopia. *Journal of Experimental Pharmacology, 13*, 807–815. https://doi.org/10.2147/JEP.S316007

Baddley, J. W. (2011, April). Clinical risk factors for invasive aspergillosis. *Medical Mycology, 49*(Supplement_1), S7–S12. https://doi.org/10.3109/13693786.2010.505204

Benedict, K., & Park, B. J. (2014). Invasive fungal infections after natural disasters. *Emerging Infectious Diseases, 20*(3), 349–355. https://doi.org/10.3201/eid2003.131230

Bhat, P., Noval, M., Doub, J. B., & Heil, E. (2020). Concurrent COVID-19 and pneumocystis jirovecii pneumonia in a severely immunocompromised 25-year-old patient. *International Journal of Infectious Diseases, 99*, 119–121. https://doi.org/10.1016/J.IJID.2020.07.061

Biran, R., Cohen, R., Finn, T., Brosh-Nissimov, T., Rahav, G., Yahav, D., Amit, S., Shachor-Meyouhas, Y., Atamna, A., Bishara, J., Ashkenazi-Hoffnung, L., Ben Zvi, H., Hershman-Sarafov, M., Maayan, S., Maor, Y., Schwartz, O., Zimhony, O., Lellouche, J., Elbaz, M., … Ben-Ami, R. (2023). Nationwide outbreak of *Candida auris* infections driven by COVID-19 hospitalizations, Israel, 2021–20221. *Emerging Infectious Diseases, 29*(7). https://doi.org/10.3201/eid2907.221888

Bongomin, F., Gago, S., Oladele, R., & Denning, D. (2017). Global and multi-national prevalence of fungal diseases—Estimate precision. *Journal of Fungi, 3*(4), 57. https://doi.org/10.3390/jof3040057

Bongomin, F., Olum, R., Nsenga, L., & Baluku, J. B. (2020). Burden of tinea capitis among children in Africa: Protocol for a systematic review and meta-analysis of observational studies, 1990–2020. *British Medical Journal Open, 10*(9), Article e041230. https://doi.org/10.1136/bmjopen-2020-041230

Bretagne, S., Sitbon, K., Botterel, F., Dellière, S., Letscher-Bru, V., Chouaki, T., Bellanger, A., Bonnal, C., Fekkar, A., Persat, F., Costa, D., Bourgeois, N., Dalle, F., Lussac-Sorton, F., Paugam, A., Cassaing, S., Hasseine, L., Huguenin, A., Guennouni, N., Mazars, E., Le Gal, S., Sasso, M., Brun, S., Cadot, L., Cassagne, C., Cateau, E., Gangneux, J., Moniot, M., Roux, A., Tournus, C., Desbois-Nogard, N., Le Coustumier, A., Moquet, O., Alanio, A., & Dromer, F. (2021). COVID-19-associated pulmonary aspergillosis, fungemia, and pneumocystosis in the intensive care unit: A retrospective multicenter observational cohort during the first french pandemic wave. *Microbiology Spectrum, 9*, e01138–21. https://doi.org/10.1128/Spectrum.01138-21

Brown, G. D., Denning, D. W., Gow, N. A. R., Levitz, S. M., Netea, M. G., & White, T. C. (2012). Hidden killers: Human fungal infections. *Science Translational Medicine, 4*(165). https://doi.org/10.1126/scitranslmed.3004404

Buitrago, M. J., Aguado, J. M., Ballen, A., Bernal-Martinez, L., Prieto, M., Garcia-Reyne, A., Garcia-Rodriguez, J., Rodriguez-Tudela, J. L., & Cuenca-Estrella, M. (2013). Efficacy of DNA amplification in tissue biopsy samples to improve the detection of invasive fungal disease. *Clinical Microbiology and Infection, 19*(6), E271–E277. https://doi.org/10.1111/1469-0691.12110

Casadevall, A., Coelho, C., & Alanio, A. (2018). Mechanisms of cryptococcus neoformans-mediated host damage. *Frontiers in Immunology, 9*. https://doi.org/10.3389/fimmu.2018.00855

Chakrabarti, A., Patel, A. K., Soman, R., & Todi, S. (2023). Overcoming clinical challenges in the management of invasive fungal infections in Low—And Middle-Income Countries (LMIC). *Expert Review of Anti-Infective Therapy, 21*(10), 1057–1070. https://doi.org/10.1080/14787210.2023.2257895

Chandley, P., Subba, P., & Rohatgi, S. (2022). COVID-19-associated mucormycosis: A matter of concern amid the SARS-CoV-2 pandemic. *Vaccines, 10*(8). https://doi.org/10.3390/vaccines10081266

Chanyachailert, P., Leeyaphan, C., & Bunyaratavej, S. (2023). Cutaneous fungal infections caused by dermatophytes and non-dermatophytes: An updated comprehensive review of epidemiology, clinical presentations, and diagnostic testing. *Journal of Fungi, 9*(6), 669. https://doi.org/10.3390/jof9060669

Chavda, V., Mishra, T., Kamaraj, S., Punetha, S., Sengupta, O., Joshi, Y., Vuppu, S., Vaghela, D., & Vora, L. (2023). Post-COVID-19 fungal infection in the aged population. *Vaccines, 11*(3), 555. https://doi.org/10.3390/vaccines11030555

Cho, S., Crenshaw, K. W., & McCall, L. (2013). Toward a field of intersectionality studies: Theory, applications, and praxis. *Signs: Journal of Women in Culture and Society, 38*(4), 785–810. https://doi.org/10.1086/669608

Choudhary, N., Panday, D., Mishra, D., Lahiri, K., Sil, A., & Chaddha, R. (2024). Over-the-counter medicine-seeking behavior in patients with dermatophyte infections across various socioeconomic strata: A cross-sectional study. *Cureus*. https://doi.org/10.7759/cureus.51686

Chowdhary, A., Sharma, C., & Meis, J. F. (2017). Candida auris:. A rapidly emerging cause of hospital-acquired multidrug-resistant fungal infections globally. *PLOS pathogens, 13*(5), e1006290. https://doi.org/10.1371/journal.ppat.1006290

Cobb, N., Papali, A., Pisani, L., Schultz, M. J., Ferreira, J. C., & COVID-LMIC Task Force and the Mahidol-Oxford Research Unit (MORU). (2021). Pragmatic recommendations for infection prevention and control practices for healthcare facilities in low—And middle-income countries during the COVID-19 pandemic. *The American Journal of Tropical Medicine and Hygiene, 104*(3_Suppl), 25–33. https://doi.org/10.4269/ajtmh.20-1009

Comella-del-Barrio, P., De Souza-Galvão, M. L., Prat-Aymerich, C., & Domínguez, J. (2021). Impact of COVID-19 on tuberculosis control. *Archivos De Bronconeumología, 57*, 5–6. https://doi.org/10.1016/j.arbres.2020.11.016

Cornely, O. A., Alastruey-Izquierdo, A., Arenz, D., Chen, S. C. A., Dannaoui, E., Hochhegger, B., Hoenigl, M., Jensen, H. E., Lagrou, K., Lewis, R. E., Mellinghoff, S. C., Mer, M., Pana, Z. D., Seidel, D., Sheppard, D. C., Wahba, R., Akova, M., Alanio, A., Al-Hatmi, A. M. S., … Chakrabarti, A. (2019). Global guideline for the diagnosis and management of mucormycosis: An initiative of the European confederation of medical mycology in cooperation with the mycoses study group education and research consortium. *The Lancet Infectious Diseases, 19*(12), e405–e421. https://doi.org/10.1016/S1473-3099(19)30312-3

Dahiya, S., Sharma, N., Punia, A., Choudhary, P., Gulia, P., Parmar V. S., & Chhillar, A. K. (2022). Antimycotic drugs and their mechanisms of resistance to Candida species. *Current Drug Targets, 23*(2), 116–125. https://doi.org/10.2174/1389450122666210719124143

Denning, D. W. (2024). Global incidence and mortality of severe fungal disease. *The Lancet Infectious Diseases*. https://doi.org/10.1016/S1473-3099(23)00692-8

Denning, D. W et al. (2017). Pulmonary and sinus fungal diseases in non-immunocompromised patients. *The Lancet Infectious Diseases, 17*(11), e357–e366. https://doi.org/10.1016/S1473-3099(17)30309-2

Denny, S., Abdolrasouli, A., Elamin, T., Gonzalo, X., Charani, E., Patel, A., Donaldson, H., Hughes, S., Armstrong-James, D., Moore, L. S., & Mughal, N. A. (2021, June). Retrospective multicenter analysis of candidaemia among COVID-19 patients during the first UK pandemic wave. *The Journal of Infection, 82*(6), 276–316. PMID: 33610684; PMCID: PMC7890346. https://doi.org/10.1016/j.jinf.2021.02.020

Diongue, K., Dembélé, B., Ndiaye, M., Seck, M. C., Diallo, M. A., Badiane, A. S., Ndiaye, D., & Ranque, S. (2023). Evaluation of knowledge and experience of fungal infections (mycoses) among clinical doctors in Senegal. *Journal of Medical Mycology, 33*(3), Article 101408. https://doi.org/10.1016/j.mycmed.2023.101408

Donnelly, J. P., Chen, S. C. Kauffman, C. A., Steinbach, W. J., Baddley, J. W., Verweij, P. E., Clancy, C. J., Wingard, J. R., Lockhart, S. R., Groll, A. H., Sorrell, T. C., Bassetti, M., Akan, H., Alexander, B. D., Andes, D., Azoulay, E., Bialek, R., Bradsher, R. W., Bretagne, S., …, & Pappas, P. G. (2020, September 15). Revision and update of the consensus definitions of invasive fungal disease from the european organization for research and treatment of cancer and the mycoses study group education and research consortium. *Clinical Infectious Diseases, 71*(6), 1367–1376. https://doi.org/10.1093/cid/ciz1008

Dudoignon, E., Chevret, S., Tsague, S., Hamane, S., Chaouat, M., Plaud, B., Vicault, E., Mebazaa, A., Legrand, M., Alanio, A., Denis, B., Dépret, F., & Dellière, S. (2024). Risk factors and outcome associated with fungal infections in patients with severe burn injury: 10-year retrospective IFI-BURN study. *Clinical Infectious Diseases, 79*(3), 682–689. https://doi.org/10.1093/cid/ciae337

Du, H., Bing, J., Hu, T., Ennis, C. L., Nobile, C. J., & Huang, G. (2020, October 22). *Candida auris*: Epidemiology, biology, antifungal resistance, and virulence. *PLoS Pathog, 16*(10), e1008921. PMID: 33091071; PMCID: PMC7581363. https://doi.org/10.1371/journal.ppat.1008921

Dupont, D., Menotti, J., Turc, J., Miossec, C., Wallet, F., Richard, J.-C., Argaud, L., Paulus, S., Wallon, M., Ader, F., & Persat, F. (2021). Pulmonary aspergillosis in critically ill patients with coronavirus disease 2019 (COVID-19). *Medical Mycology, 59*(1), 110–114. https://doi.org/10.1093/mmy/myaa078

Edwards, J. E., Schwartz, M. M., Schmidt, C. S., Sobel, J. D., Nyirjesy, P., Schodel, F., Marchus, E., Lizakowski, M., DeMontigny, E. A., Hoeg, J., Holmberg, T., Cooke, M. T., Hoover, K., Edwards, L., Jacobs, M., Sussman, S., Augenbraun, M., Drusano, M., Yeaman, M. R., … Hennessey, J. P. (2018). A fungal immunotherapeutic vaccine (NDV-3A) for treatment of recurrent vulvovaginal candidiasis—A phase 2 randomized, double-blind, placebo-controlled trial. *Clinical Infectious Diseases, 66*(12), 1928–1936. https://doi.org/10.1093/cid/ciy185

Egger, M., Bussini, L., Hoenigl, M., & Bartoletti, M. (2022). Prevalence of COVID-19-associated pulmonary aspergillosis: Critical review and conclusions. *Journal of Fungi (Basel, Switzerland), 8*(4). https://doi.org/10.3390/jof8040390

Facciolà, A., Laganà, A., Genovese, G., Romeo, B., Sidoti, S., D'Andrea, G., Raco, C., Visalli, G., & DI Pietro, A. (2023). Impact of the COVID-19 pandemic on the infectious disease epidemiology. *Journal of Preventive Medicine and Hygiene, 64*(3), E274–E282. https://doi.org/10.15167/2421-4248/jpmh2023.64.3.2904

Fekkar, A., Lampros, A., Mayaux, J., Poignon, C., Demeret, S., Constantin, J. M., Marcelin, A. G., Monsel, A., Luyt, C. E., & Blaize, M. (2021, February 1). Occurrence of invasive pulmonary fungal infections in patients with severe COVID-19 admitted to the ICU. *American Journal of Respiratory and Critical Care medicine, 203*(3), 307–317. PMID: 33480831; PMCID: PMC7874326. https://doi.org/10.1164/rccm.202009-3400OC

Feys, S., Almyroudi, M. P., Braspenning, R., Lagrou, K., Spriet, I., Dimopoulos, G., & Wauters, J. (2021). A visual and comprehensive review on COVID-19-associated pulmonary aspergillosis (CAPA). *Journal of Fungi, 7*(12), 1067. https://doi.org/10.3390/jof7121067

Gangneux, J.-P., Dannaoui, E., Fekkar, A., Luyt, C.-E., Botterel, F., De Prost, N., Tadié, J.-M., Reizine, F., Houzé, S., Timsit, J.-F., Iriart, X., Riu-Poulenc, B., Sendid, B., Nseir, S., Persat, F., Wallet, F., Le Pape, P., Canet, E., Novara, A., … Bougnoux, M.-E. (2022). Fungal infections in mechanically ventilated patients with COVID-19 during the first wave: The French multicentre MYCOVID study. *The Lancet Respiratory Medicine, 10*(2), 180–190. https://doi.org/10.1016/S2213-2600(21)00442-2

Garber, G. (2001). An overview of fungal infections. *Drugs, 61*(Supplement 1), 1–12. https://doi.org/10.2165/00003495-200161001-00001

Gillibrand, S., Kapadia, D., Watkinson, R., Issa, B., Kwaku-Odoi, C., & Sanders, C. (2024). Marginalisation and distrust in the context of the COVID-19 vaccination programme: Experiences of communities in a northern UK city region. *BMC Public Health, 24*(1), 853. https://doi.org/10.1186/s12889-024-18308-0

Glavaš Tahtler, J., Cicvarić, A., Koulenti, D., Karvouniaris, M., Bogdan, M., Kralik, K., Krajina Kmoniček, I., Grbić Mlinarević, M., & Kvolik, S. (2024). Isolation of Candida species is associated with comorbidities, prolonged mechanical ventilation, and treatment outcomes in surgical icu patients, a cross-sectional study. *Journal of Fungi, 10*(11), 743. https://doi.org/10.3390/jof10110743

Hartnett, K. P., Jackson, B. R., Perkins, K. M., Glowicz, J., Kerins, J. L., Black, S. R., Lockhart, S. R., Christensen, B. E., & Beer, K. D. (2019). A guide to investigating suspected outbreaks of mucormycosis in healthcare. *Journal of Fungi, 5*(3), 69. https://doi.org/10.3390/jof5030069

Hernández, J. L., & Buckley, C. J. (2025). *Mucormycosis.*

Hoenigl, M. (2022). When disaster strikes fungi take control. *The Lancet Respiratory Medicine, 10*(12), 1104–1106. https://doi.org/10.1016/S2213-2600(22)00268-5

Hoenigl, M., Salmanton-García, J., Walsh, T. J., Nucci, M., Neoh, C. F., Jenks, J. D., Lackner, M., Sprute, R., Al-Hatmi, A. M. S., Bassetti, M., Carlesse, F., Freiberger, T., Koehler, P., Lehrnbecher, T., Kumar, A., Prattes, J., Richardson, M., Revankar, S., Slavin, M. A., … Cornely, O. A. (2021). Global guideline for the diagnosis and management of rare mould infections: An initiative of the European confederation of medical mycology in cooperation with the international society for human and animal mycology and the American society for microbiolo. *The Lancet Infectious Diseases, 0*(0), 1–12. https://doi.org/10.1016/S1473-3099(20)30784-2

Hoenigl, M., Seidel, D., Sprute, R., Cunha, C., Oliverio, M., Goldman, G. H., Ibrahim, A. S., & Carvalho, A. (2022). COVID-19-associated fungal infections. *Nature Microbiology, 7*(8), 1127–1140. https://doi.org/10.1038/s41564-022-01172-2

Huang, S.-F., Wu, A. Y.-J., Lee, S. S.-J., Huang, Y.-S., Lee, C.-Y., Yang, T.-L., Wang, H.-W., Chen, H. J., Chen, Y. C., Ho, T.-S., Kuo, C.-F., & Lin, Y.-T. (2023). COVID-19 associated mold infections: Review of COVID-19 associated pulmonary aspergillosis and mucormycosis. *Journal of Microbiology, Immunology and Infection, 56*(3), 442–454. ISSN: 1684–1182. https://doi.org/10.1016/j.jmii.2022.12.004

https://www.who.int/india/home/emergencies/coronavirus-disease-(covid-19)/mucormycosis#:~:text=The%20incidence%20rate%20of%20mucormycosis,to%201.7%20per%20million%20population

https://www.who.int/publications/i/item/9789240060241

Jenks, J. D., Aneke, C. I., Al-Obaidi, M. M., Egger, M., Garcia, L., Gaines, T., Hoenigl, M., & Thompson, G. R. (2023). Race and ethnicity: Risk factors for fungal infections? *PLOS Pathogens, 19*(1), Article e1011025. https://doi.org/10.1371/journal.ppat.1011025

Jeong, W., Keighley, C., Wolfe, R., Lee, W. L., Slavin, M. A., Kong, D. C. M., & Chen, S.C.-A. (2019). The epidemiology and clinical manifestations of mucormycosis: A systematic review and meta-analysis of case reports. *Clinical Microbiology and Infection, 25*(1), 26–34. https://doi.org/10.1016/j.cmi.2018.07.011

Kalua, K., Zimba, B., & Denning, D. W. (2018). Estimated burden of serious fungal infections in Malawi. *Journal of Fungi (Basel, Switzerland), 4*(2). https://doi.org/10.3390/jof4020061

Kanj, A. N., Doumat, G., & Limper, A. H. (2024). Invasive pulmonary aspergillosis in other patient populations. In A. O. Soubani (Eds.), *Pulmonary aspergillosis.* Springer. https://doi.org/10.1007/978-3-031-76524-7_15

Khan, S., Bilal, H., Shafiq, M., Zhang, D., Awais, M., Chen, C., Khan, M. N., Wang, Q., Cai, L., Islam, R., & Zeng, Y. (2024, June 4). Distribution of aspergillus species and risk factors for aspergillosis in mainland china: A systematic review. *Therapeutic advances in infectious disease, 11*, 20499361241252537. PMID: 38835831; PMCID: PMC11149451. https://doi.org/10.1177/20499361241252537

Khojasteh, S., Jafarzdeh, J., Hosseini, S. A., Haghani, I., Turki, H., Aghaei Gharehbolagh, S., Abastabar, M., & Mahmoudi, S. (2022, September). *Candida auris* and COVID-19: A health threatening combination. *Current Medical Mycology, 8*(3), 44–50. PMID: 37051551; PMCID: PMC10084486. https://doi.org/10.18502/cmm.8.3.11211

Koehler, P., von Stillfried, S., Borrega, J. G, Fuchs, F., Salmanton-García, J., Pult, F., Böll, B., Eichenauer, D. A., Shimabukuro-Vornhagen, A., Kurzai, O., Boor, P., Kochanek, M., & Cornely, O. A. (2022, May 5). Aspergillus tracheobronchitis in COVID-19 patients with acute respiratory distress syndrome: A cohort study. *The European Respiratory Journal, 59*(5), 2103142. PMID: 35144992; PMCID: PMC9068972. https://doi.org/10.1183/13993003.03142-2021

Koffi, D., Bonouman, I. V., Toure, A. O., Kouadjo, F., N'Gou, M. R. E., Sylla, K., Dosso, M., & Denning, D. W. (2021). Estimates of serious fungal infection burden in Côte d'Ivoire and country health profile. *Journal of Medical Mycology, 31*(1), 101086. ISSN: 1156–5233. https://doi.org/10.1016/j.mycmed.2020.101086

Kontoyiannis, D. P., Azie, N., Franks, B., & Horn, D. L. (2014). Prospective antifungal therapy (<scp>PATH</scp>) alliance ®: Focus on mucormycosis. *Mycoses, 57*(4), 240–246. https://doi.org/10.1111/myc.12149

Kosmidis, C., & Denning, D. W. (2015, March). The clinical spectrum of pulmonary aspergillosis. *Thorax, 70*(3), 270–277. PMID: 25354514. https://doi.org/10.1136/thoraxjnl-2014-206291

Krishna, V., Bansal, N., Morjaria, J., & Kaul, S. (2022). COVID-19-associated pulmonary mucormycosis. *Journal of Fungi, 8*(7), 711. https://doi.org/10.3390/jof8070711

Kundu, R., & Singla, N. (2022). COVID-19 and plethora of fungal infections. *Current Fungal Infection Reports, 16*(2), 47–54. https://doi.org/10.1007/s12281-022-00432-2

Kung, H.-C., Huang, P.-Y., Chen, W.-T., Ko, B.-S., Chen, Y.-C., Chang, S.-C., & Chuang, Y.-C. (2018). 2016 guidelines for the use of antifungal agents in patients with invasive fungal diseases in Taiwan. *Journal of Microbiology, Immunology and Infection, 51*(1), 1–17. https://doi.org/10.1016/j.jmii.2017.07.006

Lamoth, F., Glampedakis, E., Boillat-Blanco, N., Oddo, M., & Pagani, J.-L. (2020). Incidence of invasive pulmonary aspergillosis among critically ill COVID-19 patients. *Clinical Microbiology and Infection, 26*(12), 1706–1708. https://doi.org/10.1016/j.cmi.2020.07.010

Li, Z., & Denning, D. W. (2023). The impact of corticosteroids on the outcome of fungal disease: A systematic review and meta-analysis. *Current Fungal Infection Reports, 17*(1), 54–70. https://doi.org/10.1007/s12281-023-00456-2

Liu, T., Sun, S., Zhu, X., Wu, H., Sun, Z., & Peng, S. (2025, April 11). Epidemiology, clinical characteristics, and outcome in candidemia: A retrospective five-year analysis from two tertiary general hospitals. *BMC Infectious Diseases, 25*(1), 512. PMID: 40217142; PMCID: PMC11992820. https://doi.org/10.1186/s12879-025-10908-4

Lopes, S., Soares, P., Gama, A., Pedro, A. R., Moniz, M., Laires, P., Goes, A. R., Nunes, C., & Dias, S. (2022). Association between perception of COVID-19 risk, confidence in health services and avoidance of emergency department visits: Results from a community-based survey in Portugal. *British Medical Journal Open, 12*(7), Article e058600. https://doi.org/10.1136/bmjopen-2021-058600

Loyse, A., Burry, J., Cohn, J., Ford, N., Chiller, T., Ribeiro, I., Koulla-Shiro, S., Mghamba, J., Ramadhani, A., Nyirenda, R., Aliyu, S. H., Wilson, D., Le, T., Oladele, R., Lesikari, S., Muzoora,

C., Kalata, N., Temfack, E., Mapoure, Y., … Harrison, T. S. (2019). Leave no one behind: Response to new evidence and guidelines for the management of cryptococcal meningitis in low-income and middle-income countries. *The Lancet Infectious Diseases, 19*(4), e143–e147. https://doi.org/10.1016/S1473-3099(18)30493-6

Maertens, J., Vrebos, M., & Boogaerts, M. (2001). Assessing risk factors for systemic fungal infections. *European Journal of Cancer Care, 10*(1), 56–62. https://doi.org/10.1046/j.1365-2354.2001.00241.x

Mang, S., Kaddu-Mulindwa, D., Metz, C., Becker, A., Seiler, F., Smola, S., Maßmann, A., Becker, S. L., Papan, C., Bals, R., Lepper, P. M., & Danziger, G. (2021). Pneumocystis jirovecii Pneumonia and severe acute respiratory syndrome coronavirus 2 coinfection in a patient with newly diagnosed HIV-1 infection. *Clinical Infectious Diseases, 72*(8), 1487–1489. https://doi.org/10.1093/cid/ciaa906

Merkhofer, R. M., O'Neill, M. B., Xiong, D., Hernandez-Santos, N., Dobson, H., Fites, J. S., Shockey, A. C., Wuethrich, M., Pepperell, C. S., & Klein, B. S. (2019). Investigation of genetic susceptibility to blastomycosis reveals interleukin-6 as a potential susceptibility locus. *MBio, 10*(3). https://doi.org/10.1128/mBio.01224-19

Mery, A., Sendid, B., François, N., Cornu, M., Poissy, J., Guerardel, Y., & Poulain, D. (2016). Application of mass spectrometry technology to early diagnosis of invasive fungal infections. *Journal of Clinical Microbiology, 54*(11), 2786–2797. https://doi.org/10.1128/JCM.01655-16

Miceli, M., & Maertens, J. (2015). Role of non-culture-based tests, with an emphasis on galactomannan testing for the diagnosis of invasive aspergillosis. *Seminars in Respiratory and Critical Care Medicine, 36*(05), 650–661. https://doi.org/10.1055/s-0035-1562892

Mude, W., Mwenyango, H., Preston, R., O'Mullan, C., Vaughan, G., & Jones, G. (2024). HIV testing disruptions and service adaptations during the COVID-19 pandemic: A systematic literature review. *AIDS and Behavior, 28*(1), 186–200. https://doi.org/10.1007/s10461-023-04139-4

Najeeb, H., Siddiqui, S. A., Anas, Z., Ali, S. H., Usmani, S. U. R., Jawed, F., & Jatoi, H. N. (2022). The menace of Candida auris epidemic amidst the COVID-19 pandemic: A systematic review. *Diseases, 10*(3), 58. https://doi.org/10.3390/diseases10030058

Neblett Fanfair, R., Benedict, K., Bos, J., Bennett, S. D., Lo, Y.-C., Adebanjo, T., Etienne, K., Deak, E., Derado, G., Shieh, W.-J., Drew, C., Zaki, S., Sugerman, D., Gade, L., Thompson, E. H., Sutton, D. A., Engelthaler, D. M., Schupp, J. M., Brandt, M. E., … Park, B. J. (2012). Necrotizing cutaneous mucormycosis after a Tornado in Joplin, Missouri, in 2011. *New England Journal of Medicine, 367*(23), 2214–2225. https://doi.org/10.1056/NEJMoa1204781

Ngandu, N. K., Mmotsa, T. M., Dassaye, R., Thabetha, A., Odendaal, W., Langdown, N., & Ndwandwe, D. (2022). Hospital acquired COVID-19 infections amongst patients before the rollout of COVID-19 vaccinations, a scoping review. *BMC Infectious Diseases, 22*(1), 140. https://doi.org/10.1186/s12879-022-07128-5

Oladele, R., Otu, A. A., Olubamwo, O., Makanjuola, O. B., Ochang, E., Ejembi, J. A., Irurhe, N., Ajanaku, I., Ekundayo, H. A., Olayinka, A., Atoyebi, O., & Denning, D. (2020). Evaluation of knowledge and awareness of invasive fungal infections amongst resident doctors in Nigeria. *Pan African Medical Journal, 36*. https://doi.org/10.11604/pamj.2020.36.297.23279

Osaigbovo, I. I., Ekeng, B. E., Davies, A. A., & Oladele, R. O. (2023). Mucormycosis in Africa: Epidemiology, diagnosis and treatment outcomes. *Mycoses, 66*(7), 555–562. https://doi.org/10.1111/myc.13581

Pal, R., Singh, B., Bhadada, S. K., Banerjee, M., Bhogal, R. S., Hage, N., & Kumar, A. (2021). COVID-19-associated mucormycosis: An updated systematic review of literature. *Mycoses, 64*(12), 1452–1459. https://doi.org/10.1111/myc.13338

Pasquier, G. (2023). COVID-19-associated mucormycosis in India: Why such an outbreak? *Journal De Mycologie Medicale, 33*(3), Article 101393. https://doi.org/10.1016/j.mycmed.2023.101393

Pfavayi, L. T., Denning, D. W., Baker, S., Sibanda, E. N., & Mutapi, F. (2021). Determining the burden of fungal infections in Zimbabwe. *Scientific Reports, 11*(1), 13240. https://doi.org/10.1038/s41598-021-92605-1

Prakash, H., & Chakrabarti, A. (2019). Global epidemiology of mucormycosis. *Journal of Fungi, 5*(1), 26. https://doi.org/10.3390/jof5010026

Prakash, H., & Chakrabarti, A. (2021). Epidemiology of mucormycosis in India. *Microorganisms, 9*(3), 523. https://doi.org/10.3390/microorganisms9030523

Prattes, J., Wauters, J., Giacobbe, D. R., Salmanton-García, J., Maertens, J., Bourgeois, M., Reynders, M., Rutsaert, L., Van Regenmortel, N., Lormans, P., Feys, S., Reisinger, A. C., Cornely, O. A., Lahmer, T., Valerio, M., Delhaes, L., Jabeen, K., Steinmann, J., Chamula, M., … Muñoz, P. (2022). Risk factors and outcome of pulmonary aspergillosis in critically ill coronavirus disease 2019 patients—A multinational observational study by the European Confederation of Medical Mycology. *Clinical Microbiology and Infection, 28*(4), 580–587. https://doi.org/10.1016/j.cmi.2021.08.014

Prestel, C., Anderson, E., Forsberg, K., Lyman, M., de Perio, M. A., Kuhar, D., Edwards, K., Rivera, M., Shugart, A., Walters, M., & Dotson, N. Q. (2021, January 15). *Candida auris* outbreak in a COVID-19 specialty care unit – Florida, July–August 2020. *Morbidity and Mortality Weekly Report, 70*(2), 56–57. PMID: 33444298; PMCID: PMC7808709. https://doi.org/10.15585/mmwr.mm7002e3

Pristov, K. E., & Ghannoum, M. A. (2019, July). Resistance of Candida to azoles and echinocandins worldwide. *Clinical Microbiology and Infection, 25*(7), 792–798. PMID: 30965100. https://doi.org/10.1016/j.cmi.2019.03.028

Qin, W., Guo, T., You, T., Tian, R., Cui, X., & Wang, P. (2024). Metagenomic next generation sequencing of bronchoalveolar lavage fluids for the identification of pathogens in patients with pulmonary infection: A retrospective study. *Diagnostic Microbiology and Infectious Disease, 110*(1), Article 116402. https://doi.org/10.1016/j.diagmicrobio.2024.116402

Rammaert, B., Lanternier, F., Zahar, J.-R., Dannaoui, E., Bougnoux, M.-E., Lecuit, M., & Lortholary, O. (2012). Healthcare-Associated Mucormycosis. *Clinical Infectious Diseases, 54*(suppl_1), S44–S54. https://doi.org/10.1093/cid/cir867

Rayens, E., Rayens, M. K., & Norris, K. A. (2022). Demographic and socioeconomic factors associated with fungal infection risk, United States, 2019. *Emerging Infectious Diseases, 28*(10). https://doi.org/10.3201/eid2810.220391

Richardson, M. (2009). The ecology of the Zygomycetes and its impact on environmental exposure. *Clinical Microbiology and Infection, 15*, 2–9. https://doi.org/10.1111/j.1469-0691.2009.02972.x

Rosenthal, V. D., Myatra, S. N., Divatia, J. V., Biswas, S., Shrivastava, A., Al-Ruzzieh, M. A., Ayaad, O., Bat-Erdene, A., Bat-Erdene, I., Narankhuu, B., Gupta, D., Mandal, S., Sengupta, S., Joudi, H., Omeis, I., Agha, H. M., Fathallala, A., Mohahmed, E. H., Yesiler, I., … Yin, R. (2022). The impact of COVID-19 on health care–associated infections in intensive care units in low—And middle-income countries: International Nosocomial Infection Control Consortium (INICC) findings. *International Journal of Infectious Diseases, 118*, 83–88. https://doi.org/10.1016/j.ijid.2022.02.041

Rutsaert, L., Steinfort, N., Van Hunsel, T., Bomans, P., Naesens, R., Mertes, H., Dits, H., & Van Regenmortel, N. (2020). COVID-19-associated invasive pulmonary aspergillosis. *Annals of Intensive Care, 10*(1), 71. https://doi.org/10.1186/s13613-020-00686-4

Sanyaolu, A., Okorie, C., Marinkovic, A., Patidar, R., Younis, K., Desai, P., Hosein, Z., Padda, I., Mangat, J., & Altaf, M. (2020). Comorbidity and its impact on patients with COVID-19. *SN Comprehensive Clinical Medicine, 2*(8), 1069–1076. https://doi.org/10.1007/s42399-020-00363-4

Seagle, E. E., Jackson, B. R., Lockhart, S. R., Georgacopoulos, O., Nunnally, N. S., Roland, J., Barter, D. M., Johnston, H. L., Czaja, C. A., Kayalioglu, H., Clogher, P., Revis, A., Farley, M. M., Harrison, L. H., Davis, S. S., Phipps, E. C., Tesini, B. L., Schaffner, W., Markus, T. M., & Lyman, M. M. (2022). The landscape of Candidemia during the coronavirus disease 2019 (COVID-19) pandemic. *Clinical Infectious Diseases, 74*(5), 802–811. https://doi.org/10.1093/cid/ciab562

Shishido, A. A., Mathew, M., & Baddley, J. W. (2022). Overview of COVID-19-associated invasive fungal infection. *Current Fungal Infection Reports, 16*(3), 87–97. https://doi.org/10.1007/s12281-022-00434-0

Singh, A. K., Singh, R., Joshi, S. R., & Misra, A. (2021). Mucormycosis in COVID-19: A systematic review of cases reported worldwide and in India. *Diabetes & Metabolic Syndrome: Clinical Research & Reviews, 15*(4), Article 102146. https://doi.org/10.1016/j.dsx.2021.05.019

Sipsas, N. V., & Kontoyiannis, D. P. (2008). Occupation, lifestyle, diet, and invasive fungal infections. *Infection, 36*(6), 515–525. https://doi.org/10.1007/s15010-008-8129-5

Skiada, A., Pagano, L., Groll, A., Zimmerli, S., Dupont, B., Lagrou, K., Lass-Florl, C., Bouza, E., Klimko, N., Gaustad, P., Richardson, M., Hamal, P., Akova, M., Meis, J. F., Rodriguez-Tudela, J.-L., Roilides, E., Mitrousia-Ziouva, A., & Petrikkos, G. (2011). Zygomycosis in Europe: Analysis of 230 cases accrued by the registry of the European Confederation of Medical Mycology (ECMM) working group on Zygomycosis between 2005 and 2007. *Clinical Microbiology and Infection, 17*(12), 1859–1867. https://doi.org/10.1111/j.1469-0691.2010.03456.x

Tolle, L. B., & Standiford, T. J. (2013). Danger-associated molecular patterns (<scp>DAMPs</scp>) in acute lung injury. *The Journal of Pathology, 229*(2), 145–156. https://doi.org/10.1002/path.4124

Urban, K., Chu, S., Scheufele, C., Giesey, R. L., Mehrmal, S., Uppal, P., & Delost, G. R. (2021a). The global, regional, and national burden of fungal skin diseases in 195 countries and territories: A cross-sectional analysis from the global burden of disease study 2017. *JAAD International, 2*, 22–27. https://doi.org/10.1016/j.jdin.2020.10.003

Urban, K., Chu, S., Scheufele, C., Giesey, R. L., Mehrmal, S., Uppal, P., & Delost, G. R. (2021b). The global, regional, and national burden of fungal skin diseases in 195 countries and territories: A cross-sectional analysis from the Global Burden of Disease Study 2017. *JAAD International, 2*, 22–27. https://doi.org/10.1016/j.jdin.2020.10.003

Vallabhaneni, S., Kallen, A., Tsay, S., Chow, N., Welsh, R., Kerins, J., Kemble, S. K., Pacilli, M., Black, S. R, Landon, E., Ridgway, J., Palmore, T. N., Zelzany, A., Adams, E. H., Quinn, M., Chaturvedi, S., Greenko, J., Fernandez, R., Southwick, K., …, & Chiller, T. M. (2017, January). Investigation of the first seven reported cases of *candida auris*, a globally emerging invasive, multidrug-resistant fungus—United States, May 2013–August 2016. *American Journal of Transplantation, 17*(1), 296–299. PMID: 28029734. https://doi.org/10.1111/ajt.14121

van Arkel, A. L. E., Rijpstra, T. A., Belderbos, H. N. A., van Wijngaarden, P., Verweij, P. E., & Bentvelsen, R. G. (2020). COVID-19–associated pulmonary aspergillosis. *American Journal of Respiratory and Critical Care Medicine, 202*(1), 132–135. https://doi.org/10.1164/rccm.202004-1038LE

Wang, Z., Pan, M., & Zhu, J. (2025). Global burden of reported lower respiratory system fungal infection. *Frontiers in Cellular and Infection Microbiology, 15*. https://doi.org/10.3389/fcimb.2025.1542922

Wilbourn, A. C., Tsodikov, O. V, & Garneau-Tsodikova, S. (2024). Association of COVID-19 risk factors with systemic fungal infections in hospitalized patients. medRxiv. https://doi.org/10.1101/2024.10.10.24315254

Wong, J., Lao, C., Dino, G., Donyaei, R., Lui, R., & Huynh, J. (2024). Vaccine hesitancy among immigrants: A narrative review of challenges, opportunities, and lessons learned. *Vaccines, 12*(5), 445. https://doi.org/10.3390/vaccines12050445

Chapter 9
Resilience to Disease Outbreaks in Resource-Limited Endemic Regions—A Post-COVID-19 Analysis

Peter Suwirakwenda Nyasulu, Calvin Bisong Ebai, Nebiyu Dereje Abebe, Jacques Lukenze Tamuzi, Doris Yasinti Sakala, Mosoka Fallah, Gideon Kofi Helegbe, and Fingani Annie Mphande

Abstract Infectious disease outbreaks either endemic or emerging and re-emerging infectious diseases contribute to the burden of infectious disease particularly in limited resource settings. The management of outbreaks is quite demanding given the number of cases and sometimes deaths that occur. The incidence of some disease outbreaks has risen over time and somewhat exacerbated by other emerging and re-emerging diseases of pandemic propensity. The COVID-19 pandemic challenged the already struggling health systems and affected routine public health programmes globally. There is need for endemic countries to review the successes and failures during the pandemic and identify gaps and areas that need strengthening to build resilient communities and infrastructure. The COVID-19 pandemic put enormous pressure on health systems and other infectious disease outbreaks that followed,

P. S. Nyasulu · C. B. Ebai · J. L. Tamuzi · D. Y. Sakala
Division of Epidemiology and Biostatistics, Department of Global Health, University of Stellenbosch, Cape Town, South Africa

C. B. Ebai
Department of Medical Laboratory Science, University of Bamenda, Bamenda, Cameroon

N. D. Abebe · M. Fallah
Africa Centres for Disease Control and Prevention, Addis Ababa, Ethiopia

N. D. Abebe
School of Public Health, Wachemo University, Hosainna, Ethiopia

G. K. Helegbe
Department of Biochemistry and Molecular Medicine, School of Medicine, University for Development Studies, Tamale, Ghana

F. A. Mphande (✉)
King Mongkut's Institute of Technology Ladkrabang, Bangkok, Thailand
e-mail: yadoster@gmail.com

P. S. Nyasulu
Division of Epidemiology and Biostatistics, School of Public Health, University of the Witwatersrand, Johannesburg, South Africa

F. Mphande and P. Nyasulu (eds.), *Evaluating Outbreak Potential of Infections in Tropical Climates*, https://doi.org/10.1007/978-981-95-0618-7_9

monkeypox (Mpox), cholera, and Ebola presented devastating outcomes in populations struggling with the impact of the pandemic. These infections remain endemic in some parts of the globe. Although Mpox, cholera and Ebola have a global impact, the WHO African Region remains particularly vulnerable. Insufficient health system preparedness, effects climate change, conflicts, poverty, cultural routines and norms, and epidemic propensity of the diseases remain important aspects to deal with for a better response to the outbreaks. An integrated approach including community education and empowerment are important elements to consider for a better response to outbreaks. This chapter presents a picture on the distribution, transmission, response, and the impact of the response to the outbreaks of the diseases over time and reviews disease outbreaks and their responses during and after the COVID-19 pandemic.

Keywords Outbreaks · Monkeypox (Mpox) · Cholera · Ebolavirus · Transmission · Response to outbreaks · Impact of response

List of Abbreviations

AWD	Acute watery diarrhoea
BVD	Bundibugyo virus disease
CATI	Case Area Targeted Interventions
CFR	Case fatality rate
CORT	Community outbreak response teams
EOC	Emergency Operations Centre
ETU	Ebolavirus disease treatment unit
EVD	Ebola virus disease
IDSR	Integrated Disease Surveillance Response
IPC	Infection prevention and control
LGA	Local government area
MPXV	Monkeypox virus
MVA-BN	Modified Vaccinia Ankara-Bavarian Nordic
NFP	National focal point
OCV	Oral cholera vaccine
PHEIC	Public Health Emergency of International Concern
PoE	Point of entrance
RAT	Rapid assessment tool
RCCE	Risk communication and community engagement
RRT	Rapid response team
SVD	Sudan ebolavirus disease
WASH	Water sanitation and hygiene
WHO AFRO	World Health Organization African regional Office

9.1 General Introduction

Health systems in resource-limited settings generally struggle to prepare for, respond, and sustain disease outbreaks. The COVID-19 pandemic evidently destabilized already fragile health systems further crippling health activities in the affected regions. The pandemic disrupted health service delivery, pressurized others beyond their capacities, and disrupted prevention strategies in many countries. These disruptions posed greater risks of other preventable diseases both endemic and emerging. Outbreaks from some of these diseases including monkeypox (Mpox), cholera, and Ebola were apparent during and post-COVID-19 pandemic, affecting several countries. The outbreaks profoundly influence affected resource-limited countries, leading to considerable morbidity, mortality, and disruption of daily life, healthcare systems, and economies. Children, the elderly, and individuals with pre-existing conditions are disproportionately affected by Ebola, cholera, and Mpox in most cases. Epidemics like Ebola, cholera, and Mpox can adversely affect economies by reducing productivity, interrupting trade, and increasing healthcare costs. Ebola, cholera, and Mpox outbreaks can overwhelm healthcare systems, resulting in a lack of resources and manpower. Ebola, cholera, and Mpox outbreaks have a huge impact on health systems, necessitating intensive surveillance, research, and training to manage outbreaks, enhance diagnosis, and reinforce public health infrastructure.

In resource-limited countries, emerging and re-emerging infectious diseases present a considerable public health danger, with recent outbreaks of cholera, Ebola, and Mpox resulting in severe morbidity and mortality. Ongoing difficulties such as urbanization, accelerated population development, and climate change-induced natural disasters pose a significant risk of cholera epidemics in low- and middle-income countries (LMICs). Flooding can contaminate water sources with Vibrio cholerae and disrupt sanitation systems, creating conducive conditions for disease transmission. The increasing urbanization of environments alters the behaviour of wildlife; urban squirrels display reduced vigilance and flight initiation compared to their rural counterparts, leading to increased interactions between humans and wild animals, which may be a plausible hypothesis for the emergence and re-emergence of infectious diseases such as cholera, Ebola, and Mpox (Olu et al., 2023). Resource-limited health systems affected by these outbreaks, however, took measures to mitigate the impact on the individuals, health personnel, and communities. A picture of the distribution, transmission, the health systems' response, and the impact of the responses are presented in this chapter to help inform health systems and other stakeholders on the use for future preparedness, response, and sustenance against outbreaks. Strengthening surveillance systems, augmenting access to vaccines and treatments, and expanding regional coordination are imperative measures. Furthermore, tailored risk communication must concentrate on vulnerable populations, such as people living with HIV, to improve awareness and diminish transmission rates. Furthermore, the capability of health system response and country-specific health indicators must be considered, especially in non-endemic nations. Most of these outbreaks in various countries have been and are currently managed by local governments, Ministries of Health, public health departments, and international organizations, including the WHO, the Africa Centre for Disease Control and Prevention, and the United States Centers for Disease Control (CDC). Given climate change and the region's susceptibility to infectious diseases, it is crucial to create a strong organization focused on contact tracing, active surveillance, and the enforcement of infection prevention and control measures in both healthcare settings and the community, which are vital for outbreak containment. African governments and stakeholders must acknowledge and address cholera prevention and control through a long-term developmental perspective, utilizing the existing cholera emergency preparedness and response initiatives to enhance the health, water, and sanitation systems of the affected nations (Olu et al., 2023).

9.2 Monkeypox Disease

Monkeypox now known as Mpox is a viral disease caused by the monkeypox virus (MPXV), an enveloped double-stranded DNA virus of the *Orthopoxvirus* genus in the *Poxviridae* family, which includes Variola, Cowpox, Vaccinia, and other viruses. The virus exists as two distinct clades: clade I which is subdivided into subclades Ia and Ib; and clade II which is also divided into subclades IIa and IIb. Monkeypox disease could be severe, manifesting with a characteristic rash and sometimes fever, chills, and lymphadenopathy (CDC, 2024). Historically, Mpox was first isolated in 1958 from Cynomolgus monkeys in Danish research facility in Coppenhagen Denmark (von Magnus et al., 1959). The first human case was reported 12 years later in 1970 from a 9-month-old baby in the Democratic republic of Congo. Due to the proximity with the rain forest region, the disease was mostly reported in West and Central Africa where it is still endemic in some countries up to date (Fine et al., 1988).

Exposure to the disease-causing virus has been linked to contact with animals that are reservoirs for the virus including consumption of such. Several outbreaks have been reported in the past decades. The most notable ones include the 2022 outbreak which spread to many non-endemic countries outside the African continent, with approximately 117, 663 cases reported between 2022 and 2024 (https://www.who.int/emergency/situations/monkeypox-oubreak-2022). Estimation of confirmed cases has been challenging especially in remote communities and some countries due to various limitations (Table 9.1).

Due to the varying healthcare systems, settings, and availability of resources, management of outbreaks in various countries has been varied. The variations in management of the cases and disease outcomes could be attributed to limited public health measures, persistent transmission in endemic areas as well as diversity in the circulating virus. To tackle these challenges, WHO recommends four practical aspects that could assist in combating the spread of the disease. The first recommendation is in the prompt identification of the disease-causing agents. This could

Table 9.1 Challenges and recommendations for the management of MPXV

Challenges	Recommendation
Limited public health measures	- Enhanced surveillance and timely reporting - Targeted vaccinations - Enhanced surveillance and timely response - Public engagement in high-risk areas
Persistent transmission in endemic areas	Cross-border collaboration and resource sharing
Diversity of circulating clades	Strengthen laboratory capacity

Source WHO https://www.afro.who.int/publications/regional-Mpox-bulletin-6-september-2024

be achieved through strengthening laboratory capacity in endemic countries as well as non-endemic countries with limited resources but at high risk of the disease. Secondly, collaboration and resource sharing between countries and within the various regions. This could assist in preparedness and response efforts to combat the disease. Enhanced surveillance is the third important factor which also links well with collaboration. Surveillance both local and cross-border is crucial in timely identification and reporting of outbreaks. Timely identification allows for timely response that could enhance targeted vaccination for affected communities and populations. Community engagement is the final aspect to be considered. Without cooperation from communities, it is difficult to achieve infection prevention and control. The transmission was kept under control within these sites. However, a surge in number of cases was observed prior to the COVID-19 pandemic (WHO, 2024b). These cases were soon followed by a large-scale outbreak, which unfolded across the world, driven by local, in-country transmission within previously unaffected countries. On 23 July 2022, WHO declared the outbreak a Public Health Emergency of International Concern (PHEIC). Health sector response from countries has varied in terms of resilience depending on the quantity and quality of their resources.

9.2.1 Geographical Distribution

Mpox cases have been reported in several WHO regions, including Africa, Americas, Europe, Eastern Mediterranean, South East Asia, and Western Pacific (https://worldhealthorg.shinyapps.io/mpx_global/#sec-clade-export). Prior to the pandemic, MPXV was reported predominantly on the African continent, and the United States was the only country that reported MPXV outside Africa (Brown et al., 2016) (Table 9.2).

Based on phylogenetic analysis, the Mpox virus (MPXV) is divided into two major clades. Clade I which was formerly known as the Congo Basin Clade and Clade II, which was formerly known as the West African Clade (https://www.who.int/news-room/fact-sheets/detail/Mpox). The distribution of the clades varies in the different countries with Clade I reported in Central African Republic and Sudan, while Clade Ib is reported in Angola and East Africa (Kenya, Burundi, Uganda, and United Republic of Tanzania), and in Southern Africa (Zambia). Interestingly, Clade II is

Table 9.2 Countries with confirmed cases of MPXV before the 2022 Global Outbreak

Year	Country
1970	Democratic republic of Congo, Sierra Leone
1971	Sierra Leone, Nigeria
1975–1976	Cameroon
1978	Nigeria
1981	Cote D'ivoire
1984	Central African Republic (CAR)
1987	Gabon
1990	Cameroon
1991	Gabon
2003	United States of America, Congo
2005	Sudan (Now South Sudan)
2010	CAR
2014	Sierra Leone
2015	CAR
2016	CAR
2015 to date	Sporadic outbreaks in Congo and DRC
2022	Global outbreak covering multiple WHO regions

reported in West Africa (Nigeria, Sierra Leone, Benin, Cote D'Ivoire, Ghana) and in North Africa (Morocco). Clade Ia and Ib are circulating in the Democratic Republic of Congo (DRC) and in the Congo while Clade Ia and Clade II are circulating in Cameroon (Table 9.3). As of the year 2025, Clade Ib has been reported in many countries in the WHO region, outside the endemic areas. This has been attributed to sustained human-to-human transmission with travellers spreading the disease across the regions (Vakaniaki et al., 2024).

Cross-border movements and sustained human transmission have been implicated in mixing of the sequences of Clade Ia MPVX circulating within countries in Central Africa. Similarly, Clade Ib circulating in DRC is highly transmissible and has further spread to countries within and outside the African continent, currently being reported as far as Europe, Eastern Mediterranean, South East Asia, Western Pacific, and the Americas (https://worldhealthorg.shinyapps.io/mpx_global/#sec-clade-export).

The current geographical distribution shows Clade I and II in All WHO regions while Clade I is uniquely distributed in the African region and in central African countries (Central African Republic, South Sudan, Republic of the Congo, Democratic Republic of Congo, Angola, Zambia, Zimbabwe, The People's Republic of Tanzania, and Kenya). Cameroon and South Africa have both reported Clade I and Clade II cases while Gabo has reported 2 cases with an unknown clade (https://www.cdc.gov/Mpox/outbreaks/2023/index.html#:~:text=Since%20January%201%2C%202024%2C%20the,and%20more%20than%2065%20deaths.CDC).

Table 9.3 Geographical distribution of MPXV clades between 2021 and 2024

Region	Clade Ia	Clade Ib	Clade II	Clade Ia and Ib	Clade Ia and II
Africa	***Central African Republic*** *(2021–2025)*	Angola *(2024)*	***Nigeria***	***Congo (2025)***	***Cameroon (2024)***
	South Sudan *(2022–2023)*	Zambia *(2025)*	Sierra Leone *(2024)*	***Democratic Republic of Congo*** *(2024, 2025)*	
		Burundi *(2024)*	Benin *(2024)*		
		Kenya *(2024)*	Cote D'Ivoire *(2024)*		
		Uganda *(2024)*	Liberia *(2024)*		
		United Republic of Tanzania *(2025)*	Ghana *(2024)*		
		Congo *(2024, 2025)*	Morroco *(2024)*		
Western Pacific		China *(2025)*			
		Thailand *(2024)*			
		Belgium *(2024)*			
Europe		Sweden *(2024)*			
		United Kingdom *(2024, 2025)*			
		France *(2024)*			
		Germany *(2024, 2025)*			
South East Asia		India *(2024)*			
Eastern Mediterranean		Pakistan *(2024)*			
		Oman *(2024)*			
		Qatar			

(continued)

Table 9.3 (continued)

Region	Clade Ia	Clade Ib	Clade II	Clade Ia and Ib	Clade Ia and II
		United Arab Emirates *(2024)*			
Americas		Brazil *(2024)*			
		United States of America *(2024, 2025)*			

In bold—Endemic Countries
In bold—Endemic Countries and transmission in the last 12 months

MPVX clade I was further divided into Clade Ia and Clade Ib and these have been reported to occur in combination either Clade Ia and Clade Ib as well as Clade Ia and Clade II (Fig. 9.1).

Clade Ia: Confirmed cases of MPXV have been reported in South Sudan post-pandemic between July 2022 and 2023, while CAR had reported cases during the pandemic, since 2021 to date.

Clade Ib: Confirmed case reports have increased post-pandemic between 2023 and October 2024 and have plateaued with sporadic increase in December 2024 and January 2025.

Clade II: Confirmed cases were reported in Nigeria pre- and post-pandemic from 2021 to 2025, while Sierra Leone registered cases between 2021 and 2023. Liberia

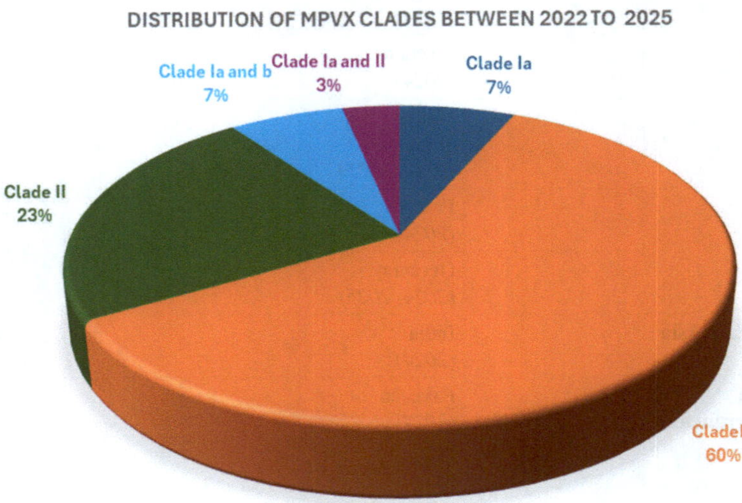

Fig. 9.1 MPXV clade distribution in confirmed cases between 2022 and 2025

registered cases between 2022 and 2025, Cote D'Ivoire between 2024 and 2025, Morocco and Benin 2023, and Ghana from 2022 to 2023.

As of April 2025, active MPVX outbreaks are reported in Central Africa (Central African Republic, South Sudan, Republic of the Congo, Democratic Republic of Congo, Angola, Zambia, Zimbabwe, The People's Republic of Tanzania, and Kenya.

However, even prior to the COVID-19 pandemic, cases of the disease were recorded in non-endemic settings including the United States, the United Kingdom, Denmark, Israel, and some parts of Asia. In the United States, 71 cases were recorded in 2003, two others were recorded in 2021; between 2018 and 2021, 7 cases were reported in the United Kingdom. More cases were reported in the endemic areas. In 2017, 122 cases were confirmed in Nigeria adding to the several cases in outbreaks reported in the Democratic Republic of Congo between 1981 and 2017. As of October 2022, monkeypox was reported from 13 Africa Union (AU) Member States (MS): Benin, Cameroon, Central African Republic, Congo, Democratic Republic of Congo, Egypt, Ghana, Liberia, Morocco, Mozambique, Nigeria, Sudan, and South Africa. Prior to 2022, the following 11 countries had historically reported cases of monkeypox: Benin, Cameroon, Central African Republic, Congo, Côte d'Ivoire, DRC, Gabon, Liberia, Nigeria, Sierra Leone, and South Sudan. Between January and May 2022, the Democratic Republic of Congo was the country that reported the greatest number of suspected monkeypox cases, with 1, 284 cases and 58 deaths reported to WHO.

In July 2022, following consultation of the Emergency Committee convened under the International Health Regulations (IHR, 2005), the WHO Director-General declared the Mpox multicounty outbreak to be a Public Health Emergency of International Concern. In line with the IHR, WHO issued temporary recommendations to support countries and guide a coordinated global response, including global Mpox surveillance guidance. Following this declaration, a global surveillance was put in place.

The African Region contributed 1.2% of the globally reported cases (869 of 73,437) and almost 50% (13 of 29) of the global deaths. The three countries that have reported the highest cumulative number of cases in the region are Nigeria (61%), the Democratic Republic of the Congo (23%), and Ghana (12%). Together, these countries account for 96% of all confirmed cases in the region. More than half (61%) of confirmed cases in the WHO African Region were males, with a median age of 27 years and an interquartile range of 13–36 years. A total of 13 deaths have been reported from the region, from Nigeria (7), Ghana (4), and Cameroon (2).

Furthermore, from 1 January 2022 through 30 November 2023, a cumulative total of 92 783 laboratory-confirmed cases of Mpox, including 171 deaths, were reported to WHO from 116 countries in all six WHO Regions (Table 9.2). A total of 906 new cases were reported in November, which represents a 26% increase compared to the number of new cases reported during the previous month. Most cases in November 2023 were reported from the Region of the Americas (34%) and from the European Region (29%). During the 2022 outbreak, the Americas and Europe recorded the highest number of confirmed cumulative cases compared to Africa, where the disease is endemic in some countries (Fig. 9.2).

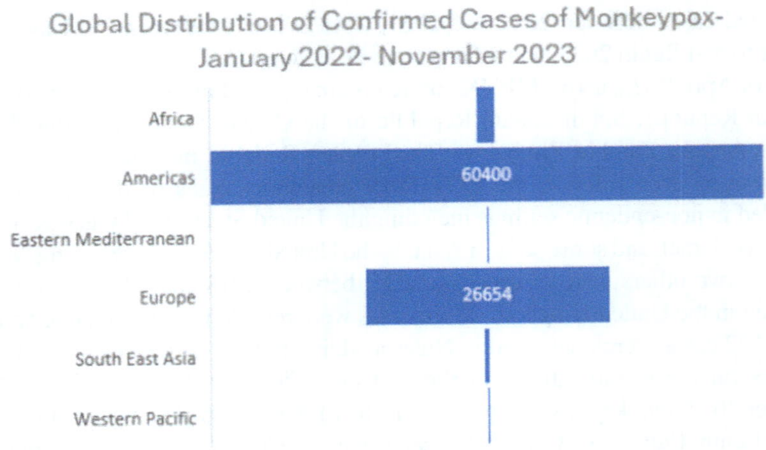

Fig. 9.2 Global distribution of confirmed cases of MPXV during the global outbreak (*Source* WHO, Mpox Multi-country external situation reports no. 38, published 28 September 2024 [WHO, n.d.])

9.2.1.1 Central and East Africa

In Burundi, on 25 July 2024, the Ministry of Health of Burundi declared an outbreak of Mpox following the confirmation of three cases. As of 17 August 2024, there were 545 alerts of Mpox cases since the outbreak declaration, 474 suspected cases (86.9%) were investigated, 358 were tested, 142 (39.7%) tested positive for MPXV and confirmed clade Ib MPXV. No deaths were reported as of 17 August. Males accounted for 55.6% of the cases and females for 44.4%. Children under the age of five years made up 28.9% of the cases, followed by those aged from 11 to 20 years (20.4%), and those aged from 21 to 30 years (18.3%).

In Kenya, on 29 July 2024, the Ministry of Health confirmed a case of Mpox near the border with Tanzania. As of 13 August, a total of 14 suspected cases had been identified, one case had tested positive for MPXV Clade Ib, 12 suspected cases had tested negative. This is the first Mpox case ever identified in Kenya. No deaths were reported as of 13 August.

In Rwanda, on 24 July 2024, IHR National Focal Point (NFP) for Rwanda notified WHO of two laboratory-confirmed Mpox cases in Rwanda, and on 27 July, the Ministry of Health declared an outbreak of Mpox in the country. These are the first confirmed Mpox cases ever identified in Rwanda. As of 7 August 2024, four cases were confirmed through sequencing analysis to be of Clade Ib.

In Uganda, in June and early July 2024, Uganda enhanced surveillance for Mpox disease along the border with the Democratic Republic of the Congo considering reported increasing cases in the neighbouring country. Six suspected cases were identified on 11 July, two of which tested positive for MPXV Clade Ib on 15 July. Investigations revealed that transmission occurred outside Uganda and no secondary transmission has been linked to the two cases as of 12 August 2024. By the same date, 39 suspected cases had been reported. No deaths were reported as of 20 August.

Sudan reported its first monkeypox case from Khartoum State on 22 May 2022. Due to limited testing capacity, in June, fifteen samples were shipped and 14 confirmed positive all clade 1 in a reference laboratory in Germany. In mid-June, PCR test kits were received to facilitate molecular testing. More cases were confirmed over time. Children less than 5 years old were predominantly affected. Epidemiological-linked cases in West and North Darfur reported exposure to animals (wild pigs and squirrels respectively).

In Cameroon, as of 1 January to 30 April 2024, there were 23 suspected cases of Mpox, with five confirmed cases (four males and one female) and two deaths (40% CFR). Genomic sequencing of these cases identified clade II as the responsible variant. Over the years, Cameroon is the only country to have reported both clades I and II MPXV. In 2024 the confirmed MPXV cases were distributed across three regions: Northwest ($n = 2$), Southwest ($n = 2$), and Littoral ($n = 1$). This highlights the potential for regional spread.

In the Republic of Congo, on 23 April 2024, the government declared a national Mpox epidemic. Genomic sequencing of MPXV samples confirmed clade I, like those found in neighbouring Democratic Republic of Congo. From 1 January to 30 May 2024, the Republic of Congo reported 19 confirmed and 10 probable Mpox cases.

9.2.1.2 West Africa

Nigeria and DRC have reported significant number of Mpox cases in the African region. Persistent transmission of Mpox within the countries due to Mpox being endemic in these countries has contributed to the high number of cases (https://www.afro.who.int/publications/regional-Mpox-bulletin-6-september-2024).

In Côte d'Ivoire, in July 2024, two non-fatal cases of Mpox were confirmed. No epidemiological link between these first two cases was identified. As of 7 August 2024, seven Mpox cases had been confirmed in. The country previously reported Mpox, but no cases had been notified since the start of the multi-country outbreak in 2022. The newly detected cases in 2024 belong to clade II MPXV.

In Nigeria, on 26 September 2017, WHO was alerted to a suspected outbreak of monkeypox in Yenagoa Local Government Area (LGA) in Bayelsa State, Nigeria. The index cluster was reported in a family. All of whom developed similar symptoms of fever and generalized skin rash over a period of four weeks. Epidemiological investigations into the cluster showed that all infected cases had a contact with monkey about a month prior to onset. From the onset of the outbreak in September 2017 through 15 September 2018, there were 269 suspected cases including 115 confirmed cases, seven deaths were recorded, four of which were in patients with a pre-existing immunocompromised condition. The most affected age group was 21–40 years and 79% of the confirmed cases were males. In 2018, there were 76 cases reported, 37 confirmed and two deaths. Genetic sequencing suggests multiple introductions of the monkeypox virus (MPXV) into the population with evidence of human-to-human transmission. The isolates were closely related to the West African, Nigerian 1971 strain.

In the Democratic Republic of Congo, on December 2022, the DRC declared a national outbreak of Mpox, and an incident management system was put in place by February 2023, based on the increasing number of reported cases. An outbreak was later reported in the non-endemic South Kivu province, driven by sexual contact transmission, a new variant of clade I MPXV was described. It carries predominantly APOBEC3-type mutations, indicating adaptation of the virus due to circulation among humans. Additionally, the variant carries gene deletions that affect diagnostics in the DRC. In 2024, as of 26 May, a total of 7 851 Mpox cases were reported in the country, including 384 deaths (Case Fatality Rate (CFR) 4.9%).

9.2.1.3 South Africa

From 1 January to 6 June 2024, five confirmed Mpox cases were reported in South Africa, all of whom were men aged between 35 and 39 years old. All five specimens were sequenced and identified to be clade IIb MPXV. Two other cases were reported in Gauteng province, and a cluster of three cases in KwaZulu-Natal province. The cases in these two clusters did not report any international travel history. Four of the five men were initiated into treatment with tecovirimat provided by WHO from the limited reserve for compassionate use, upon request of the Government of South Africa. The severity of all the cases identified in persons with immune suppressions suggests less severe cases are not being identified, tested, or reported.

9.2.2 Transmission and Risk Factors for MPVX

Reports prior to the discovery of human Mpox in 1970 showed a sustained transmission of the virus among animal reservoirs in Central and West Africa (Gessian et al., 2022). Spillovers from 1970 right up to 2017, from sporadic occurrences led to human infections especially in rural communities. Human-to-human transmission occurred and spread to other countries from 2018 to 2021 (Fig. 9.3).

The virus is primarily transmitted from person to person through direct contact with infected lesions and bodily fluids. This can be mainly through close contact with someone who has Mpox, including members of a household. Close contact includes skin-to-skin (such as touching or sex) and mouth-to-mouth or mouth-to-skin contact (such as kissing), and it can also include being face-to-face with someone (such as talking or breathing close to one another, which can generate infectious respiratory droplets) (Fig. 9.3). People with multiple sexual partners are at higher risk of acquiring Mpox. Transmission can also be through contaminated objects such as clothing or linen, needle injuries in health care, or in community settings such as tattoo parlours (WHO, 2024a). During pregnancy or birth, the virus may be passed to the baby. Contracting Mpox during pregnancy can be dangerous for the foetus

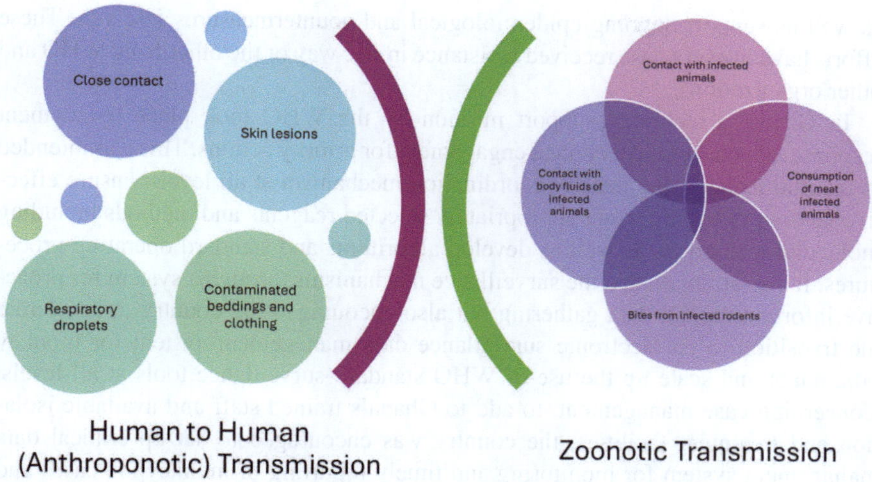

Fig. 9.3 Transmission of MPXV, anthroponotic and zoonotic transmission

or newborn infant and can lead to loss of the pregnancy, stillbirth, death of the newborn, or complications for the parent. A systematic review including 31 articles revealed that Interaction with infected animals, HIV infection, other sexually transmitted infections, unprotected sexual activities, contact with an infected person, identification as men who have sex with men, and having multiple sexual partners were associated with increased Mpox infection risk. Conversely, smallpox vaccination was associated with a significantly reduced risk of Mpox infection (Ugwu et al., 2025). In a study to analyze data from a global surveillance of Mpox cases reported by WHO Member States, through the global surveillance system from 1 January 2022, to 29 January 2023, the findings showed that most of the cases were transmitted via sexual exposure (Schafer et al., 2023). The advent of the clade 1b variant of Mpox has transformed the virus into a global health hazard, forcing the World Health Organization to designate it a public health emergency. Clade 1b is characterized by heightened transmissibility. This type has spread fast from its core in the Democratic Republic of Congo to neighbouring African countries and beyond, with verified cases in Europe and Asia (Ugwu et al., 2025).

9.2.3 *Response to Monkeypox Outbreaks—Success and Challenges*

Public health responses to EVD outbreaks have been activated by countries to coordinate comprehensive case finding, contact tracing, laboratory investigation, supported isolation, clinical management, implementation of infection prevention and control measures, risk communication, community engagement, and vaccination activities, as well as support ongoing epidemiological and countermeasures research. These efforts have in every case received assistance in one way or the other from WHO and other organizations.

In Ghana, a technical support mission by the WHO took place to augment response, advocacy, and technical engagement for priority actions. This was intended to institutionalize "one health" coordination mechanism at all levels, ensure effective laboratory testing using appropriately selected reagents and methods including molecular techniques as well as develop algorithms and standard operating procedures. It also strengthened the surveillance mechanisms through a system for proactive information and data gathering but also encouraged the country to accelerate the transition to an electronic surveillance data management system for monkey pox, adapt and scale up the use of WHO standard surveillance tools at all levels. Concerning case management, to add to Ghana's trained staff and available isolation and treatment facilities, the country was encouraged to set up clinical data management system for monitoring and timely reporting of monkeypox cases and their prevailing co-morbidities; to leverage existing infectious disease centres for COVID-19 to cover other severe clinical syndromes; and to strengthen the capacity at PHC facilities to identify and manage MPX. In the same way, to add to Ghana's existing partnerships for Risk communication and community engagement (RCCE), they were encouraged to use available opportunities to scale up RCCE for monkeypox (e.g. tailoring to high-risk groups).

In Sudan, a total of three joint One Health monkeypox outbreak response missions were carried out by the Federal Ministry of Health to strengthen the monkeypox response in the country. Also, together with the State Ministries a state level monkeypox preparedness and response plans with the technical support of WHO were developed.

In Burundi, the national Emergency Operations Centre (EOC) was activated, with support from WHO, a surveillance system put in place, investigation and testing of suspected cases, and contact tracing for confirmed cases. However, the resources were limited and not sufficient for total surveillance, testing, and isolation of cases. Case management consisted of syndromic treatment of Mpox. RCCE activities were to advise the population on protecting themselves from contracting the disease.

Kenya, Cote D'Ivoire, Rwanda, and Uganda:

Following the confirmation of the Mpox case in Kenya, the Ministry of Health took various response measures, including activation of Public Health emergency operations, establishment of incident management teams, drafting of national Mpox response plan and case management guidelines, and contact tracing of all patients' contacts. Surveillance in all highways was heightened to identify all exposed individuals and any other unidentified cases. Mpox case definition was developed and shared with all counties. Cross-border communication and monitoring was ongoing, and Rapid Response Teams were deployed to support affected counties with detailed investigations. Public sensitization on hygiene, Emergency Hotline Numbers were provided for the public. The Ministry of Health issued advisories to the health workers and the public, risk communication messages were developed and disseminated to the public and at the Points of Entry (PoEs). Similar measures were taken in Cote D'Ivoire, Ruanda, and Uganda. But additionally, Rwanda reinforced RCCE by audio and video spots development on Mpox outbreak. They equally translated Mpox awareness materials at PoEs. Social media assets on Mpox awareness and social media influencer engagement on Mpox awareness were initiated.

In Cameroon, Mpox is a priority disease. The surveillance strategy involves case-based surveillance under the Integrated Disease Surveillance and Response (IDSR) strategy implemented in 2002, with immediate notification of suspected cases. Before the implementation of Mpox surveillance system, only five confirmed cases of human Mpox were documented in Cameroon. Many outbreaks have gone undocumented due to delays in sample collection and submission.

The DRC witnessed continued development of the Mpox outbreak and high incidence in endemic areas with high case fatality. The geographic expansion to previously unaffected areas, the appearance of a novel strain of clade I MPXV, the observed sustained community transmission driven by sexual transmission and other forms of close physical contact in the eastern part of the country, resource constraints to respond over such a wide geographic area, limited public awareness of Mpox, the insufficient availability of treatment kits and lack of vaccines, multiple competing public health priorities, and insecurity are among the challenges faced by intervention efforts there. Based on the situation, WHO assesses that the risk associated with Mpox in the DRC remains high. In the DRC, where the highest number of cases was recorded, in addition to the measures put in place by the other states, the Ministry of Health also carried out some other activities. Clade-specific PCR assays were initiated especially to detect the novel strain of Mpox (MPXV) in the country. A clinical trial was also started to assess the clinical efficacy of tecovirimat for the treatment of patients with Mpox. Following the authorization of temporary use of the vaccines LC16 and MVA-BN vaccines for emergency response by the national immunization technical advisory group, work was also underway to develop vaccination strategies for emergency response and to initiate clinical vaccine studies to address knowledge gaps for Mpox vaccines, including continuing immunogenicity, efficacy, and safety studies. Outbreak response in South Africa included contact-tracing and clinician training. It is important to note that there is extensive travel between South Africa and the Democratic Republic of Congo, linked to commercial and professional activity between the two countries.

The WHO African Regional Office (AFRO) reviewed and expanded the regional incident management support team to ensure that Member States receive the necessary support for managing the Mpox outbreak. A critical meeting held in South Africa discussed urgent measures to address the rising number of Mpox cases. It also proposed a review of the regional risk assessment given the acute situation. WHO engaged in technical coordination meetings with the Africa Centres for Disease Control and Prevention (Africa CDC) to develop a joint Mpox taskforce. Additionally, both organizations agreed on actions to accelerate the operational response, particularly in strengthening the technical working group on vaccines and enhancing cross-border readiness and surveillance. An Infection Prevention and Control (IPC) Rapid Assessment Tool (RAT) for health facilities was developed and disseminated to countries that are experiencing an active outbreak of Mpox, to rapidly assess IPC and WASH capacities to care for Mpox patients safely in health facilities.

9.2.4 *Impact of Interventions*

According to the WHO, interventions like strengthened surveillance, early outbreak detection, community engagement, access to vaccines and diagnostics, and robust infection prevention and control (IPC) measures in healthcare settings have significantly impacted the control of monkeypox outbreaks, helping to mitigate transmission and limit the spread of the virus, particularly by targeting high-risk groups and adapting strategies to local contexts. Some of the impacts recorded include;

- Reductions in sexual partners and contact tracing/isolation which prevented transmission,
- Vaccination's effect varied across areas due to the programmes' timing and coverage, with Mpox infections prevented,
- The ability to recognize monkeypox symptoms and the willingness to take ill family members to the hospital were significantly increased,
- People's self-reported experience of Mpox highlighted the role of stigma and discrimination in increasing the emotional distress produced by the physical symptoms of the illness,
- Temporary adaptations of people's sexual behaviour to manage their risk,
- In contrast, the willingness to deter some high-risk behaviours, such as eating animal carcasses found in the forest, remained fundamentally unchanged.

Monkeypox disease remains endemic in several parts of the globe with the possibility of spreading to non-endemic areas. The spread of the virus is entwined with daily lives and cultural practices. Preparedness and effective combating of the disease require the involvement of communities to ensure acceptability and proper implementation of measures. Efforts to mitigate the dissemination of the current clade 1b Mpox must encompass improved surveillance, prompt diagnosis, and immunization, especially among high-risk groups.

9.3 Cholera

9.3.1 *Introduction*

Cholera is an acute diarrheal infection caused by consuming food or water contaminated with the bacterium *Vibrio cholerae*. There are over 200 serogroups of *Vibrio cholerae*, but only two, O1 and O139, are responsible for most cholera outbreaks. The O1 serogroup has two biotypes: El Tor and classical. Access to safe water, basic sanitation, and hygiene is essential to prevent cholera and other waterborne diseases. Most people with cholera have mild or moderate diarrhoea and can be treated with oral rehydration solution (ORS). However, the disease can progress rapidly, so starting treatment quickly is vital to save lives. Patients with severe disease need intravenous fluids, oral rehydration solutions (ORS), and antibiotics. Countries need strong epidemiological and laboratory surveillance to swiftly detect, monitor outbreaks, and guide responses. Effectively, since 1817 and until now, cholera remains a global challenge to public health and an indicator of inequity and lack of social development (Hassan & Nellums, 2021). Endemic areas continue to suffer outbreaks while the spread continues to non-endemic areas. The disease has remained a serious problem to health systems because of its epidemic propensity and lethality. African countries have suffered several outbreaks with increased incidence and death rates caused probably by health systems overstretched by other health challenges including COVID-19 pandemic.

9.3.2 Geographical Distribution of Cholera Outbreaks

Cholera continues to be endemic globally and a serious challenge even to the most equipped health systems. The first pandemic was recorded in the nineteenth century. Since then, seven pandemics have killed millions of people worldwide. The first six pandemics all seem to have originated in Bangladesh and are thought to be due to the infection of the Classical O1 biotype. The current (seventh) pandemic which started in Indonesia in 1961 continues to affect populations worldwide increasing in burden and spreading to non-endemic areas. It was initially caused by the O1 El Tor biotype; the 0139-biotype appeared in 1992. A cumulative total of 838 315 cases were notified to the WHO during 2004–2008, whereas 676 651 cases were reported during 2000–2004; this represents a 24% increase in the number of cases reported between 2000 and 2004. Climate and other factors that drive cholera transmission are multifaceted and complex. Notably, El Niño, a climate phenomenon characterized by abnormal warming of the Pacific Ocean leading to significant changes in weather conditions worldwide, has been linked to increases in cholera cases. Reduced rainfall due to El Niño can result in water scarcity and insufficient access to clean water sources, forcing vulnerable communities to use contaminated water and reduce proper hygiene practices (handwashing). Meanwhile, heavy rainfall and flooding associated with El Niño can lead to contamination of drinking water sources and disrupt sanitation infrastructures (Makuntima et al., 2023).

During the twentieth century, cholera outbreaks were recorded in Haiti, Yemen, Nigeria, The Democratic Republic of Congo, Dominican Republic, Egypt, Somalia, Bangladesh, Pakistan, the Philippines, China, Ghana, and Cameroon. Just before the COVID-19 pandemic expanded to Europe, cholera outbreaks occurred in Belgium, Chechia, France, Germany, Spain, Sweden, and the United Kingdom. Nine countries from the same continent reported other outbreaks during COVID-19 (2019–2021).

In 2019, a total of 117,167 deaths due to cholera were recorded globally with 92,790 (79.2%) occurring in the WHO African region.

The African region is experiencing high transmission of cholera, particularly in east and southern Africa. Since 2021, there have been recurrent and sometimes prolonged outbreaks that have affected 17 countries. Currently, the main countries of concern are Zambia, Malawi, and Zimbabwe. Democratic Republic of Congo, Ethiopia, Mozambique, and Tanzania are also reporting active outbreaks.

Countries in West, Central, and Southern Africa have witnessed high case fatality rates (2.5%). The affected areas are insecure with limited response capacity. This is worsened by droughts and floods due to El Nino which lead to population displacement and limited access to safe water. The workforce is also overstretched by other health emergencies like COVID-19, Ebola, and Mpox. Countries under monitoring here included Nigeria, Cameroon, Malawi, and The Democratic Republic of Congo. In the horn of Africa, Kenya, Ethiopia, and Somalia have witnessed about 36 million displaced people due to climate changes, increase refugees, and internally displaced people. Kenya has witnessed a second outbreak of cholera since 2022. Ethiopia has recorded increase in cases with high CFR, with fear of spread because of drought and ongoing conflict. Somalia is going through a prolonged outbreak which is aggravated by malnutrition caused by droughts.

In 2023, cholera outbreaks occurred in many countries, including South Africa, Ethiopia, Haiti, and Mozambique. The World Health Organization (WHO) classified the global cholera resurgence as a grade 3 emergency, its highest internal level for emergencies. Worldwide, cholera cases increased by 13% in 2023, from 473 000 in 2022 to more than 535 000 in 2023, according to an epidemiological report by the WHO. The cases were reported in 45 countries, up from 44 in 2022. Kenya, Mozambique, and Ethiopia reported their outbreaks between August and October 2022, while Burundi, Zambia, the United Republic of Tanzania, South Africa, Zimbabwe, and South Sudan reported cholera outbreaks between January and March 2023 (Table 9.4).

Table 9.4 Some cholera outbreaks in Africa before the COVID-19 pandemic

Year	Country
2014	South Sudan
2015	DRC, Tanzania (twice)
2016	Tanzania
2017	Kenya (twice), Zambia
2018	The Democratic Republic of Congo (DRC), Mozambique, The United Republic of Tanzania

9.3.3 Transmission of Cholera

Cholera can be spread by drinking water or eating food contaminated with cholera bacteria, *Vibrio cholerae.* It can spread quickly through the faecal-oral route especially in areas where sewage and drinking water aren't adequately treated. The bacteria can also live in brackish (slightly salty) and coastal waters. Eating raw shellfish like shrimp and crab from contaminated water bodies can be a source of cholera. Large outbreaks are often related to contaminated water supplies or food from street vendors. Increased urbanization causes strain on water and sanitation systems; this can also compromise disposal of human waste and facilitate the spread of the disease. Healthcare personnel treating cholera patients, cholera response workers, and travellers to an area where cholera is present are among those who are easily exposed. In some areas, transmission is enhanced by open defecation, displacement of populations, conflicts that fragilize health systems and natural disasters including floods and droughts. About 1 in 10 people will develop severe symptoms of cholera that can be life-threatening. Cholera can be fatal for up to 50 per cent of people with severe disease. The interaction between *Vibrio cholerae* and phytoplacton and zooplankton blooms due to the confluence of rain and nutrients colonized can potentially act as a vehicle of disease transmission, as in the case of cholera. This hypothesis may be proven by endemic cholera in the African Great Lakes Region (AGLR). These environmental changes, which were observed in Lakes Victoria, Malawi (another African Great Lake, also known as Lake Nyasa), and Tanganyika, could have affected the dynamics of cholera (Bompangue et al., 2011).

9.3.4 Response to Outbreaks

Most health systems are usually overwhelmed by cholera disease outbreaks. In a situation of rapid spread, the strategies and facilities put in place are generally inadequate and will require assistance. This assistance has in many cases come from WHO, UNICEF, International Red Cross, and others. The WHO supports states during outbreaks. The assistance is usually by providing supplies, training, and technical support to countries. It also advocates for improved water and sanitation systems and promotes the use of oral cholera vaccines. To respond to an outbreak, it must be investigated, confirmed, response organized, monitored, do risk communication and community engagement, empower health facilities for case management, and administer oral cholera vaccine.

In the past years, UNICEF has strengthened the use of cholera response teams in various countries (Haiti, Yemen, Zimbabwe, Mozambique, DR Congo). These teams deliver a Case Area Targeted Interventions (CATI) in affected communities which are effective in contributing to reduce the local transmission of cholera. The UNICEF guideline focuses on Community Outbreak Response Teams (CORT) which are different from Rapid Response Teams (RRT), used in the framework of the

Integrated Disease Surveillance Response (IDSR) by Ministry of Health-led teams intervening at the onset of an outbreak by;

- Conducting field investigations to verify and confirm the outbreak.
- Managing cases through surveillance and reporting.
- Exploring possible sources of contamination and identifying risk factors, to assess the risk of the spread and the potential impact of the disease on the community.

The operational guideline and toolkit by UNICEF focus specifically on the activities provided at household and community level once an outbreak has been confirmed. These are mainly water, sanitation, and hygiene (WASH) control measures aiming to limit the spread of the disease in affected households and in surrounding neighbours, also known as Case Area Targeted Interventions (CATI). Thus, a CORT mostly aims to implement a CATI.

However, depending on the context, it can also deliver a case cluster-based intervention, integrate health-related activities, and initiate a wider WASH community response. The model includes the tools and resources required to facilitate the set-up, implementation, training and capacity building, data-collection, analysis and reporting, and monitoring and evaluation for these teams. The CORTs are established and trained teams, usually made up of three to four people from government partners or non-governmental organizations (NGOs). These teams act as an integral part of a national government's alert and response strategy for cholera. As much as possible they should be led by the national government or built on existing outbreak surveillance and response mechanisms, with support from UNICEF when required.

Alternatively, community-based volunteers can be trained and equipped to deliver similar response within their community. Such government leadership and complementarity with civil society and local actors allow for a long-term transition when external funding is limited, and when outbreak ends. CORTs' responsibilities can in some settings include health-related activities, such as oral chemoprophylaxis.

9.3.5 Impact of Interventions on Cholera Transmission

The dynamics of cholera outbreaks are becoming increasingly complex, driven by factors that transcend borders such as mass displacement, natural disasters, civil unrest, military conflict, and climate change. Recent severe floods across Central and West Africa, as well as South East Asia, have intensified cholera transmission, with several countries continuing to report surges in cases.

Cholera is surging globally. While the triggers for cholera outbreaks such as poverty and conflict are enduring, today countries face a growing threat of climate change. Extreme climate events like floods, cyclones, and droughts further reduce the access to clean water and create an ideal environment for cholera to thrive. As of 14 October 2024, the global stockpile of Oral Cholera Vaccine (OCV) is depleted, with no remaining doses available. Although more doses are expected in the coming weeks, this shortage poses significant challenges to outbreak response efforts and hampers efforts to control the spread of the disease.

A Global Review of the various models done by UNICEF in 2019 highlighted the added value of such flexible systems for supporting cholera response and prevention activities in the different countries where it has been used. A series of existing studies and evidence supports the rationale for targeted responses. This is how the CATI model of UNICEF was designed and implemented in outbreak settings in Haiti, Yemen, Zimbabwe, and Mozambique. Evidence proves that early case detection and treatment act as key control measures in reducing cholera incidence and fatality rates. The early establishment and prompt use of CORTs enables a speedy response so that control measures can stay ahead of the epidemic curve. There is also evidence proving the relationship between the relative risk of cholera transmission and proximity of households with confirmed cases. The closer a household to a confirmed case, the greater the chances of being infected.

Some of the strategies for cholera intervention include,

- Promoting handwashing with soap, and treatment of water, can achieve significant protection for the household contacts of cholera patients.
- Early targeted response interventions are more resource efficient than mass interventions against cholera.

From the Haiti cholera outbreak, a systematic review to assess the effectiveness of CATIs was conducted over a three-year period from 1 January 2015 to 31 December 2017 in one administrative department of Haiti, revealed the following outcome key findings:

- The sooner the first correct response was implemented by the response teams, the lower the number of suspected cholera cases.
- The quicker the response by the teams, the shorter the duration of outbreaks.

Emphasize a policy of cholera vaccination in endemic areas, prior to the cholera season.

- This demonstrates that by responding using targeted interventions delivered by specialized teams, it is possible to reduce or contain transmission in households and communities.

Communities should be reminded of basic hygienic behaviours. These include the need to always wash hands with soap after defecation and before handling food or eating, as well as safe preparation and conservation of food. Strengthening surveillance and early warning systems are important measures to allow detection of the first cases in an outbreak and to put in place control measures as quickly as possible.

9.3.6 Conclusion

Although the cholera situation is under control in some areas, the incidence has been seen to rise in some. In December 2024, the WHO African Region reported 19 659 new cholera cases across 14 countries, marking a 67% increase compared with November. During this period, the highest number of cases were from South Sudan (12 897), Ghana, and the Democratic Republic of the Congo (1814). Several predisposing factors such as natural disasters and climate change have continued to fuel the pandemic in the African region. Ongoing conflicts in some countries including Cameroon, Sudan, DRC, and others have made some affected communities inaccessible to response teams. In addition, concurrent health challenges like COVID-19, Ebola, Mpox, measles, wild polio, and other health exigencies as well as poor hygiene, unavailability of safe water, rural–urban migration and cross-border movements have served as driving factors to cholera outbreaks. Animal handlers are susceptible to developing infectious diseases and frequently spread such infections to others. Regular monitoring of these individuals is crucial for averting developing infectious disease outbreaks. To improve early warning systems and emerging infectious disease epidemic identification, proactive animal handler surveillance can be a significant addition to hospital surveillance. Interventions beyond the health sector through engagement with partners across other sectors are vital. The development and implementation of multi-sectoral cholera control plans is a useful mechanism to bring together all relevant sectors and forge lines of communication and coordination that are valuable for cholera control.

9.4 Ebola Virus Disease

9.4.1 Introduction

Ebola virus disease (EVD), formerly known as Ebola haemorrhagic fever, is a severe, usually fatal illness affecting humans and non-human primates. Infection with four of the six known species of the Ebola virus genus causes human illness, respectively named, (Zaire) Ebola virus disease (EVD), Sudan virus disease (SVD), Bundibugyo virus disease (BVD), and Taï Forest virus disease. The disease was originally identified in 1976, when two SVD and EVD outbreaks occurred practically concurrently in South Sudan and near the Ebola River in the Democratic Republic of Congo (DRC). Since then, sporadic outbreaks have occurred in the DRC, Uganda, South Sudan, Congo, and Gabon, with most cases caused by the Zaire ebolavirus, several by Sudan ebolavirus, and two in the DRC by Bundibugyo ebolavirus, resulting in less than 2,500 confirmed cases and mortality rates ranging from 50 to 90% of Ebola patients. Further EVD and SVD outbreaks have been recorded between 2017 and 2022, with two reported in 2022 from the DRC (EVD) and one now continuing in Uganda (SVD).

9.4.2 Geographical Distribution

Ebolavirus was first discovered in 1976, the first Ebolavirus disease (EVD) outbreaks occurred in remote villages in Central Africa, near tropical rainforests. The 2014–2016 outbreak in West Africa has been the largest and most complex outbreak since the discovery. There were more cases and deaths in this outbreak than all others combined. It spread between countries, starting in Guinea then moving across land borders to Sierra Leone and Liberia between December 2013 and June 2016, with over 28,616 suspected cases and 11,310 deaths reported to the World Health Organization. Although outbreaks have been reported in other regions, the African Region has recorded the largest outbreaks with the highest case fatality rates. Some species have been more recurrent in outbreaks than others. Some areas have witnessed outbreaks with different species of viruses. The SVD for instance has been detected in eight outbreaks, five in Uganda in 2000, 2011, twice in 2012 and 2022; and three in Sudan. However, the Zaire ebolavirus has been the most recurrent in outbreaks, detected in outbreaks in the West Africa, central and East Africa. On the other hand, Uganda witnessed Bundibugyo virus outbreaks in 2007 and Zaire Ebola virus outbreaks in 2019 (Table 9.5).

9.4.3 Mode of Transmission

The virus is transmitted to humans from wild animals (such as fruit bats, porcupines, and non-human primates) and then spreads in the human population through direct contact with the blood, secretions, organs, or other bodily fluids of infected people, and with surfaces and materials (e.g. bedding, clothing) contaminated with these fluids. The average EVD case fatality rate is around 50% varying from 25 to 90% in past outbreaks. The incubation period is from 2 to 21 days.

The dynamics of transmission in endemic areas of Africa are different from other regions. In endemic areas especially in forest regions, the drivers of transmission include contact with infected animals especially hunters (enzootic), close personal contact with families, contact of health personnel with patients during care, people attending funerals of infected deceased, and use of contaminated syringes and needles. This is exacerbated by the presence of other disease outbreaks like measles. On the other hand, outbreaks reported elsewhere are mainly due to accidental inoculation from a contaminated needle, contact with animals by laboratory workers, visit to endemic areas, health care workers returning to home country after volunteering in an outbreak.

It can be difficult to clinically distinguish EVD from other infectious diseases such as malaria, typhoid fever, and meningitis. A range of diagnostic tests have been developed to confirm the presence of the virus. Infected people can only spread the disease when they become symptomatic. Symptoms of EVD can be sudden and include fever, fatigue, muscle pain, headache, and sore throat. This is followed by

Table 9.5 Outbreaks of Ebola from 1976 to 2022

Year	Country	Species	Cases	Deaths (%)
1976	United Kingdom	*Zaire ebolavirus*	1	0
	Sudan	*Sudan ebolavirus*	284	151 (53.0)
	DRC	*Zaire ebolavirus*	318	280 (88.0)
1977	DRC	*Zaire ebolavirus*	1	1 (100)
1979	Sudan	*Sudan ebolavirus*	34	22 (65.0)
1989	The Philippines	*Reston ebolavirus* (does not cause illness in humans)	3	0 (0.0)
	USA	*Reston ebolavirus* (does not cause illness in humans)	4 asymptomatic	0 (0.0)
1994	Cote D'Ivoire	*Taï Forest ebolavirus*	1	0 (0.0)
	Gabon	*Zaire ebolavirus*	51	31 (61.0)
1995	DRC	*Zaire ebolavirus*	315	254 (81.0)
1996	Russia	*Zaire ebolavirus*	1	1 (100)
	South Africa	*Zaire ebolavirus*	2	1 (50.0)
	Gabon (fall)	Zaire ebolavirus	60	45 (75.0)
	Gabon (spring)	*Zaire ebolavirus*	31	21 (68.0)
2000	Uganda	*Sudan ebolavirus*	425	224 (53.0)
2001	DRC	*Zaire ebolavirus*	59	44 (75.0)
	Gabon	*Zaire ebolavirus*	65	53 (81)
2003	DRC	*Zaire ebolavirus*	35 (Nov-Dec)	29 (83)
	DRC	*Zaire ebolavirus*	143	128 (89)
2004	Russia	*Zaire ebolavirus*	1	1 (100)
	Sudan	*Sudan ebolavirus*	17	7 (41)
2005	DRC	*Zaire ebolavirus*	12	10 (83)
2007	Uganda	*Bundibugyo ebolavirus1*	131	42 (32)
	DRC	*Zaire ebolavirus*	264	187 (71)
2008	DRC	*Zaire ebolavirus*	32	15 (47)
	Philippines	*Reston ebolavirus* (does not cause illness in humans)	6	0 (0)
2011	Uganda	*Sudan ebolavirus*	1	1 (100)
2012	Uganda	*Sudan ebolavirus*	6	3 (50)
	DRC	*Bundibugyo ebolavirus*	38	13 (34)
	Uganda	*Sudan ebolavirus*	11	4 (36)
2014	DRC	*Zaire ebolavirus*	69	49 (71)
	Guinea, Liberia, Sierra Leone	*Zaire ebolavirus*	28,610	11,308 (39)
	Italy	*Zaire ebolavirus*	1	0 (0)

(continued)

Table 9.5 (continued)

Year	Country	Species	Cases	Deaths (%)
	Mali	*Zaire ebolavirus*	8	6 (75)
	Nigeria	*Zaire ebolavirus*	20	8 (40)
	Senegal	*Zaire ebolavirus*	1	0 (0)
	Spain	*Zaire ebolavirus*	1	0 (0)
	United Kingdom	*Zaire ebolavirus*	1	0 (0)
	USA	*Zaire ebolavirus*	4	1 (25)
2017	DRC	*Zaire ebolavirus*	8	4 (50)
2018	DRC	*Zaire ebolavirus*	3,470	2,287 (66)
	DRC	*Zaire ebolavirus*	54	33 (61)
2020	DRC	*Zaire ebolavirus*	130	55(42.3)
2021	DRC	*Zaire ebolavirus*	11	9 (82)
	DRC	*Zaire ebolavirus*	12	6 (50)
	Guinea	*Zaire ebolavirus*	23	12 (52.2)
2022	Uganda	*Sudan ebolavirus*	164	55 (34)
	DRC	*Zaire ebolavirus*	1	1 (100)
	DRC	*Zaire ebolavirus*	5	5 (100)

Source Izudi and Bajunirwe 2024

vomiting, diarrhoea, rash, symptoms of impaired kidney and liver function, and in some cases internal and external bleeding (e.g. oozing from the gums, blood in the stools). The people at risk of contracting EVD include hunters, healthcare workers, those in close contact with infected people, and those who have direct contact with the bodies of the deceased as part of burial ceremonies.

9.4.4 Response to Outbreaks

Response to Ebolavirus disease requires an integrated response to prevent transmission, treat cases, and ensure epidemiological surveillance and adequate preparedness in the event of a new outbreak.

Prevention of transmission should be targeted at animal to human, human to human in communities and in health facilities. Prevention of animal to human transmission requires education of hunters and other people who contact animals. Prevention in homes and communities is ensured through education of the masses. In some areas, risk communication and health education through community mobilization activities and meetings yield satisfactory results. Radio broadcasts were used to deliver accurate and timely messages to the local population about EVD spread and prevention. At the level of the health facilities, transmission was halted in some cases almost immediately once proper protective measures were taken, such as the use of face masks, gloves, and gowns for healthcare personnel. Factors that helped stop the spread of the Ebola virus and limit the size of some outbreaks included: (1) a high suspicion of haemorrhagic fever by clinical staff at the outset, (2) the correct use of personal protective equipment and barrier methods to protect hospital staff, and (3) the ability to rapidly confirm Ebola virus through laboratory testing in-country.

The management of cases requires supportive care sometimes in Ebola treatment units (ETU). This includes rehydration with oral or intravenous fluids and treatment of specific symptoms which improved survival of Ebola virus disease patients. A range of potential treatments including blood products, immune therapies, and drug therapies are currently being evaluated.

Several international partners have been involved in the response to outbreaks. The Centres for Disease Control (CDC) and the Public Health Agency of Canada (PHAC) provided laboratory support through a field laboratory in Isiro Health Zone, as well as through the CDC/UVRI (Uganda Virus Research Institute) laboratory in Uganda. Teams from international agencies, including CDC, WHO, MSF (Doctors without Borders), and USA, supported the Ministries of Public Health in epidemiological, diagnostic, clinical, and communications efforts to respond to the outbreaks in DRC and elsewhere. The responses sometimes faced challenging logistical obstacles, including the remoteness of the area and limited services. Mobile diagnostic laboratories provided testing of samples in the affected areas. International partners in collaboration with state health personnel coordinated activities and provided technical guidance related to laboratory testing, contact tracing, infection control, border health screening, data management, risk communication and health education, vaccination, and logistics. Identification of cases was sometimes difficult because of weak surveillance and fragile public health infrastructure. Poor infection control measures and strained health care systems also contribute to the devastation of outbreaks.

In the 2018–2020 Ebola outbreak in DRC, the first-ever multi-drug randomized control trial was conducted to evaluate the effectiveness and safety of drugs used in the treatment of Ebola patients under an ethical framework developed in consultation with experts in the field and the DRC. Two monoclonal antibodies (Inmazeb and Ebanga) were approved for the treatment of Zaire ebolavirus (Ebolavirus) infection in adults and children by the US Food and Drug Administration in late 2020. Also, the Ervebo vaccine has been shown to be effective in protecting people from the species Zaire ebolavirus and is recommended by the Strategic Advisory Group of Experts on Immunization as part of a broader set of Ebola outbreak response tools. In December 2020, the vaccine was approved by the US Food and Drug Administration and prequalified by WHO for use in individuals 18 years of age and older (except for pregnant and breastfeeding women) for protection against Ebola virus disease caused by Zaire Ebola virus. In May 2020, the European Medicines Agency recommended granting marketing authorization for a 2-component vaccine called Zabdeno-and-Mvabea for individuals 1 year and older. The vaccine is delivered in 2 doses: Zabdeno is administered first and Mvabea is given approximately 8 weeks later as a second dose. This prophylactic 2-dose regimen is therefore not suitable for an outbreak response where immediate protection is necessary.

Implementing ring vaccination during an outbreak alongside conventional Ebola management strategies. Ring vaccination is effective, operationally efficient, and conserves doses compared to population immunization, making it feasible for teams working in insecure environments (Muyembe et al., 2024).

9.4.5 Impact of Interventions

It is likely that the creation of Ebolavirus Treatment Units (ETU) for isolation of patients reduces the spread of the disease. Opened in Monrovia during the largest West African outbreak, did contribute to reducing transmission and boosting morale. It played a crucial role in treating and isolating patients and likely helped to reduce case fatality rates. It is however important to introduce them early enough.

The use of home hygiene kits to reduce transmission in households was another strategy explored and implemented as an intervention but may have greater utility in rural areas given their limited access to other facilities.

Laboratories provided important information to the ETUs for the diagnosis, isolation, and discharge of their patients and tests confirmed the presence of EVD in new areas. But the impact of the laboratories on transmission was limited in some areas for two important reasons: laboratory capacity was very limited, meaning that testing was not widespread.

Social mobilization and safe burial teams had a significant impact on reducing transmission. Social mobilization activities appeared to be succeeding in changing population knowledge and attitudes towards EVD. This was remarkable and seems to represent the most important aspect of the response. Sometimes, traditional beliefs and the resistance to cremation led to the continuance of unsafe burials in some areas. Efforts to trace the contacts are good but could be hampered by a variety of difficulties. Gaps in the flow of information between case finders, the laboratories, the ETUs, the safe burial teams, and County Health Teams.

The two Zaire Ebola vaccines that have been granted licenses since 2019 and 2020 are only partially effective against the Zaire Ebola virus, which causes the bulk of outbreaks and was developed in response to the worst Ebola epidemic in history, which lasted from 2014 to 2016, in West Africa. Only candidate vaccines are available for the Sudan Ebola virus, and trials in the Ugandan outbreak are being done.

9.5 Conclusion

Globally, the EBV disease CFR is heterogeneous but higher in countries within SSA than those outside. The CFR has declined over the years, climaxing at 76% in 2003 and stabilizing at around 61% between 2014 and 2022. Although new treatments and vaccines for the Zaire virus are emerging, access to these promising interventions remains a challenge. In addition, there is a need to develop similar interventions for other strains; in the absence of such treatments, the health systems' preparedness and rapid response to outbreaks will be crucial to reduce significant morbidity and mortality. It seems likely that interventions had reinforcing effects on each other, but that behaviour changes were the core driver of the epidemic decline. Future efforts to strengthen health systems should focus on building community capabilities and local leadership, and not simply on building more physical infrastructure.

References

Brown, K., & Leggat, P. A. (2016). Human monkeypox: current state of knowledge and implications for the future. *Tropical medicine and infectious disease, 1*(1), 8.https://doi.org/10.3390/tropicalmed1010008

CDC. (2024). https://africacdc.org/news-item/mpox-situation-in-africa/

Fine, P. E. M., Jezek, Z., Grab, B., & Dixon, H. (1988). The transmission potential of monkeypox virus in human populations. *International Journal of Epidemiology, 17*(3), 643–650. https://doi.org/10.1093/ije/17.3.643

Hassan, O. B., & Nellums, L. B. (2021). Cholera during COVID-19: The forgotten threat for forcibly displaced populations. *Eclinical Medicine., 32,* Article 100753. https://doi.org/10.1016/j.eclinm.2021.100753

Izudi, J., & Bajunirwe, F. (2024). Case fatality rate for Ebola disease, 1976–2022: A meta-analysis of global data. *Journal of Infection and Public Health, 17*(1), 25–34. https://doi.org/10.1016/j.jiph.2023.10.020

Laurenson-Schafer, H., Sklenovská, N., Hoxha, A., Kerr, S. M., Ndumbi, P., Fitzner, J., Almiron, M., de Sousa, A. L., Briand, S., Cenciarelli, O., Colombe, S., Doherty, M., Fall, I. S., García-Calavaro, C., Haussig, J. M., Kato, M., Mahamud, A. R., Morgan, O. W., Nabeth, P., Naiene, J, D., Navegantes, W. A., Ogundiran, O., Okot, C., Pebody, R., Matsui, T., Ramírez, H. L.-G., Smallwood, C., Tasigchana, R. F. P., Vaughan, A. M., Williams, G. S., WHO Mpox Surveillance and Analytics team, Mala, P. O., Lewis, R. F., Pavlin, B, I., de Waroux, O. L. P. (2023). Description of the first global outbreak of Mpox: An analysis of global surveillance data. *Lancet Glob Health, 11*(7), e1012–23.

Makuntima, N. T., Bompangue, D., Moore, S., de Richemond, N. M., Vandevelde, T., Mwamba, D., Colwell, R., & Muyembe, J. J. (2023, Dec). Cholera resurgence potentially induced by the consequences of climate in the El Niño phenomenon: An urgent call for strengthened cholera elimination in Africa. *The Pan African Medical Journal, 4*(46), 96. https://doi.org/10.11604/pamj.2023.46.96.42258.PMID:38405090;PMCID:PMC10891368

Nkoko, B. D., Giraudoux, P., Plisnier, P. D., Tinda, A. M., Piarroux, M., Sudre, B., Horion, S., Tamfum, J. -J. M., Ilunga, B. K., & Piarroux, R. (2011, Nov). Dynamics of cholera outbreaks in Great Lakes region of Africa, 1978–2008. *Emerging Infectious Diseases, 17*(11), 2026–2034.

Olu, O. O., Usman, A., Ameda, I. M., Ejiofor, N., Mantchombe, F., Chamla, D., & Nabyonga-Orem, J. (2023, Nov). The Chronic Cholera situation in Africa: Why are African countries unable to Tame the well-known Lion? *Health Serv Insights., 14*(16), 11786329231211964. https://doi.org/10.1177/11786329231211964.PMID:38028119;PMCID:PMC10647958

Ugwu, C. L. J., Bragazzi, N. L., Wu, J., Kong, J. D., Asgary, A., Orbinski, J., & Woldegerima, W. A. (2025, Feb). Risk factors associated with human Mpox infection: A systematic review and meta-analysis. BMJ Glob Health, 10(2), e016937. https://doi.org/10.1136/bmjgh-2024-016937

Vakaniaki, E.H., Kacita, C., Kinganda-Lusamaki, E., O'Toole, Á., Wawina-Bokalanga, T., Mukadi-Bamuleka, D., Amuri-Aziza, A., Malyamungu-Bubala, N., Mweshi-Kumbana, F., Mutimbwa-Mambo, L., Belesi-Siangoli, F., Mujula, Y., Parker, E., Muswamba-Kayembe, P. C., Nundu, S.

S., Lushima, R. S., Makangara-Cigolo, J. C., Mulopo-Mukanya, N., Pukuta-Simbu, E., Akil-Bandali, P., Kavunga, H., Abdramane, O., Brosius, I., Bangwen, E., Vercauteren, K., Sam-Agudu, N. A., Mills, E. J., Tshiani-Mbaya, O., Hoff, N. A., Rimoin, A. W., Hensley, L. E., Kindrachuk, J., Baxter, C., de Oliveira, T., Ayouba, A., Peeters, M., Delaporte, E., Ahuka-Mundeke, S., Mohr, E. L., Sullivan, N. J., Muyembe-Tamfum, J. J., Nachega, J. B., Rambaut, A., Liesenborghs, L., & Mbala-Kingebeni, P. (2024). Sustained human outbreak of a new MPXV clade I lineage in eastern Democratic Republic of the Congo. *Nat Med., 30*, 2791–2795. https://doi.org/10.1038/s41591-024-03130-3

von Magnus, P., Andersen, E. K., Petersen, K. B., & Birch-Andersen, A. (1959). A pox-like disease in cynomolgus monkeys. *Acta Pathologica Et Microbiologica Scandinavica, 46*, 156–176.

WHO—Director-general's statement on the report of the meeting of the IHR 2005 emergency committee regarding the multi-country monkeypox outbreak.

World Health Organization. Global Mpox Trends. (2024a). Regional Mpox Bulletin: September 2024. World Health Organization. Regional office for Africa.

World Health Organization. Regional Office for Africa. (2024b). Monthly regional Cholera Bulletin: December 2024. World Health Organization. Regional office for Africa. https://iris.who.int/handle/10665/380302

Chapter 10
Human Mobility, Migration and Ebola Virus Disease Spread and Response in Resource-Limited Settings in Africa

Mulekya Francis Bwambale, Christine Chawhanda, Fingani Annie Mphande, and Peter Suwirakwenda Nyasulu

Abstract This chapter examines the impact of human mobility and migration on the transmission of Ebola, as well as the lessons learned and best practices in responding to Ebola Virus Disease (EVD) outbreaks. It focuses on cross-border surveillance, risk communication, community engagement, and health systems strengthening in resource-limited settings in Africa. Drawing from both published and grey literature, this chapter discusses how migration and human movement models can provide valuable predictions of EVD invasion in resource-poor settings in Africa, particularly in areas with limited mobility data. In addition, it highlights the challenges encountered during and after the epidemic. The authors conclude by proposing key interventions to enhance community engagement, improve surveillance, develop robust early-warning systems, refine predictive models, and coordinate national, cross-border, and regional public health responses. These measures aim to prevent, detect, and respond effectively to EVD epidemics.

M. F. Bwambale (✉)
School of Public Health, Makerere University, Kampala, Uganda
e-mail: francisbmf@gmail.com

International Organisation for Migration (IOM), Juba, South Sudan

Department of Research and Innovations, Faculty of Public Health, Nursing and Midwifery, Uganda Christian University - Kagando University College, Kasese, Uganda

C. Chawhanda · P. S. Nyasulu
School of Public Health, Faculty of Health Sciences, University of the Witwatersrand, Johannesburg, South Africa

C. Chawhanda
Department of Community and Social Development, Faculty of Social and Behavioural Sciences, University of Zimbabwe, Harare, Zimbabwe

F. A. Mphande
Faculty of Medicine, King Mongkut's Institute of Technology Ladkrabang, Bangkok, Thailand

P. S. Nyasulu
Division of Epidemiology and Biostatistics, Department of Global Health, Faculty of Medicine and Health Sciences, University of Stellenbosch, Cape Town, South Africa

F. Mphande and P. Nyasulu (eds.), *Evaluating Outbreak Potential of Infections in Tropical Climates*, https://doi.org/10.1007/978-981-95-0618-7_10

Abbreviations

PoE Point of entry
PoC Point of contact
EVD Ebola virus disease
CDC Centres for Disease Control and Prevention
DRC Democratic Republic of Congo

> Ebola has exposed the extreme weaknesses of our institutions as governments, countries which are affected were found totally unprepared,
>
> Graça Machel, the widow of former South African President Nelson Mandela, 2014.

10.1 History of Ebola Outbreaks

Ebolaviruses have consistently emerged as a significant public health threat in Africa, with major outbreaks causing high mortality rates and challenging containment efforts across the continent. Ebolaviruses were first described in 1976 near the Ebola River in the Democratic Republic of the Congo (formerly Zaire) (Report of an International Commission, 1978). Since then, ebolaviruses have periodically emerged, infecting individuals in various African countries. Major EVD outbreaks have occurred mainly in West and East Africa, encompassing countries such as South Sudan, DRC, Gabon, Uganda, Guinea, Liberia, Ivory Coast, Sierra Leone, and Nigeria. The EVD outbreak in Guinea, Liberia, and Sierra Leone was unprecedented in its sheer magnitude and the emergence of EBOV outside the Congo basin. The effect of the outbreak is profound; as of March 27, 2016, a total of 28,646 EVD cases and 11,323 deaths had been documented. The most recent Ebola Virus Disease (EVD) outbreaks occurred in Cote d'Ivoire (1994), Uganda (2022), and the Democratic Republic of Congo (2022). Isolated cases have also been documented in South Africa, USA, UK, and Italy. Further details on past EVD outbreaks by country and year can be found on the CDC website, which also includes information on ongoing outbreaks (CDC data https://www.cdc.gov/vhf/ebola/history/distribution-map.html).

It should be noted that Sub-Saharan Africa continues to face significant challenges in controlling EVD, with negligible changes observed in case fatality rates. Zaire ebolavirus, Bundibugyo ebolavirus, and Sudan ebolavirus are the three species responsible for most Ebola disease outbreaks in Africa. Historically, case fatality rates have ranged from 25 to 90%, averaging approximately 50%. For instance, the largest Ebola outbreak in 2000 in Gulu, Uganda associated with Sudan virus, caused 425 cases (224 fatal) (Breman et al., 2016; Towner et al., 2004).

Zaire ebolavirus is the most lethal species, often causing outbreaks in the DRC. This species was linked to the 2014–2016 outbreak in West Africa (Guinea, Liberia,

Sierra Leone), which remains the largest Ebola disease outbreak to date with more than 28,600 cases. In addition, it was associated with the 2018–2020 outbreak in DRC where a few cases were reported in Uganda. Other significant outbreaks of Zaire ebolavirus have resulted in hundreds of cases in DRC and Gabon. Smaller outbreaks of this species have also occurred in the Republic of the Congo and South Africa (Houlihan et al., 2017; Kamorudeen et al., 2020).

Sudan ebolavirus, with a fatality rate of 50 per cent, has caused multiple outbreaks in Uganda and regions near the border between South Sudan and DRC. Bundibugyo ebolavirus, identified in 2007, has been associated with two outbreaks: one in the DRC and the other near the border of DRC and Uganda. Taï Forest ebolavirus was responsible for a single case reported in Côte d'Ivoire in 2014 (Singh et al., 2017). The historical burden of EVD and the ongoing risk of new infections underscore the importance of international collaboration and research to develop preventive measures and robust healthcare systems to mitigate the future occurrence and impacts of this deadly disease.

10.1.1 Ebola Virus and Human Mobility and Threat to Global Security

Human mobility is an important driver of geographic spread of infectious pathogens. However, detailed information about human movements during outbreaks is difficult to obtain and may not be available during future epidemics. Current literature indicates that increased migration and human mobility have the potential to exacerbate the spread of EVD epidemics, posing a threat to global health security (Fig. 10.1).

Beyond migration, factors contributing to the global spread of EVD and other infectious diseases include changes in human behaviour, weak health systems, and changing geographic distributions of disease vectors. In regard to cross-border dynamics, Ebola pandemics pose continuous threats to global health security, with countries having fragile health systems in Africa being particularly vulnerable to emerging infectious diseases. Hence, understanding the migration context of the Ebola epidemic is crucial for reinforcing cross-border surveillance health systems, implementing mitigation measures, and preventing disease importation (Duah et al., 2023). The likelihood of EVD transmission in a location where an infectious individual travels can also be influenced by local factors such as population density and contact patterns. Additionally, increased human mobility through porous borders has been hypothesised to contribute significantly to the severity of past EVD outbreaks (Duah et al., 2023).

The requisite contextual domains such as environmental factors reflect the complexities and levels of awareness that are critical to understanding a human mobility associated with EBV epidemics and applying innovative strategies to improve quality outcomes. Experts note disparities in infrastructure at points of entry/exit, with airports better equipped than ground crossings and seaports. They observed

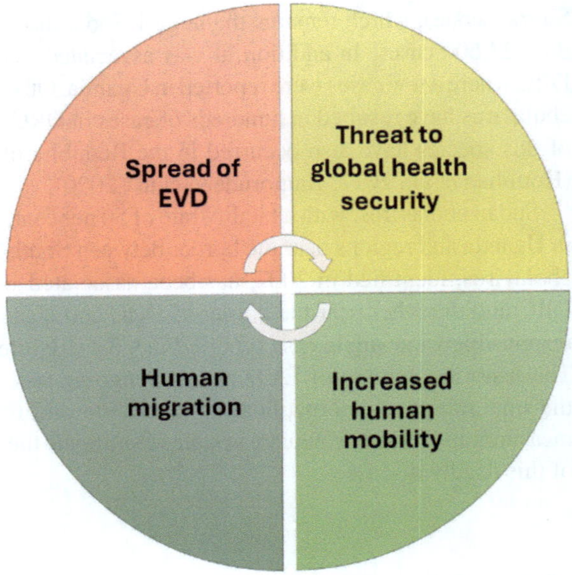

Fig. 10.1 Increased human mobility and migration could pose a threat through the spread of EBV and global security

gaps in risk communication and community engagement at borders. The free movement protocol adds logistical and administrative challenges for health screenings due to language barriers and fake documents among migrants crossing borders (Duah et al., 2023). Past literature suggests factors affecting disease transmission and the complexity of PoE facilities make this consideration important.

10.2 Models for Mitigating Cross-Border Spread of Ebola

Mathematical models of Ebola virus disease dynamics play a crucial role in understanding how new strains of ebolavirus can cross borders, whether through either mutation or the continuous and impulsive immigration of infectives. Current mathematical analysis of the models shows that when the immigration of infectives is continuous, the new strain invades a country if its invasion reproduction number is greater than one. Modelling studies by Djiomba and Nyabadza (2023) suggest that controlled movements by closing borders to stop people across countries that have had Ebola outbreaks are practically impossible (Diane Djiomba Njankou & Nyabadza, 2023).

In a country such as the DRC, which has experienced multiple Ebola outbreaks, scholars have proposed methods to estimate the proportionate volume of travellers that points-of-care (POC) or points-of-entry (PoE) screening measures that can assess based on their location (Duah et al., 2023; Huber et al., 2022). In these studies, a model-based approach has been investigated and applied to mitigate the risk of disease translocation associated with ground-level population mobility during outbreaks (Huber et al., 2022). This research has demonstrated that mobility models and simple spatial techniques can help identify potential locations for health screening at newly placed POCs or existing POEs during public health emergencies, based on expected human movement patterns. While mathematical models provide valuable frameworks for understanding disease dynamics, it is crucial to approach their findings with caution and to consider the broader context of public health, ethical implications, and the complexities of human behavior.

In addition to mathematical models, human behaviour models have been found to explain the link between EVD spread and human mobility. These models provide valuable insights into how human behaviour can influence the transmission of infectious diseases and underscore their significance in formulating and designing control measures (Huber et al., 2022). The studies predominantly used data from Seirra Leone and Liberia. Nevertheless, one of the limitations of these behaviour models is their inability to incorporate human mobility as a modifying or explanatory factor.

10.3 Factors Contributing to Crossborder Spread of Ebola Disease

The spread of Ebola disease remains a pressing public health challenge, driven by various interconnected factors that exacerbate its spread across affected regions. Among the multiple factors contributing to the spread of the Ebola disease, migration and travel are particularly significant. Two possible explanations have been suggested: the international travel of infectious individuals or their contacts, and the movement of people across borders in affected countries (Findlater & Bogoch, 2018). In West Africa, research has highlighted that proximity to transportation networks, particularly lengths of roads and rivers near spillover sites, is correlated with the number of Ebola cases in the first 100 days of an outbreak. Effective and early management and containment efforts along these networks can greatly support in mitigating transmission and spread (Gonzalez et al., 2023). To address this global emergency, the World Health Organization (WHO) and relevant stakeholders have developed a package of interventions aimed to reduce the caseload (number of cases) in affected countries. Consequently, educating the public about preventive measures during travel and ensuring preparedness from authorities can notably mitigate the risk of transmission of Ebola disease transmission across within and international borders (Saurabh & Prateek, 2017).

The challenges posed by weak surveillance systems and poor public health infrastructure have contributed to the difficulty of controlling Ebola outbreak in resource-limited settings, facilitating its quick spread to neighbouring countries. Inadequate surveillance, recognition of suspected cases, and Ebola diagnosis coupled with mobility of human populations and extensive urban transmission, further complicate the situation. In addition, the community's insufficient general understanding about the disease has created an unprecedented opportunity for transmission (Spengler et al., 2016). As a result, these interconnected factors not only exacerbate existing outbreaks but also facilitate the rapid cross-border spread of the virus, amplifying the public health crisis in the region.

10.4 Lessons, Challenges, and Experiences

10.4.1 Challenges in Cross-Border Response

Geography has been found to hinder Ebola virus disease (EVD) response efforts. Porous borders in East and West Africa allow easy cross-border movement, complicating contact training as infected individuals cross undetected (Kaawa-Mafigiri et al., 2021). Poor road infrastructure and the rainy season further hamper transportation of people and supplies, thereby jeopardising effective response and containment of the disease (Office of Inspector General, U.S. Agency for International Development, 2018). The 2014–2016 West Africa EVD epidemic highlighted profound limitations in preparedness and coordination for emerging infectious diseases among national and international responders. The international response to Ebola was poorly coordinated, and the World Health Organization (WHO) delayed releasing an Ebola response plan until the disease spread internationally (Jacobsen et al., 2016). Response teams faced challenges due to inadequate inter-agency structures and processes, leading to unclear roles and coordination difficulties (Office of Inspector General, U.S. Agency for International Development, 2018). This led to difficulties in defining clear responsibilities, and capabilities for the EVD responders.

The fragmented international response to the Ebola outbreak highlights significant shortcomings in global health governance and crisis management. Moreover, the lack of inter-agency structures exacerbated the inefficiencies in responding to the epidemic. This highlights the importance of having well-defined protocols and communication channels in place prior to an outbreak, ensuring that all actors—whether governmental, non-governmental, or international—are aligned in their objectives and understanding of their roles.

In addition, challenges related to preparedness and coordination, disseminating information about the EVD presented several difficulties for both migrants, non-migrants, and responders. In West Africa, incorrect information about Ebola transmission, prevention, and treatment created confusion during the initial phase of the outbreak. The relationship between local populations and international responders is critical during outbreaks of infectious diseases, such as Ebola. As noted in the studies by Jacobsen et al. and Wilkinson and Leach, confusion and lack of clear communication can foster mistrust, complicating efforts to control and manage the outbreak (Jacobsen et al., 2016; Wilkinson & Leach, 2015). This mistrust can lead to increased transmission of the virus, as individuals may be less likely to seek medical help, adhere to health advisories, or cooperate with containment measures.

The recent findings from the Mubende district outbreak in Uganda further reinforce this observation. Kabami et al. and Ninsiima and Lesley et al. illustrate that similar dynamics persisted in this more recent context (Kabami et al., 2024; Ninsiima et al., 2024). The perceived shortcomings of international responses—ranging from cultural insensitivity to inadequate engagement with local communities—contribute to scepticism and resistance towards health interventions. This is particularly concerning in regions where previous responses to health crises may have been viewed as ineffective or exploitative. To mitigate these issues, it is essential for responders to engage local communities in the response process actively. Building trust requires transparent communication, culturally competent care, and the integration of local knowledge and practices into response strategies.

In the United States, frequent updates to CDC guidelines for quarantining travellers instilled fear among migrants and the non-migrants (Gonsalves & Staley, 2014; Jacobsen et al., 2016). International organisations play a key role in devising global health policies, possess extensive medical knowledge, and have the resources needed to respond to global pandemics. As such, they are recognised and trusted by national governments. However, they often lack sufficient understanding of local contexts, which can lead to a lack of trust from citizens. Consequently, gaining trust from local communities, including migration-impacted communities can become a major challenge for Ebola responders. Local responders are often viewed as more relatable and credible, and they may possess a better understanding of the socio-cultural dynamics at play. Collaborative efforts that merge international expertise with local insights can create a more effective and holistic approach to outbreak response.

The presence of language barriers and cultural differences can significantly hinder effective healthcare responses during cross-border epidemics. In the context of Ebola outbreaks, responders from various nations faced substantial challenges in communicating with local communities that spoke different languages and dialects. As highlighted by Richards and UNICEF, these language differences complicated essential activities such as health education, contact tracing, and case management, all of which are crucial for controlling disease transmission (Richards, 2020).

Moreover, cultural practices in West African nations, shaped by deep-rooted traditions and beliefs, presented additional hurdles in executing formal medical protocols. As noted by multiple researchers (Ascuntar, 2020; Kemp, 2020; Mugamba, Nanyondo, & Millard, 2020; Richards et al., 2016; Shin & Yeo, 2020), the isolation of Ebola patients for quarantine or hospitalisation often conflicted with local customs and societal norms. As a result, communities were sometimes resistant to adhering to public health directives, viewing such practices as infringements on personal and communal beliefs rather than necessary health measures. This scenario underscores the importance of incorporating cultural competency into health interventions and ensuring that communication efforts are tailored to suit local contexts.

During Ebola outbreaks, health practices that involve behaviour change have been found to be slow to gain acceptance and faced resistance, as family members can continue to care for the sick loved ones and practice funeral rituals such as washing the deceased. These actions have been identified as major risk factors for community transmission (Ascuntar, 2020; Mugamba et al., 2020; Richards et al., 2016;

Shin & Yeo, 2020). This resistance is attributed to the cultural traditions in which the deceased are believed to become ancestors who protect their families. The practice of isolating sick patients and the deceased from their relatives in an Ebola centre is therefore considered unacceptable.

The intersection of culture, religion, and healthcare is a critical factor in managing public health crises, such as Ebola Virus Disease (EVD). Culture and religion have been found to hinder effective EVD treatment and prevention. For instance, refugees in West African countries often consult faith-healers or traditional healers instead of medical professionals, which perpetuated disease transmission in refugee settlement camps (Shin & Yeo, 2020). This highlights the need for culturally tailored response mechanisms in refugee settings and across border communities.

10.5 Experiences in Cross-Border Ebola Response

10.5.1 Experiences of Migrants

Uncontrolled cross-border population movement has increased vulnerability to Ebola disease spread, complicating contact tracing as infected migrants can cross borders undetected (Breman et al., 2016; Kaawa-Mafigiri et al., 2021). Consequently, migrants have faced stigma and discrimination and have been profiled as disease transmitters, resulting in some migrants being reluctant to disclose their travel history or symptoms (Bedson et al., 2020; Rajapakse & Dixit, 2020; Rwagasore et al., 2023; UNICEF, 2021).

10.5.2 Experiences of Host Communities

Host communities situated near porous borders face heightened exposure risks (Kaawa-Mafigiri et al., 2021). Tailoring public health messages to local languages and addressing cultural practices like funerals enhances community acceptance of the response (Ascuntar, 2020; Kemp, 2020; Mugamba et al, 2020; Richards et al., 2016; Shin & Yeo, 2020). In addition, empowering communities as response partners boosts ownership of containment measures (Bedson et al., 2020).

10.5.3 Experiences of Responders

National and international responders encountered coordination due to differing national response structures and language barriers (Rwagasore et al., 2023). These factors can negate the trust between responders and the population, with cultural sensitivity playing a key role in building community trust over time (Bedson et al., 2020). The safety of responders was a major concern in high-risk border areas with inadequate local infrastructure, as geographical factors hindered effective response (Kaawa-Mafigiri et al., 2021). The Ebola epidemic has highlighted lived experiences specific to both national and cross-border responses among key stakeholders. Therefore, addressing vulnerabilities, cultural competence, and coordinated partnerships has emerged as an important lesson for strengthening future preparedness. Technology remains a useful tool for facilitating data and resource sharing to support national, cross-border, multi-country efforts (Konyndyk, 2019).

10.5.4 Lessons from Cross-Border Ebola Response Experience

The cross-border movement of animal pathogens poses a significant public health risk. About 60% of the emerging infectious diseases, over the past several decades, are zoonotic (Jacobsen et al., 2016). For example, Ebola transmission is linked to bushmeat consumption and bat exposure (Bausch & Schwarz, 2014). Preventing such zoonotic diseases before they are transmitted to humans is critical in controlling the epidemic and requires collaborative efforts on surveillance, reporting, and trade regulation than dwelling on reactive approaches. Proactive surveillance for zoonotic infections and wildlife must be a global public health priority to improve local and international responses to epidemics.

Experience has demonstrated the need of coordinated, multi-country planning and regional action to address cross-border epidemics (Rwagasore et al., 2023; Ryan et al., 2022). Effective cross-border collaboration and regional coordination of preparedness and response efforts to Ebola outbreaks has proved to be crucial in managing cross-border transmission of Ebola outbreaks. This was epitomised by the cross-border collaboration of Uganda, Rwanda, and DRC which facilitated cross-border surveillance, sharing of information, and timely detection of cross-border transmission of the disease (Ryan et al., 2022).

Collaboration between Priority 1 countries (Burundi, Rwanda, South Sudan, and Uganda) and Priority 2 countries (Angola, Tanzania, Zambia, and Kenya) with the DRC enhanced cross-border management of EVD, which could have impacted the health and economic security of neighbouring African countries if not contained (UNICEF, 2021). It was observed that border communities are sites of epidemic transmission as most of them have porous borders, with populations crossing mainly through informal or illegal points of entry/exit, thereby increasing the risk of infectious diseases and other health issues (Kaawa-Mafigiri et al., 2021).

Vulnerability in border communities remains high, and during epidemics, they are often blamed for disease outbreaks (Kaawa-Mafigiri et al., 2021). Public health campaigns should avoid targeting these border communities with blame and hate.

These communities need to be regularly engaged to strengthen cross-border communities in epidemic preparedness. Risk communication must consider their vulnerability, as blanket messaging can lead to information fatigue, especially among vulnerable migrants who face barriers to health-promoting behaviours (Bedson et al., 2020; Kemp, 2020; Rwagasore et al., 2023; UNICEF, 2021).

A recurrent theme identified in the lessons learnt from EVD preparedness and response in countries bordering the DRC EVD outbreaks, as well as from Uganda's experience, is the need for short-term interventions rather than sustainable investments in strengthening systems for health security (Ryan et al., 2022). Joint operational plans, joint surveillance, training, and resource sharing have been found to be effective in harmonising response efforts across international borders. Thus, the lessons learnt from the outbreaks highlight the benefits of EVD preparedness in the countries bordering the DRC, which were at high risk of cross-border transmission during the DRC's recurrent EVD outbreaks. However, conflict and insecurity have been documented as factors that hampered collaboration in South Sudan, particularly around the South Sudan/DRC border. Due to a history of conflict and marginalisation of groups in Uganda, it was recommended not to involve the military in epidemic response as their involvement can be misinterpreted by the majority.

Building trust between communities and responders has been found to be crucial for an effective cross-border Ebola outbreak response (Bedson et al., 2020). Investing time to understanding local contexts and empowering migration-impacted border communities significantly increases acceptance of control measures amidst initial resistance. Addressing misinformation and involving migrants and host communities has been found to be essential in responding to EVD. (Bedson et al, 2020). The role of technology has been highlighted as it facilitated cross-border coordination, especially when travel restrictions limited physical meetings. Teleconferencing often enabled regular communication and strategy reviews across borders (Konyndyk, 2019). Tools such as Epi Info supported joint data collection, analysis, and response planning across agencies from different countries. Community involvement is critical in building trust and fostering a sense of ownership when responding to EVD, (Bedson et al, 2020; Mafigiri & Schmidt-Sane, 2019).

Measures such as contact tracing, safe burials, and border screening proved more effective when communities comprehended their role in limiting cross-border transmission rather than perceiving it as an external imposition (National Ebola Response Centre, 2019). The Ebola epidemic has underscored the necessity for integrated, cross-border public health responses to address challenges posed by human mobility.

During the Ebola epidemic in West Africa, it became evident that survivors experience ongoing mental and psychological health issues. Comprehensive support is essential for addressing the medical and psychosocial challenges encountered by Ebola survivors. In addition, regular monitoring and assistance are necessary to reduce the risk of further Ebola transmission (McPake et al., 2015; Spengler et al., 2016) (http://www.who.int/csr/disease/ebola/one-year-report/introduction/en/). One key takeaway from West Africa was that disease outbreaks often progress more quickly than the funds allocated to respond to them, necessitating the need of establishing rapid response funding mechanism to ensure immediate availability of funding to jump-start outbreak response initiatives.

The Ugandan experiences of 2000/2001 and 2023 demonstrate that responses to an Ebola outbreak can be significant, but potentially disproportionate to the actual danger presented. A key objective for any future outbreak control strategy should be to prevent excessive fear, which is expected to reduce stigma and other negative outcomes. In this regard, the importance of transparency in the provision of public information, and critically, being perceived as transparent, cannot be overemphasised (Kinsman, 2012).

In conclusion, the interplay of human mobility and migration is critical in understanding the transmission dynamics of Ebola disease in resource-limited settings across Africa. The historical context of EVD outbreaks reveals deep-seated inadequacies in public health infrastructure, which must be urgently addressed to enhance epidemic preparedness. The experiences and lessons drawn from past experiences underscore the importance of fostering partnerships between border communities, governments, and international organizations to create a cohesive and adaptive response framework. A unified, trust-based response and robust cross border health system is essential for protecting public health and community resilience against future EVD outbreaks and other infectious diseases.

References

Ascuntar, M. (2020). Community first: The key to stopping the Ebola epidemic—Humanitarian Practice Network. *Humanitarian Practice Network*. Retrieved from https://odihpn.org/publication/community-first-the-key-to-stopping-the-ebola-epidemic/

Bausch, D. G., & Schwarz, L. (2014). Outbreak of Ebola virus disease in Guinea: Where ecology meets economy. *PLOS Neglected Tropical Diseases, 8*(7), Article e3056. https://doi.org/10.1371/JOURNAL.PNTD.0003056

Bedson, J., Jalloh, M. F., Pedi, D., Bah, S., Owen, K., Oniba, A., & Hébert-Dufresne, L. (2020). Community engagement in outbreak response: Lessons from the 2014–2016 Ebola outbreak in Sierra Leone. *BMJ Global Health, 5*(8). https://doi.org/10.1136/BMJGH-2019-002145

Breman, J. G., Heymann, D. L., Lloyd, G., McCormick, J. B., Miatudila, M., Murphy, F. A., & Johnson, K. M. (2016). Discovery and description of Ebola Zaire virus in 1976 and relevance to the West African epidemic during 2013–2016. *The Journal of Infectious Diseases, 214*(Suppl 3), S93. https://doi.org/10.1093/INFDIS/JIW207

Cohen, N. J. (2016). Travel and border health measures to prevent the international spread of Ebola. *MMWR Supplements, 65*.

Diane Djiomba Njankou, S., & Nyabadza, F. (2023). Modeling the potential influence of economic migration on Ebola virus disease transmission dynamics. *Frontiers in Applied Mathematics and Statistics, 9*. https://doi.org/10.3389/fams.2023.1024571

Duah, J. K., Dotun-Olujinmi, O., Johnson, J. A., & Greenhill, R. G. (2023). Points of entry dynamics: Understanding the cross-border threats for Ebola virus disease and COVID-19 in Ghana using a logic model approach. *Journal of Public Health in Africa, 14*(4), 7. https://doi.org/10.4081/jphia.2023.2264

Findlater, A., & Bogoch, I. I. (2018). Human mobility and the global spread of infectious diseases: A focus on air travel. *Trends in Parasitology, 34*(9), 772–783.

Gonsalves, G., & Staley, P. (2014). Panic, paranoia, and public health—The AIDS epidemic's lessons for Ebola. *New England Journal of Medicine, 371*(25), 2348–2349. https://doi.org/10.1056/NEJMP1413425/SUPPL_FILE/NEJMP1413425_DISCLOSURES.PDF

Gonzalez, A., Nikparvar, B., Matson, M. J., Seifert, S. N., Ross, H. D., Munster, V., & Bharti, N. (2023). Human movement and transmission dynamics early in Ebola outbreaks. *MedRxiv*. https://doi.org/10.1101/2023.12.18.23300175

Houlihan, C. F., McGowan, C. R., Dicks, S., Baguelin, M., Moore, D. A. J., Mabey, D., & Glynn, J. R. (2017). Ebola exposure, illness experience, and Ebola antibody prevalence in international responders to the West African Ebola epidemic 2014–2016: A cross-sectional study. *PLOS Medicine, 14*(5), Article e1002300. https://doi.org/10.1371/JOURNAL.PMED.1002300

Huber, C., Watts, A., Thomas-Bachli, A., McIntyre, E., Tuite, A., Khan, K., & Merrill, R. D. (2022). Using spatial and population mobility models to inform outbreak response approaches in the Ebola affected area, Democratic Republic of the Congo, 2018–2020. *Spatial and Spatio-Temporal Epidemiology, 44*, Article 100558. https://doi.org/10.1016/J.SSTE.2022.100558

Jacobsen, K. H., Aguirre, A. A., Bailey, C. L., Baranova, A. V., Crooks, A. T., Croitoru, A., & Agouris, P. (2016). Lessons from the Ebola outbreak: Action items for emerging infectious disease preparedness and response. *EcoHealth, 13*(1), 200–212. https://doi.org/10.1007/s10393-016-1100-5

Kaawa-Mafigiri, D., Kato, F., & Schmidt-Sane, M. (2021). *TDDA briefing key considerations for epidemic response and preparedness in uganda tackling deadly diseases in Africa: Key considerations for epidemic response and preparedness in Uganda.*

Kabami, Z., Ario, A. R., Harris, J. R., Ninsiima, M., Ahirirwe, S. R., Ocero, J. R. A., & Nabadda, S. (2024). Ebola disease outbreak caused by the Sudan virus in Uganda, 2022: A descriptive epidemiological study. *The Lancet Global Health, 12*(10), e1684–e1692. https://doi.org/10.1016/S2214-109X(24)00260-2

Kamorudeen, R. T., Adedokun, K. A., & Olarinmoye, A. O. (2020). Ebola outbreak in West Africa, 2014–2016: Epidemic timeline, differential diagnoses, determining factors, and lessons for future response. *Journal of Infection and Public Health, 13*(7), 956–962. https://doi.org/10.1016/j.jiph.2020.03.014

Kemp, E. (2020). *Humanitarian exchange special feature responding to Ebola in the Democratic Republic of Congo 02 | Responding to Ebola in the Democratic Republic of Congo*. www.elrha.org/r2hc.

Kinsman, J. (2012). "A time of fear": Local, national, and international responses to a large Ebola outbreak in Uganda. *Globalization and Health, 8*(1), 1–12. https://doi.org/10.1186/1744-8603-8-15/FIG.S/2

Konyndyk, J. (2019). *Struggling with scale: Ebola's lessons for the next pandemic CGD BRIEF*. https://www.unicef.org/esa/sanitation-and-hygiene

Mafigiri, D. K., & Schmidt-Sane, M. (2019). Strengthening community linkages to Ebola virus disease (EVD) outbreak preparedness in Uganda.

McPake, B., Witter, S., Ssali, S., Wurie, H., Namakula, J., & Ssengooba, F. (2015). Ebola in the context of conflict affected states and health systems: Case studies of Northern Uganda and Sierra Leone. *Conflict and Health, 9*(1), 1–9. https://doi.org/10.1186/S13031-015-0052-7/TABLES/1

Mugamba, S., Nanyondo, J., & Millard, M. (2020). *Community engagement: The key to successful Ebola research*. https://odihpn.org/publication/community-engagement-the-key-to-successful-ebola-research/

Ninsiima, L. R., Mor, S. M., Romano, J. S., Namakula, L. N., Kankya, C., Kungu, J., & Nyakarahuka, L. (2024). Perceived drivers of the Ebola virus disease outbreak in Mubende and Kassanda districts, Uganda: A qualitative study. *BMJ Public Health, 2*(2), Article e001267. https://doi.org/10.1136/BMJPH-2024-001267

Rajapakse, N., & Dixit, D. (2020). Human and novel coronavirus infections in children: A review. *Paediatrics and International Child Health, 1–20*,. https://doi.org/10.1080/20469047.2020.1781356

Richards, F. O., Klein, R. E., de León, O., Mendizábal-Cabrera, R., Morales, A. L., Cama, V., & Rizzo, N. (2016). A Knowledge, attitudes and practices survey conducted three years after halting ivermectin mass treatment for onchocerciasis in Guatemala. *PLoS Neglected Tropical Diseases*. https://doi.org/10.1371/journal.pntd.0004777

Richards, P. (2020). Ebola and COVID-19 in Sierra Leone: Comparative lessons of epidemics for society. *Journal of Global History, 15*(3), 493–507. https://doi.org/10.1017/S1740022820000303

Rwagasore, E., Nsekuye, O., El-Khatib, Z., Kabeja, A., Mucunguzi, V. H., Nizeyimana, P., & Muvunyi, C. M. (2023). Lessons learned from Sudan Ebola virus disease (SUDV) preparedness in Rwanda: A comprehensive review and way forward. *Journal of Epidemiology and Global Health, 13*(3), 528–538. https://doi.org/10.1007/S44197-023-00133-0/FIG.S/6

Ryan, C. S., Belizaire, M. R. D., Nanyunja, M., Olu, O. O., Ahmed, Y. A., Latt, A., & Talisuna, A. O. (2022). Sustainable strategies for Ebola virus disease outbreak preparedness in Africa: A case study on lessons learnt in countries neighbouring the Democratic Republic of the Congo. *Infectious Diseases of Poverty, 11*(1). https://doi.org/10.1186/S40249-022-01040-5,

Saurabh, S., & Prateek, S. (2017). Role of contact tracing in containing the 2014 Ebola outbreak: A review. *African Health Sciences, 17*(1), 225–236. https://doi.org/10.4314/ahs.v17i1.28

Shin, Y. A., & Yeo, J. (2020). Response to Ebola Virus outbreak in a refugee camp. In *Cultural competency for emergency and crisis management* (pp. 197–209). https://doi.org/10.4324/9780367321888-14

Singh, R. K., Dhama, K., Malik, Y. S., Ramakrishnan, M. A., Karthik, K., Khandia, R., ... & Joshi, S. K. (2017). Ebola virus–Epidemiology, diagnosis, and control: Threat to humans, lessons learnt, and preparedness plans–An update on its 40 year's journey. *Veterinary Quarterly, 37*(1), 98–135.

Spengler, J. R., Estrada-Peña, A., Garrison, A. R., Schmaljohn, C., Spiropoulou, C. F., Bergeron, É., & Bente, D. A. (2016). A chronological review of experimental infection studies of the role of wild animals and livestock in the maintenance and transmission of Crimean-Congo hemorrhagic fever virus. *Antiviral Research, 135*, 31–47. https://doi.org/10.1016/j.antiviral.2016.09.013

Towner, J. S., Rollin, P. E., Bausch, D. G., Sanchez, A., Crary, S. M., Vincent, M., & Nichol, S. T. (2004). Rapid diagnosis of Ebola hemorrhagic fever by reverse transcription-PCR in an outbreak setting and assessment of patient viral load as a predictor of outcome. *Journal of Virology, 78*(8), 4330–4341. https://doi.org/10.1128/JVI.78.8.4330-4341.2004

UNICEF. (2021). UNICEF eastern and southern Africa. In *Sanitation and hygiene* (p. 11). https://www.unicef.org/esa/reports/ebola-virus-disease

Wilkinson, A., & Leach, M. (2015). Briefing: Ebola–myths, realities, and structural violence. *African Affairs, 114*(454), 136–148. https://doi.org/10.1093/AFRAF/ADU080

Bibliography

Chapter 1

Abela-Ridder, B., Knopf, L., Martin, S., Taylor, L., Torres, G., & De Balogh, K. (2016). 2016: The beginning of the end of rabies? *The Lancet. Global Health, 4*(11), e780–e781. https://doi.org/10.1016/S2214-109X(16)30245-5

Acharya, K. P., Acharya, N., Phuyal, S., Upadhyaya, M., & Lasee, S. (2020). One-health approach: A best possible way to control rabies. *One Health (Amsterdam, Netherlands), 10*, 100161. https://doi.org/10.1016/j.onehlt.2020.100161

Akinsulie, O. C., Adebowale, O. O., Adesola, R. O., Banwo, O. G., Idris, I., Ogunleye, S. C., Fasakin, O., Bakre, A., Oladapo, I. P., Aliyu, V. A., Waniwa, E. O., Fasiku, O., Joshi, M., & Olorunshola, M. (2024). Holistic application of the one health approach in the prevention and control of rabies: Plausible steps towards achieving the 2030 vision in Africa. *One Health Outlook, 6*(1), 22. https://doi.org/10.1186/s42522-024-00108-6

Amani, A., Abela, B., Biey, J., Traore, T., & Impouma, B. (2024). Accelerating rabies elimination in Africa by 2030. *Lancet (London, England)*. https://doi.org/10.1016/S0140-6736(24)02141-X

Aptriana, C. D., Sudarnika, E., Basri, C., Indrawan, D., Daryono, J., & Suseno, P. P. (2024). Assessment of the burden of rabies in one health approach control program in Ketapang District Indonesia: Using zDALY. *Preventive Medicine Reports, 45*, 102838. https://doi.org/10.1016/j.pmedr.2024.102838

Ashwini, M. A., Pattanaik, A., & Mani, R. S. (2024). Recent updates on laboratory diagnosis of rabies. *The Indian Journal of Medical Research, 159*(1), 48–61. https://doi.org/10.4103/ijmr.ijmr_131_23

Athingo, R., Tenzin, T., Shilongo, A., Hikufe, E., Shoombe, K. K., Khaiseb, S., van der Westhuizen, J., Letshwenyo, M., Torres, G., & Mettenleiter, T. C. (2020). Fighting dog-mediated rabies in Namibia—Implementation of a rabies elimination program in the Northern communal areas. *Tropical Medicine and Infectious Disease, 5*(1), 12.

Ben Nasrallah, C., Abroug, H., Ghoul, M., Grira, S., Ben Fredj, M., Kacem, M., Dhouib, W., Zemni, I., Bouanene, I., & Belguith Sriha, A. (2024). Rabies epidemiology in the central of Tunisia: A call for a one-health approach. *European Journal of Public Health, 34*(Supplement_3), ckae144–1081.

CDC. (2024). *Information for diagnostic laboratories*. https://www.cdc.gov/rabies/php/laboratories/diagnostic.html

CDC-Africa. (2023). *World Rabies Day 2023 Campaign: "All for 1 One Health for All."* https://africacdc.org/news-item/world-rabies-day-2023-campaign-all-for-1-one-health-for-all/

F. Mphande and P. Nyasulu (eds.), *Evaluating Outbreak Potential of Infections in Tropical Climates*, https://doi.org/10.1007/978-981-95-0618-7

Coetzer, A., Sabeta, C. T., Markotter, W., Rupprecht, C. E., & Nel, L. H. (2014). Comparison of biotinylated monoclonal and polyclonal antibodies in an evaluation of a direct rapid immunohistochemical test for the routine diagnosis of rabies in southern Africa. *PLoS Neglected Tropical Diseases, 8*(9), e3189. https://doi.org/10.1371/journal.pntd.0003189

da Costa, I. A., Gatambire, A. C., Tivane, A. R., Chicanequisso, M. V., Chilengue, I., Ali, S., Rossetto, É., Baltazar, C., Chongo, I., & Inlamea, O. F. (2023). Evaluation of rabies surveillance system using the one health approach-Mozambique, 2020–2021. *American Journal of Field Epidemiology, 1*(4 (Supplement)), S20–S20.

Dürr, S., Naïssengar, S., Mindekem, R., Diguimbye, C., Niezgoda, M., Kuzmin, I., Rupprecht, C. E., & Zinsstag, J. (2008). Rabies diagnosis for developing countries. *PLoS Neglected Tropical Diseases, 2*(3), e206. https://doi.org/10.1371/journal.pntd.0000206

FAO. (2024). *One health approach to rabies*. https://www.fao.org/one-health/areas-of-work/rabies/en

Fooks, A. R., Banyard, A. C., Horton, D. L., Johnson, N., McElhinney, L. M., & Jackson, A. C. (2014). Current status of rabies and prospects for elimination. *Lancet (London, England), 384*(9951), 1389–1399. https://doi.org/10.1016/S0140-6736(13)62707-5

Franka, R., Smith, T. G., Dyer, J. L., Wu, X., Niezgoda, M., & Rupprecht, C. E. (2013). Current and future tools for global canine rabies elimination. *Antiviral Research, 100*(1), 220–225. https://doi.org/10.1016/j.antiviral.2013.07.004

Freuling, C. M., van der Westhuizen, J., Khaiseb, S., Tenzin, T., & Müller, T. (2023). From field tests to molecular tools—Evaluating diagnostic tests to improve rabies surveillance in Namibia. *Viruses, 15*(2), 371.

Hampson, K., Coudeville, L., Lembo, T., Sambo, M., Kieffer, A., Attlan, M., Barrat, J., Blanton, J. D., Briggs, D. J., Cleaveland, S., Costa, P., Freuling, C. M., Hiby, E., Knopf, L., Leanes, F., Meslin, F.-X., Metlin, A., Miranda, M. E., Müller, T., … Dushoff, J. (2015). Correction: Estimating the global burden of endemic canine rabies. *PLoS Neglected Tropical Diseases, 9*(5), e0003786. https://doi.org/10.1371/journal.pntd.0003786

Haselbeck, A. H., Rietmann, S., Tadesse, B. T., Kling, K., Kaschubat-Dieudonné, M. E., Marks, F., Wetzker, W., & Thöne-Reineke, C. (2021). Challenges to the fight against rabies-the landscape of policy and prevention strategies in Africa. *International Journal of Environmental Research and Public Health, 18*(4). https://doi.org/10.3390/ijerph18041736

Hobbs, E. C., Colling, A., Gurung, R. B., & Allen, J. (2021). The potential of diagnostic point-of-care tests (POCTs) for infectious and zoonotic animal diseases in developing countries: Technical, regulatory and sociocultural considerations. *Transboundary and Emerging Diseases, 68*(4), 1835–1849. https://doi.org/10.1111/tbed.13880

Kardjadj, M., & Ben-Mahdi, M. H. (2019). Epidemiology of dog-mediated zoonotic diseases in Algeria: A one health control approach. *New Microbes and New Infections, 28*, 17–20. https://doi.org/10.1016/j.nmni.2019.01.001

Léchenne, M., Naïssengar, K., Lepelletier, A., Alfaroukh, I. O., Bourhy, H., Zinsstag, J., & Dacheux, L. (2016). Validation of a rapid rabies diagnostic tool for field surveillance in developing countries. *PLoS Neglected Tropical Diseases, 10*(10), e0005010. https://doi.org/10.1371/journal.pntd.0005010

Léchenne, M., Traore, A., Hattendorf, J., Kallo, V., Oussiguere, A., Tetchi, M., Moyengar, R., Traore, A. K., Moto, D. D., & Ngandolo, R. (2021). Increasing rabies data availability: The example of a one health research project in Chad, Côte d'Ivoire and Mali. *Acta Tropica, 215*, 105808.

Lembo, T., Niezgoda, M., Velasco-Villa, A., Cleaveland, S., Ernest, E., & Rupprecht, C. E. (2006). Evaluation of a direct, rapid immunohistochemical test for rabies diagnosis. *Emerging Infectious Diseases, 12*(2), 310.

Mani, R. S., & Madhusudana, S. N. (2013). Laboratory diagnosis of human rabies: Recent advances. *The Scientific World Journal, 2013*(1), 569712.

Mani, R. S., & Willoughby, R. E. (2017). Human rabies in South Asia. In S. K. Singh (Ed.), *Neglected tropical diseases—South Asia* (pp. 349–371). Springer International Publishing. https://doi.org/10.1007/978-3-319-68493-2

Marston, D. A., Jennings, D. L., MacLaren, N. C., Dorey-Robinson, D., Fooks, A. R., Banyard, A. C., & McElhinney, L. M. (Directors). (2019, July 10). *Pan-lyssavirus real time RT-PCR for rabies diagnosis* (Issue 149) [Video recording]. https://doi.org/10.3791/59709

Minghui, R., Stone, M., Semedo, M. H., & Nel, L. (2018). New global strategic plan to eliminate dog-mediated rabies by 2030. *The Lancet. Global Health, 6*(8), e828–e829. https://doi.org/10.1016/S2214-109X(18)30302-4

Müller, T., Demetriou, P., Moynagh, J., Cliquet, F., Fooks, A. R., Conraths, F. J., Mettenleiter, T. C., & Freuling, C. M. (2012). Rabies elimination in Europe: A success story. In *Rabies Control: Towards Sustainable Prevention at the Source, Compendium of the OIE Global Conference on Rabies Control, Incheon-Seoul, 7–9 September 2011, Republic of Korea* (pp. 31–44).

Nel, L. H. (2013). Discrepancies in data reporting for rabies, Africa. *Emerging Infectious Diseases, 19*(4), 529–533. https://doi.org/10.3201/eid1904.120185

Nel, L. H., & Rupprecht, C. E. (2007). Emergence of lyssaviruses in the old world: The case of Africa. *Current Topics in Microbiology and Immunology, 315*, 161–193. https://doi.org/10.1007/978-3-540-70962-6

Nyasulu, P. S., Weyer, J., Tschopp, R., Mihret, A., Aseffa, A., Nuvor, S. V., Tamuzi, J. L., Nyakarahuka, L., Helegbe, G. K., Ntinginya, N. E., Gebreyesus, M. T., Doumbia, S., Busse, R., & Drosten, C. (2021). Rabies mortality and morbidity associated with animal bites in Africa: A case for integrated rabies disease surveillance, prevention and control: A scoping review. *BMJ Open, 11*(12), e048551. https://doi.org/10.1136/bmjopen-2020-048551

Otu, A., Effa, E., Meseko, C., Cadmus, S., Ochu, C., Athingo, R., Namisango, E., Ogoina, D., Okonofua, F., & Ebenso, B. (2021). Africa needs to prioritize one health approaches that focus on the environment, animal health and human health. *Nature Medicine, 27*(6), 943–946. https://doi.org/10.1038/s41591-021-01375-w

Patrick, E. M., Bjorklund, B. M., Kirby, J. D., Nelson, K. M., Chipman, R. B., & Rupprecht, C. E. (2019). Enhanced rabies surveillance using a direct rapid immunohistochemical test. *JoVE, 146*, e59416. https://doi.org/10.3791/59416

Shafaati, M., Akbarpour, S., Saied, A. A., & Choudhary, O. P. (2023). Tackling rabies by one health approach: Pitfalls on the road to global eradication. *New Microbes and New Infections, 52*, 101098. https://doi.org/10.1016/j.nmni.2023.101098

Sheikh, K. A., Ramos-Alvarez, M., Jackson, A. C., Li, C. Y., Asbury, A. K., & Griffin, J. W. (2005). Overlap of pathology in paralytic rabies and axonal Guillain-Barré syndrome. *Annals of Neurology, 57*(5), 768–772. https://doi.org/10.1002/ana.20482

Sreenivasan, N., Li, A., Shiferaw, M., Tran, C. H., Wallace, R., Blanton, J., Knopf, L., Abela-Ridder, B., & Hyde, T. (2019). Overview of rabies post-exposure prophylaxis access, procurement and distribution in selected countries in Asia and Africa, 2017–2018. *Vaccine, 37*(Suppl 1), A6–A13. https://doi.org/10.1016/j.vaccine.2019.04.024

Talbi, C., Holmes, E. C., de Benedictis, P., Faye, O., Nakouné, E., Gamatié, D., Diarra, A., Elmamy, B. O., Sow, A., Adjogoua, E. V., Sangare, O., Dundon, W. G., Capua, I., Sall, A. A., & Bourhy, H. (2009). Evolutionary history and dynamics of dog rabies virus in western and central Africa. *The Journal of General Virology, 90*(Pt 4), 783–791. https://doi.org/10.1099/vir.0.007765-0

Velasco-Villa, A., Escobar, L. E., Sanchez, A., Shi, M., Streicker, D. G., Gallardo-Romero, N. F., Vargas-Pino, F., Gutierrez-Cedillo, V., Damon, I., & Emerson, G. (2017). Successful strategies implemented towards the elimination of canine rabies in the Western Hemisphere. *Antiviral Research, 143*, 1–12.

Vigilato, M. A., Cosivi, O., Knöbl, T., Clavijo, A., & Silva, H. M. (2013). Rabies update for Latin America and the Caribbean. *Emerging Infectious Diseases, 19*(4), 678.

Vigilato, M. A. N., Molina-Flores, B., Del Rio Vilas, V. J., Pompei, J. C., & Cosivi, O. (2018). Canine rabies elimination: Governance principles. *Revue Scientifique et Technique (International Office of Epizootics), 37*(2), 703–709. https://doi.org/10.20506/rst.37.2.2859

WHO. (2025). *The global health observarory.* https://www.who.int/data/gho/data/themes/topics/rabies

WHO Expert Consultation on Rabies. Second report. (2013). *World Health Organization Technical Report Series, 982*, 1–139, back cover.

WHO/Africa. (2024). *Rabies.* https://www.afro.who.int/health-topics/rabies

Willoughby, R. E. (2015). Rabies: Rare human infection–common questions. *Infectious Disease Clinics, 29*(4), 637–650.

World Health Organization. (2018a). *International partnership to address human-animal-environment health risks gets a boost.* https://www.who.int/news/item/30-05-2018-international-partnership-to-address-human-animal-environment-health-risks-gets-a-boost

World Health Organization. (2018b). *WHO expert consultation on rabies: Third report* (Vol. 1012). World Health Organization.

World Health Organization. (2024a). *Global Health Observatory (2024)—Processed by our world in data. "Reported deaths from rabies"*. World Health Organization, "Global Health Observatory." https://ourworldindata.org/grapher/reported-rabies-deaths

World Health Organization. (2024b). *Rabies.* https://www.who.int/news-room/fact-sheets/detail/rabies/

Yang, D.-K., Cho, I. S., & Kim, H. H. (2018). *Strategies for controlling dog-mediated human rabies in Asia: Using "One Health" principles to assess control programmes for rabies.* https://www.cdc.gov/hantavirus/hfrs/index.html#:~:text=Suggested%20Reading-,What%20is%20hemorrhagic%20fever%20with%20renal%20syndrome%3F,hemorrhagic%20fever%2C%20and%20nephropathia%20epidemica (15 September 2022).

Chapter 2

Acuna, R., Cifuentes-Munoz, N., Marquez, C. L., Bulling, M., Klingstrom, J., Mancini, R., Lozach, P. Y., & Tischler, N. D. (2014). Hantavirus Gn and Gc glycoproteins self-assemble into virus-like particles. *Journal of Virology, 88*(4), 2344–2348. https://doi.org/10.1128/JVI.03118-13

Al-Salem, W., Moraga, P., Ghazi, H., Madad, S., & Hotez, P. J. (2021). The emergence and transmission of COVID-19 in European countries, 2019–2020: A comprehensive review of timelines, cases and containment. *International Health, 13*(5), 383–398. https://doi.org/10.1093/inthealth/ihab037

Ali, H. S., Drewes, S., Weber de Melo, V., Schlegel, M., Freise, J., Groschup, M. H., Heckel, G., & Ulrich, R. G. (2015a). Complete genome of a Puumala virus strain from Central Europe. *Virus Genes, 50*(2), 292–298. https://doi.org/10.1007/s11262-014-1157-6

Antoine, M., Langlois, M. E., Bres, E., Rabeyrin, M., Reynes, J. M., & Deeb, A. (2021). Imported haemorrhagic fever with renal syndrome caused by Dobrava-Belgrade hantavirus in France. *Clinical Kidney Journal, 14*(3), 1014–1016. https://doi.org/10.1093/ckj/sfaa006

Antonen, J., Leppanen, I., Tenhunen, J., Arvola, P., Makela, S., Vaheri, A., & Mustonen, J. (2013). A severe case of Puumala hantavirus infection successfully treated with bradykinin receptor antagonist icatibant. *Scandinavian Journal of Infectious Diseases, 45*(6), 494–496. https://doi.org/10.3109/00365548.2012.755268

Arai, S., Gu, S. H., Baek, L. J., Tabara, K., Bennett, S. N., Oh, H. S., Takada, N., Kang, H. J., Tanaka-Taya, K., Morikawa, S., Okabe, N., Yanagihara, R., & Song, J. W. (2012). Divergent ancestral lineages of newfound hantaviruses harbored by phylogenetically related crocidurine shrew species in Korea. *Virology, 424*(2), 99–105. https://doi.org/10.1016/j.virol.2011.11.013

Arai, S., Kikuchi, F., Bawm, S., Son, N. T., Lin, K. S., Tu, V. T., Aoki, K., Tsuchiya, K., Tanaka-Taya, K., Morikawa, S., Oishi, K., & Yanagihara, R. (2019). Molecular phylogeny of mobatviruses (hantaviridae) in Myanmar and Vietnam. *Viruses, 11*(3). https://doi.org/10.3390/v11030228

Arai, S., Nguyen, S. T., Boldgiv, B., Fukui, D., Araki, K., Dang, C. N., Ohdachi, S. D., Nguyen, N. X., Pham, T. D., Boldbaatar, B., Satoh, H., Yoshikawa, Y., Morikawa, S., Tanaka-Taya, K.,

Yanagihara, R., & Oishi, K. (2013). Novel bat-borne hantavirus, Vietnam. *Emerging Infectious Diseases, 19*(7), 1159–1161. https://doi.org/10.3201/eid1907.121549

Arai, S., Ohdachi, S. D., Asakawa, M., Kang, H. J., Mocz, G., Arikawa, J., Okabe, N., & Yanagihara, R. (2008). Molecular phylogeny of a newfound hantavirus in the Japanese shrew mole (Urotrichus talpoides). *Proceedings National Academy of Sciences United States America, 105*(42), 16296–16301. https://doi.org/10.1073/pnas.0808942105

Arai, S., Taniguchi, S., Aoki, K., Yoshikawa, Y., Kyuwa, S., Tanaka-Taya, K., Masangkay, J. S., Omatsu, T., Puentespina, R., Jr., Watanabe, S., Alviola, P., Alvarez, J., Eres, E., Cosico, E., Quibod, M., Morikawa, S., Yanagihara, R., & Oishi, K. (2016). Molecular phylogeny of a genetically divergent hantavirus harbored by the Geoffroy's rousette (Rousettus amplexicaudatus), a frugivorous bat species in the Philippines. *Infection, Genetics and Evolution, 45*, 26-32. https://doi.org/10.1016/j.meegid.2016.08.008

Asikainen, K., Hanninen, T., Henttonen, H., Niemimaa, J., Laakkonen, J., Andersen, H. K., Bille, N., Leirs, H., Vaheri, A., & Plyusnin, A. (2000). Molecular evolution of puumala hantavirus in Fennoscandia: Phylogenetic analysis of strains from two recolonization routes, Karelia and Denmark. *Journal of General Virology, 81*(Pt 12), 2833–2841. https://doi.org/10.1099/0022-1317-81-12-2833

Aude Lalis The First Identification of Tula Hantavirus in Iran. Malaria Control & Elimination 2020, 9.

Avsic-Zupanc, T., Nemirov, K., Petrovec, M., Trilar, T., Poljak, M., Vaheri, A., & Plyusnin, A. (2000). Genetic analysis of wild-type Dobrava hantavirus in Slovenia: Co-existence of two distinct genetic lineages within the same natural focus. *Journal of General Virology, 81*(Pt 7), 1747–1755. https://doi.org/10.1099/0022-1317-81-7-1747

Avsic-Zupanc, T., Xiao, S. Y., Stojanovic, R., Gligic, A., van der Groen, G., & LeDuc, J. W. (1992). Characterization of Dobrava virus: A Hantavirus from Slovenia, Yugoslavia. *Journal of Medical Virology, 38*(2), 132–137. https://doi.org/10.1002/jmv.1890380211

Baygildina, A. A. (2014). Modern ideas about the pathogenesis of hemorrhagic fever with renal syndrome/A.A. Baygildina. *Medical Bulletin of Bashkortostan, 9*(1), 98–108.

Bennett, S. N., Gu, S. H., Kang, H. J., Arai, S., & Yanagihara, R. (2014). Reconstructing the evolutionary origins and phylogeography of hantaviruses. *Trends in Microbiology, 22*(8), 473–482. https://doi.org/10.1016/j.tim.2014.04.008

Bergstedt Oscarsson, K., Brorstad, A., Baudin, M., Lindberg, A., Forssen, A., Evander, M., Eriksson, M., & Ahlm, C. (2016). Human Puumala hantavirus infection in northern Sweden; Increased seroprevalence and association to risk and health factors. *BMC Infectious Diseases, 16*(1), 566. https://doi.org/10.1186/s12879-016-1879-2

Bi, Z., Formenty, P. B., & Roth, C. E. (2008). Hantavirus infection: A review and global update. *Journal of Infection in Developing Countries, 2*(1), 3–23. https://doi.org/10.3855/jidc.317

Binder, F., Reiche, S., Roman-Sosa, G., Saathoff, M., Ryll, R., Trimpert, J., Kunec, D., Hoper, D., & Ulrich, R. G. (2020). Isolation and characterization of new Puumala orthohantavirus strains from Germany. *Virus Genes, 56*(4), 448–460. https://doi.org/10.1007/s11262-020-01755-3

Boudreau, E. F., Josleyn, M., Ullman, D., Fisher, D., Dalrymple, L., Sellers-Myers, K., Loudon, P., Rusnak, J., Rivard, R., Schmaljohn, C., & Hooper, J. W. (2012). A Phase 1 clinical trial of Hantaan virus and Puumala virus M-segment DNA vaccines for hemorrhagic fever with renal syndrome. *Vaccine, 30*(11), 1951–1958. https://doi.org/10.1016/j.vaccine.2012.01.024

Brummer-Korvenkontio, M., Manni, T., Ukkonen, S., & Vaheri, A. (1986). Detection of hemagglutination-inhibiting antibodies in patients with nephropathia epidemica and Korean hemorrhagic fever by using Puumala virus cell culture antigen. *Journal of Infectious Diseases, 153*(5), 997–998. https://doi.org/10.1093/infdis/153.5.997-a

Brummer-Korvenkontio, M., Vaheri, A., Hovi, T., von Bonsdorff, C. H., Vuorimies, J., Manni, T., Penttinen, K., Oker-Blom, N., & Lahdevirta, J. (1980). Nephropathia epidemica: Detection of antigen in bank voles and serologic diagnosis of human infection. *Journal of Infectious Diseases, 141*(2), 131–134. https://doi.org/10.1093/infdis/141.2.131

Cao, S., Ma, J., Cheng, C., Ju, W., & Wang, Y. (2016). Genetic characterization of hantaviruses isolated from rodents in the port cities of Heilongjiang, China, in 2014. *BMC Veterinary Research, 12*, 69. https://doi.org/10.1186/s12917-016-0695-7

Carey, D. E., Reuben, R., Panicker, K. N., Shope, R. E., & Myers, R. M. (1971). Thottapalayam virus: A presumptive arbovirus isolated from a shrew in India. *Indian Journal of Medical Research, 59*(11), 1758–1760. https://www.ncbi.nlm.nih.gov/pubmed/5169031

Casals, J., Henderson, B. E., Hoogstraal, H., Johnson, K. M., & Shelokov, A. (1970). A review of Soviet viral hemorrhagic fevers, 1969. *Journal of Infectious Diseases, 122*(5), 437–453. https://doi.org/10.1093/infdis/122.5.437

Centers for Disease Control and Prevention Cleaning Up after Rodents|Rodents|CDC. Available online: https://www.cdc.gov/rodents/prevent_infestations/clean_up.html#:~:text=Clean%20up%20rodent%20urine%20and,or%20droppings%20and%20cleaning%20product (15 September 2022).

Centers for Disease Control and Prevention Facts about Hantaviruses. What You Need to Know to Prevent the Disease Pulmonary Syndrome (HPS). Available online: https://www.cdc.gov/hantavirus/pdf/hps_brochure.pdf (23 August 2022).

Centers for Disease Control and Prevention Technical/Clinical Information: HPS Treatment—Hantavirus. Available online: https://www.cdc.gov/hantavirus/technical/hps/treatment.html (12 July 2022).

Chandy, S., Abraham, S., & Sridharan, G. (2008). Hantaviruses: An emerging public health threat in India? A review. *Journal of Biosciences, 33*(4), 495–504. https://doi.org/10.1007/s12038-008-0068-x

Chandy, S., Mitra, S., Sathish, N., Vijayakumar, T. S., Abraham, O. C., Jesudason, M. V., Abraham, P., Yoshimatsu, K., Arikawa, J., & Sridharan, G. (2005). A pilot study for serological evidence of hantavirus infection in human population in south India. *Indian Journal of Medical Research, 122*(3), 211–215. https://www.ncbi.nlm.nih.gov/pubmed/16251777

Chappell, J. G., Tsoleridis, T., Onianwa, O., Drake, G., Ashpole, I., Dobbs, P., Edema, W., Kumi-Ansah, F., Bennett, M., Tarlinton, R. E., Ball, J. K., & McClure, C. P. (2020). Retrieval of the complete coding sequence of the UK-endemic tatenale orthohantavirus reveals extensive strain variation and supports its classification as a novel species. *Viruses, 12*(4). https://doi.org/10.3390/v12040454

Chen, H. X., & Qiu, F. X. (1993). Epidemiologic surveillance on the hemorrhagic fever with renal syndrome in China. *Chinese Medical Journal (England), 106*(11), 857–863. https://www.ncbi.nlm.nih.gov/pubmed/7908258

Chen, H. X., Luo, Z. Z., & Zhang, J. J. (2002). Hantavirus vaccine efficacy evaluation working group. Large scale field evaluation on vaccines of hemorrhagic fever with renal syndrome in China. *Chinese Journal of Epidemiology, 23*, 145–147.

Cheng, L. F., Wang, F., Zhang, L., Yu, L., Ye, W., Liu, Z. Y., Ying, Q. K., Wu, X. A., Xu, Z. K., & Zhang, F. L. (2016). Incorporation of GM-CSF or CD40L enhances the immunogenicity of Hantaan virus-like particles. *Frontiers in Cellular and Infection Microbiology, 6*, 185. https://doi.org/10.3389/fcimb.2016.00185

Chin, C., Chiueh, T. S., Yang, W. C., Yang, T. H., Shih, C. M., Lin, H. T., Lin, K. C., Lien, J. C., Tsai, T. F., Ruo, S. L., Nichol, S. T., Ksiazek, T. G., Rollin, P. E., Peters, C. J., Wu, T. N., & Shen, C. Y. (2000). Hantavirus infection in Taiwan: The experience of a geographically unique area. *Journal of Medical Virology, 60*(2), 237–247. https://doi.org/10.1002/(sici)1096-9071(200002)60:2%3c237::aid-jmv21%3e3.0.co;2-b

Cho, H. W., & Howard, C. R. (1999). Antibody responses in humans to an inactivated hantavirus vaccine (Hantavax). *Vaccine, 17*(20–21), 2569–2575. https://doi.org/10.1016/s0264-410x(99)00057-2

Cho, H. W., Howard, C. R., & Lee, H. W. (2002). Review of an inactivated vaccine against hantaviruses. *Intervirology, 45*(4–6), 328–333. https://doi.org/10.1159/000067925

Choi, K. H. (2012). Viral polymerases. *Advances in Experimental Medicine and Biology, 726*, 267–304. https://doi.org/10.1007/978-1-4614-0980-9

Choi, S., & Ki, M. (2020). Estimating the reproductive number and the outbreak size of COVID-19 in Korea. *Epidemiology and Health, 42*, e2020011. https://doi.org/10.4178/epih.e2020011

Chu, Y. K., Gligic, A., Tomanovic, S., Bozovjc, B., Obradovic, M., Woo, Y. D., An, C. N., Kim, H., Jiang, Y. S., Park, S. C., et al. (1999). A field efficacy trial of inactivated Hantaan Virus Vaccine (Hantavax(TM)) against Hemorrhagic Fever with Renal Syndrome (HFRS) in the endemic areas of Yugoslavia from 1996 to 1998. *Journal of the Korean Society of Virology, 29*, 55–64.

Chu, Y. K., Jennings, G. B., & Schmaljohn, C. S. (1995). A vaccinia virus-vectored Hantaan virus vaccine protects hamsters from challenge with Hantaan and Seoul viruses but not Puumala virus. *Journal of Virology, 69*(10), 6417–6423. https://doi.org/10.1128/JVI.69.10.6417-6423.1995

Clement, J., Maes, P., Muthusethupathi, M., Nainan, G., & van Ranst, M. (2006). First evidence of fatal hantavirus nephropathy in India, mimicking leptospirosis. *Nephrology, Dialysis, Transplantation, 21*(3), 826–827. https://doi.org/10.1093/ndt/gfi334

Connolly-Andersen, A. M., Rasmuson, J., Oman, M., & Ahlm, C. (2018). Mesenteric vein thrombosis following platelet transfusion in a patient with hemorrhagic fever with renal syndrome: A case report. *TH Open, 2*(3), e261–e264. https://doi.org/10.1055/s-0038-1669456

Dantas, J. R., Okuno, Y., Asada, H., Tamura, M., Takahashi, M., Tanishita, O., Takahashi, Y., Kurata, T., & Yamanishi, K. (1986). Characterization of glycoproteins of viruses causing hemorrhagic fever with renal syndrome (HFRS) using monoclonal antibodies. *Virology, 151*(2), 379–384. https://doi.org/10.1016/0042-6822(86)90058-9

Daud, N. H., Kariwa, H., Tanikawa, Y., Nakamura, I., Seto, T., Miyashita, D., Yoshii, K., Nakauchi, M., Yoshimatsu, K., Arikawa, J., & Takashima, I. (2007). Mode of infection of Hokkaido virus (Genus Hantavirus) among grey red-backed voles, Myodes rufocanus, in Hokkaido, Japan. *Microbiology and Immunology, 51*(11), 1081–1090. https://doi.org/10.1111/j.1348-0421.2007.tb04003.x

de Carvalho Nicacio, C., Gonzalez Della Valle, M., Padula, P., Bjorling, E., Plyusnin, A., & Lundkvist, A. (2002). Cross-protection against challenge with Puumala virus after immunization with nucleocapsid proteins from different hantaviruses. *Journal of Virology, 76*(13), 6669–6677. https://doi.org/10.1128/jvi.76.13.6669-6677.2002

de Oliveira, R. C., Guterres, A., Fernandes, J., D'Andrea, P. S., Bonvicino, C. R., & de Lemos, E. R. (2014). Hantavirus reservoirs: Current status with an emphasis on data from Brazil. *Viruses, 6*(5), 1929–1973. https://doi.org/10.3390/v6051929

de Vries, A., Vennema, H., Bekker, D. L., Maas, M., Adema, J., Opsteegh, M., van der Giessen, J. W. B., & Reusken, C. (2016). Characterization of Puumala hantavirus in bank voles from two regions in the Netherlands where human cases occurred. *Journal of General Virology, 97*(7), 1500–1510. https://doi.org/10.1099/jgv.0.000481

Dearing, M. D., & Dizney, L. (2010). Ecology of hantavirus in a changing world. *Annals of the New York Academy of Sciences, 1195*, 99–112. https://doi.org/10.1111/j.1749-6632.2010.05452.x

Dheerasekara, K., Sumathipala, S., & Muthugala, R. (2020). Hantavirus infections-treatment and prevention. *Current Treatment Options in Infectious Diseases, 12*(4), 410–421. https://doi.org/10.1007/s40506-020-00236-3

Dong, G. M., Han, L., An, Q., Liu, W. X., Kong, Y., & Yang, L. H. (2005). Immunization effect of purified bivalent vaccine to haemorrhagic fever with renal syndrome manufactured from primary cultured hamster kidney cells. *Chinese Medical Journal (England), 118*(9), 766–768. https://www.ncbi.nlm.nih.gov/pubmed/15899141

Dong, Y., Ma, T., Zhang, X., Ying, Q., Han, M., Zhang, M., Yang, R., Li, Y., Wang, F., Liu, R., & Wu, X. (2019). Incorporation of CD40 ligand or granulocyte-macrophage colony stimulating factor into Hantaan virus (HTNV) virus-like particles significantly enhances the long-term immunity potency against HTNV infection. *Journal of Medical Microbiology, 68*(3), 480–492. https://doi.org/10.1099/jmm.0.000897

Dunst, R., Mettang, T., & Kuhlmann, U. (1998). Severe thrombocytopenia and response to corticosteroids in a case of nephropathia epidemica. *American Journal of Kidney Diseases, 31*(1), 116–120. https://doi.org/10.1053/ajkd.1998.v31.pm9428461

Dzagurova, T. K., Siniugina, A. A., Ishmukhametov, A. A., Egorova, M. S., Kurashova, S. S., Balovneva, M. V., Deviatkin, A. A., Tkachenko, P. E., Leonovich, O. A., & Tkachenko, E. A. (2020). Pre-clinical studies of inactivated polyvalent HFRS vaccine. *Frontiers in Cellular and Infection Microbiology, 10*, 545372. https://doi.org/10.3389/fcimb.2020.545372

Easterbrook, J. D., & Klein, S. L. (2008). Corticosteroids modulate Seoul virus infection, regulatory T-cell responses and matrix metalloprotease 9 expression in male, but not female, Norway rats. *Journal of General Virology, 89*(Pt 11), 2723–2730. https://doi.org/10.1099/vir.0.2008/03715-0

Elgh, F., Linderholm, M., Wadell, G., Tarnvik, A., & Juto, P. (1998). Development of humoral cross-reactivity to the nucleocapsid protein of heterologous hantaviruses in nephropathia epidemica. *FEMS Immunology and Medical Microbiology, 22*(4), 309–315. https://doi.org/10.1111/j.1574-695X.1998.tb01220.x

Elwell, M. R., Ward, G. S., Tingpalapong, M., & LeDuc, J. W. (1985). Serologic evidence of Hantaan-like virus in rodents and man in Thailand. *Southeast Asian Journal of Tropical Medicine and Public Health, 16*(3), 349–354. https://www.ncbi.nlm.nih.gov/pubmed/3938073

Escutenaire, S., Chalon, P., Heyman, P., Van der Auwera, G., van der Groen, G., Verhagen, R., Thomas, I., Karelle-Bui, L., Vaheri, A., Pastoret, P. P., & Plyusnin, A. (2001). Genetic characterization of Puumala hantavirus strains from Belgium: Evidence for a distinct phylogenetic lineage. *Virus Research, 74*(1–2), 1–15. https://doi.org/10.1016/s0168-1702(00)00224-0

Escutenaire, S., & Pastoret, P. P. (2001). Hantavirus infection epidemiology in Belgium. *Bulletin et Memoires de L'academie Royale de Medecine de Belgique, 156*(1–2), 137–144; discussion 144–136. https://www.ncbi.nlm.nih.gov/pubmed/11697188 (Epidemiologie de l'infection par hantavirus en Belgique).

Fang, L. Z., Zhao, L., Wen, H. L., Zhang, Z. T., Liu, J. W., He, S. T., Xue, Z. F., Ma, D. Q., Zhang, X. S., Zhang, Y., & Yu, X. J. (2015). Reservoir host expansion of hantavirus, China. *Emerging Infectious Diseases, 21*(1), 170–171. https://doi.org/10.3201/eid2101.140960

Fougeroux, C., Goksoyr, L., Idorn, M., Soroka, V., Myeni, S. K., Dagil, R., Janitzek, C. M., Sogaard, M., Aves, K. L., Horsted, E. W., Erdogan, S. M., Gustavsson, T., Dorosz, J., Clemmensen, S., Fredsgaard, L., Thrane, S., Vidal-Calvo, E. E., Khalife, P., Hulen, T. M., … Sander, A. F. (2021). Capsid-like particles decorated with the SARS-CoV-2 receptor-binding domain elicit strong virus neutralization activity. *Nature Communications, 12*(1), 324. https://doi.org/10.1038/s41467-020-20251-8

Furuta, Y., Komeno, T., & Nakamura, T. (2017). Favipiravir (T-705), a broad spectrum inhibitor of viral RNA polymerase. *Proceedings of the Japan Academy: Series B, Physical and Biological Sciences, 93*(7), 449–463. https://doi.org/10.2183/pjab.93.027

Garanina, S. B., Platonov, A. E., Zhuravlev, V. I., Murashkina, A. N., Yakimenko, V. V., Korneev, A. G., & Shipulin, G. A. (2009). Genetic diversity and geographic distribution of hantaviruses in Russia. *Zoonoses and Public Health, 56*(6–7), 297–309. https://doi.org/10.1111/j.1863-2378.2008.01210.x

Ge, X. Y., Yang, W. H., Pan, H., Zhou, J. H., Han, X., Zhu, G. J., Desmond, J. S., Daszak, P., Shi, Z. L., & Zhang, Y. Z. (2016). Fugong virus, a novel hantavirus harbored by the small oriental vole (Eothenomys eleusis) in China. *Journal of Virology, 13*, 27. https://doi.org/10.1186/s12985-016-0483-9

Geldmacher, A., Schmaler, M., Kruger, D. H., & Ulrich, R. (2004). Yeast-expressed hantavirus Dobrava nucleocapsid protein induces a strong, long-lasting, and highly cross-reactive immune response in mice. *Viral Immunology, 17*(1), 115–122. https://doi.org/10.1089/088282404322875511

Geldmacher, A., Skrastina, D., Petrovskis, I., Borisova, G., Berriman, J. A., Roseman, A. M., Crowther, R. A., Fischer, J., Musema, S., Gelderblom, H. R., Lundkvist, A., Renhofa, R., Ose, V., Kruger, D. H., Pumpens, P., & Ulrich, R. (2004). An amino-terminal segment of hantavirus nucleocapsid protein presented on hepatitis B virus core particles induces a strong and highly cross-reactive antibody response in mice. *Virology, 323*(1), 108–119. https://doi.org/10.1016/j.virol.2004.02.022

GenBank. https://www.ncbi.nlm.nih.gov/nuccore/NC_055632.1. Accessed 20 January 2024.

Gralinski, L. E., & Menachery, V. D. (2020). Return of the Coronavirus: 2019-nCoV. *Viruses, 12*(2). https://doi.org/10.3390/v12020135

Gu, S. H., Lim, B. K., Kadjo, B., Arai, S., Kim, J. A., Nicolas, V., Lalis, A., Denys, C., Cook, J. A., Dominguez, S. R., Holmes, K. V., Urushadze, L., Sidamonidze, K., Putkaradze, D., Kuzmin, I. V., Kosoy, M. Y., Song, J. W., & Yanagihara, R. (2014). Molecular phylogeny of hantaviruses harbored by insectivorous bats in Cote d'Ivoire and Vietnam. *Viruses, 6*(5), 1897–1910. https://doi.org/10.3390/v6051897

Gu, S. H., Nicolas, V., Lalis, A., Sathirapongsasuti, N., & Yanagihara, R. (2013). Complete genome sequence and molecular phylogeny of a newfound hantavirus harbored by the Doucet's musk shrew (Crocidura douceti) in Guinea. *Infection, Genetics and Evolution, 20*, 118–123. https://doi.org/10.1016/j.meegid.2013.08.016

Guang, M. Y., Liu, G. Z., & Cosgriff, T. M. (1989). Hemorrhage in hemorrhagic fever with renal syndrome in China. *Reviews of Infectious Diseases, 11*(Suppl 4), S884-890. https://doi.org/10.1093/clinids/11.supplement_4.s844

Guénet, J. L., Orth, A., & Bonhomme, F. (2012). Origins and phylogenetic relationships of the laboratory mouse.

Guo, W. P., Lin, X. D., Wang, W., Tian, J. H., Cong, M. L., Zhang, H. L., Wang, M. R., Zhou, R. H., Wang, J. B., Li, M. H., Xu, J., Holmes, E. C., & Zhang, Y. Z. (2013). Phylogeny and origins of hantaviruses harbored by bats, insectivores, and rodents. *PLoS Pathogens, 9*(2), e1003159. https://doi.org/10.1371/journal.ppat.1003159

Gupta, D., Sahoo, A. K., & Singh, A. (2020). Ivermectin: Potential candidate for the treatment of Covid 19. *The Brazilian Journal of Infectious Diseases, 24*(4), 369–371. https://doi.org/10.1016/j.bjid.2020.06.002

Hall, P. R., Hjelle, B., Brown, D. C., Ye, C., Bondu-Hawkins, V., Kilpatrick, K. A., & Larson, R. S. (2008). Multivalent presentation of antihantavirus peptides on nanoparticles enhances infection blockade. *Antimicrobial Agents and Chemotherapy, 52*(6), 2079–2088. https://doi.org/10.1128/AAC.01415-07

Hall, P. R., Leitao, A., Ye, C., Kilpatrick, K., Hjelle, B., Oprea, T. I., & Larson, R. S. (2010). Small molecule inhibitors of hantavirus infection. *Bioorganic & Medicinal Chemistry Letters, 20*(23), 7085–7091. https://doi.org/10.1016/j.bmcl.2010.09.092

Hautala, T., Sironen, T., Vapalahti, O., Paakko, E., Sarkioja, T., Salmela, P. I., Vaheri, A., Plyusnin, A., & Kauma, H. (2002). Hypophyseal hemorrhage and panhypopituitarism during Puumala Virus infection: Magnetic resonance imaging and detection of viral antigen in the hypophysis. *Clinical Infectious Diseases, 35*(1), 96–101. https://doi.org/10.1086/340859

Holmes, E. C., & Zhang, Y. Z. (2015). The evolution and emergence of hantaviruses. *Current Opinion in Virology, 10*, 27–33. https://doi.org/10.1016/j.coviro.2014.12.007

Hooper, J. W., Custer, D. M., Smith, J., & Wahl-Jensen, V. (2006). Hantaan/Andes virus DNA vaccine elicits a broadly cross-reactive neutralizing antibody response in nonhuman primates. *Virology, 347*(1), 208–216. https://doi.org/10.1016/j.virol.2005.11.035

Hooper, J. W., Custer, D. M., Thompson, E., & Schmaljohn, C. S. (2001). DNA vaccination with the Hantaan virus M gene protects Hamsters against three of four HFRS hantaviruses and elicits a high-titer neutralizing antibody response in Rhesus monkeys. *Journal of Virology, 75*(18), 8469–8477. https://doi.org/10.1128/jvi.75.18.8469-8477.2001

Huggins, J. W., Hsiang, C. M., Cosgriff, T. M., Guang, M. Y., Smith, J. I., Wu, Z. O., LeDuc, J. W., Zheng, Z. M., Meegan, J. M., Wang, Q. N., et al. (1991). Prospective, double-blind, concurrent, placebo-controlled clinical trial of intravenous ribavirin therapy of hemorrhagic fever with renal syndrome. *The Journal of Infectious Diseases, 164*(6), 1119–1127. https://doi.org/10.1093/infdis/164.6.1119

Hussein, I., Haseeb, A., Haque, A., & Mir, M. A. (2011). Recent advances in hantavirus molecular biology and disease. *Advances in Applied*.

ICTV Current ICTV Taxonomy Release. Available online: https://ictv.global/taxonomy. Accessed 8 August 2022.

Jameson, L., Taori, S., Atkinson, B., Levick, P., Featherstone, C., Van Der Burgt, G., McCarthy, N., Hart, J., Osborne, J., & Walsh, A. (2013). Pet rats as a source of hantavirus in England and Wales, 2013. *Eurosurveillance, 18*(9), 20415.

Ji, T., Chen, H. L., Xu, J., Wu, L. N., Li, J. J., Chen, K., & Qin, G. (2020). Lockdown contained the spread of 2019 novel Coronavirus disease in Huangshi City, China: Early epidemiological findings. *Clinical Infectious Diseases, 71*(6), 1454–1460. https://doi.org/10.1093/cid/ciaa390

Jiang, H., Du, H., Wang, L. M., Wang, P. Z., & Bai, X. F. (2016). Hemorrhagic fever with renal syndrome: Pathogenesis and clinical picture. *Frontiers in Cellular and Infection Microbiology, 6*, 1. https://doi.org/10.3389/fcimb.2016.00001

Jiang, H., Zheng, X., Wang, L., Du, H., Wang, P., & Bai, X. (2017). Hantavirus infection: A global zoonotic challenge. *Virologica Sinica, 32*(1), 32–43. https://doi.org/10.1007/s12250-016-3899-x

Jiang, J. F., Zhang, W. Y., Wu, X. M., Zhang, P. H., & Cao, W. C. (2007). Soochong virus and Amur virus might be the same entities of hantavirus. *Journal of Medical Virology, 79*(11), 1792–1795. https://doi.org/10.1002/jmv.20957

Johnson, K. M. (2001). Hantaviruses: History and overview. *Current Topics in Microbiology and Immunology, 256*, 1–14. https://doi.org/10.1007/978-3-642-56753-7

Jonsson, C. B., Figueiredo, L. T., & Vapalahti, O. (2010). A global perspective on hantavirus ecology, epidemiology, and disease. *Clinical Microbiology Reviews, 23*(2), 412–441. https://doi.org/10.1128/CMR.00062-09

Jung, J., Ko, S. J., Oh, H. S., Moon, S. M., Song, J. W., & Huh, K. (2018). Protective effectiveness of inactivated hantavirus vaccine against hemorrhagic fever with renal syndrome. *Journal of Infectious Diseases, 217*(9), 1417–1420. https://doi.org/10.1093/infdis/jiy037

Jung, Y. T., & Kim, G. R. (1995). Genomic characterization of M and S RNA segments of hantaviruses isolated from bats. *Acta Virologica, 39*(4), 231–233. https://www.ncbi.nlm.nih.gov/pubmed/8825306

Kabwe, E., Davidyuk, Y., Shamsutdinov, A., Garanina, E., Martynova, E., Kitaeva, K., Malisheni, M., Isaeva, G., Savitskaya, T., Urbanowicz, R. A., Morzunov, S., Katongo, C., Rizvanov, A., & Khaiboullina, S. (2020). Orthohantaviruses, emerging zoonotic pathogens. *Pathogens, 9*(9). https://doi.org/10.3390/pathogens9090775

Kariwa, H., Yoshimatsu, K., & Arikawa, J. (2007a). Hantavirus infection in East Asia. *Comparative Immunology, Microbiology and Infectious Diseases, 30*(5–6), 341–356. https://doi.org/10.1016/j.cimid.2007.05.011

Kariwa, H., Yoshimatsu, K., & Arikawa, J. (2007b). Hantavirus infection in East Asia. *Comparative Immunology, Microbiology and Infectious Diseases, 30*(5–6), 341–356.

Khalil, H., Hornfeldt, B., Evander, M., Magnusson, M., Olsson, G., & Ecke, F. (2014). Dynamics and drivers of hantavirus prevalence in rodent populations. *Vector Borne and Zoonotic Diseases, 14*(8), 537–551. https://doi.org/10.1089/vbz.2013.1562

Kikuchi, F., Arai, S., Hejduk, J., Hayashi, A., Markowski, J., Markowski, M., Rychlik, L., Khodzinskyi, V., Kamiya, H., Mizutani, T., Suzuki, M., Sikorska, B., Liberski, P. P., & Yanagihara, R. (2023). Phylogeny of Shrew- and Mole-Borne Hantaviruses in Poland and Ukraine. *Viruses, 15*(4). https://doi.org/10.3390/v15040881

Kikuchi, F., Senoo, K., Arai, S., Tsuchiya, K., Son, N. T., Motokawa, M., Ranorosoa, M. C., Bawm, S., Lin, K. S., Suzuki, H., Unno, A., Nakata, K., Harada, M., Tanaka-Taya, K., Morikawa, S., Suzuki, M., Mizutani, T., & Yanagihara, R. (2021). Rodent-borne orthohantaviruses in Vietnam, Madagascar and Japan. *Viruses, 13*(7). https://doi.org/10.3390/v13071343

Kim, G. R., Lee, Y. T., & Park, C. H. (1994). A new natural reservoir of hantavirus: Isolation of hantaviruses from lung tissues of bats. *Archives of Virology, 134*(1–2), 85–95. https://doi.org/10.1007/BF01379109

Kim, J. A., Kim, W. K., No, J. S., Lee, S. H., Lee, S. Y., Kim, J. H., Kho, J. H., Lee, D., Song, D. H., Gu, S. H., Jeong, S. T., Park, M. S., Kim, H. C., Klein, T. A., & Song, J. W. (2016). Genetic diversity and reassortment of Hantaan virus tripartite RNA genomes in nature, the Republic of Korea. *PLoS Neglected Tropical Diseases, 10*(6), e0004650. https://doi.org/10.1371/journal.pntd.0004650

Klasse, P. J., & Sattentau, Q. J. (2002). Occupancy and mechanism in antibody-mediated neutralization of animal viruses. *Journal of General Virology, 83*(Pt 9), 2091–2108. https://doi.org/10.1099/0022-1317-83-9-2091

Klempa, B. (2018). Reassortment events in the evolution of hantaviruses. *Virus Genes, 54*(5), 638–646. https://doi.org/10.1007/s11262-018-1590-z

Klempa, B., Avsic-Zupanc, T., Clement, J., Dzagurova, T. K., Henttonen, H., Heyman, P., Jakab, F., Kruger, D. H., Maes, P., Papa, A., Tkachenko, E. A., Ulrich, R. G., Vapalahti, O., & Vaheri, A. (2013). Complex evolution and epidemiology of Dobrava-Belgrade hantavirus: Definition of genotypes and their characteristics. *Archives of Virology, 158*(3), 521–529. https://doi.org/10.1007/s00705-012-1514-5

Klempa, B., Witkowski, P. T., Popugaeva, E., Auste, B., Koivogui, L., Fichet-Calvet, E., Strecker, T., Ter Meulen, J., & Kruger, D. H. (2012). Sangassou virus, the first hantavirus isolate from Africa, displays genetic and functional properties distinct from those of other murinae-associated hantaviruses. *Journal of Virology, 86*(7), 3819–3827. https://doi.org/10.1128/JVI.05879-11

Koletzki, D., Biel, S. S., Meisel, H., Nugel, E., Gelderblom, H. R., Kruger, D. H., & Ulrich, R. (1999). HBV core particles allow the insertion and surface exposure of the entire potentially protective region of Puumala hantavirus nucleocapsid protein. *Biological Chemistry, 380*(3), 325–333. https://doi.org/10.1515/BC.1999.044

Krautkramer, E., & Zeier, M. (2014). Old world hantaviruses: Aspects of pathogenesis and clinical course of acute renal failure. *Virus Research, 187*, 59–64. https://doi.org/10.1016/j.virusres.2013.12.043

Kruger, D. H., Figueiredo, L. T., Song, J. W., & Klempa, B. (2015). Hantaviruses–globally emerging pathogens. *Journal of Clinical Virology, 64*, 128–136. https://doi.org/10.1016/j.jcv.2014.08.033

Kruger, D. H., Schonrich, G., & Klempa, B. (2011). Human pathogenic hantaviruses and prevention of infection. *Human Vaccines, 7*(6), 685–693. https://doi.org/10.4161/hv.7.6.15197

Kruger, D. H., Ulrich, R., & Lundkvist, A. A. (2001). Hantavirus infections and their prevention. *Microbes and Infection, 3*(13), 1129–1144. https://doi.org/10.1016/s1286-4579(01)01474-5

Kuhn, J. H., & Schmaljohn, C. S. (2023). A brief history of Bunyaviral Family Hantaviridae. *Diseases, 11*(1). https://doi.org/10.3390/diseases11010038

Kukkonen, S. K., Vaheri, A., & Plyusnin, A. (2005). L protein, the RNA-dependent RNA polymerase of hantaviruses. *Archives of Virology, 150*(3), 533–556. https://doi.org/10.1007/s00705-004-0414-8

Kurita, J., Sugawara, T., & Ohkusa, Y. (2021). Estimated effectiveness of school closure and voluntary event cancellation as COVID-19 countermeasures in Japan. *Journal of Infection and Chemotherapy, 27*(1), 62–64. https://doi.org/10.1016/j.jiac.2020.08.012

Kutanan, W., Kampuansai, J., Brunelli, A., Ghirotto, S., Pittayaporn, P., Ruangchai, S., Schroder, R., Macholdt, E., Srikummool, M., Kangwanpong, D., Hubner, A., Arias, L., & Stoneking, M. (2018). New insights from Thailand into the maternal genetic history of Mainland Southeast Asia. *European Journal of Human Genetics, 26*(6), 898–911. https://doi.org/10.1038/s41431-018-0113-7

Laenen, L., Vergote, V., Calisher, C. H., Klempa, B., Klingstrom, J., Kuhn, J. H., & Maes, P. (2019). Hantaviridae: Current classification and future perspectives. *Viruses, 11*(9). https://doi.org/10.3390/v11090788

Laenen, L., Vergote, V., Kafetzopoulou, L. E., Wawina, T. B., Vassou, D., Cook, J. A., Hugot, J. P., Deboutte, W., Kang, H. J., Witkowski, P. T., Koppen-Rung, P., Kruger, D. H., Lickova, M., Stang, A., Strieskova, L., Szemes, T., Markowski, J., Hejduk, J., Kafetzopoulos, D., … Maes, P. (2018). A novel hantavirus of the European mole, Bruges virus, is involved in frequent Nova virus coinfections. *Genome Biology and Evolution, 10*(1), 45–55. https://doi.org/10.1093/gbe/evx268

Laine, O., Leppanen, I., Koskela, S., Antonen, J., Makela, S., Sinisalo, M., Vaheri, A., & Mustonen, J. (2015). Severe Puumala virus infection in a patient with a lymphoproliferative disease treated with icatibant. *Infectious Diseases (London), 47*(2), 107–111. https://doi.org/10.3109/00365548.2014.969304

Latus, J., Kitterer, D., Segerer, S., Artunc, F., Alscher, M. D., & Braun, N. (2015). Severe thrombocytopenia in hantavirus-induced nephropathia epidemica. *Infection, 43*(1), 83–87. https://doi.org/10.1007/s15010-014-0699-9

Lee, H. W., Baek, L. J., & Johnson, K. M. (1982). Isolation of Hantaan virus, the etiologic agent of Korean hemorrhagic fever, from wild urban rats. *Journal of Infectious Diseases, 146*(5), 638–644. https://doi.org/10.1093/infdis/146.5.638

Lee, H. W., Lee, P. W., & Johnson, K. M. (1978). Isolation of the etiologic agent of Korean Hemorrhagic fever. *Journal of Infectious Diseases, 137*(3), 298–308. https://doi.org/10.1093/infdis/137.3.298

Lee, S. H., Kim, W. K., No, J. S., Kim, J. A., Kim, J. I., Gu, S. H., Kim, H. C., Klein, T. A., Park, M. S., & Song, J. W. (2017). Dynamic circulation and genetic exchange of a Shrew-borne Hantavirus, Imjin virus, in the Republic of Korea. *Science and Reports, 7*, 44369. https://doi.org/10.1038/srep44369

Leopardi, S., Drzewniokova, P., Baggieri, M., Marchi, A., Bucci, P., Bregoli, M., De Benedictis, P., Gobbo, F., Bellinati, L., Citterio, C., Monne, I., Pastori, A., Zamperin, G., Palumbo, E., Festa, F., Castellan, M., Zorzan, M., D'Ugo, E., Zucca, P., Terregino, C., & Magurano, F. (2022). Identification of Dobrava-Belgrade Virus in Apodemus flavicollis from North-Eastern Italy during enhanced mortality. *Viruses, 14*(6). https://doi.org/10.3390/v14061241

Li, Z., Zeng, H., Wang, Y., Zhang, Y., Cheng, L., Zhang, F., Lei, Y., Jin, B., Ma, Y., & Chen, L. (2017). The assessment of Hantaan virus-specific antibody responses after the immunization program for hemorrhagic fever with renal syndrome in northwest China. *Human Vaccines & Immunotherapeutics, 13*(4), 802–807. https://doi.org/10.1080/21645515.2016.1253645

Lim, J. T., Dickens, B. S. L., Chew, L. Z. X., Choo, E. L. W., Koo, J. R., Aik, J., Ng, L. C., & Cook, A. R. (2020). Impact of sars-cov-2 interventions on dengue transmission. *PLoS Neglected Tropical Diseases, 14*(10), e0008719. https://doi.org/10.1371/journal.pntd.0008719

Linderholm, M., & Elgh, F. (2001). Clinical characteristics of hantavirus infections on the Eurasian continent. *Current Topics in Microbiology and Immunology, 256*, 135–151. https://doi.org/10.1007/978-3-642-56753-7

Ling, J., Sironen, T., Voutilainen, L., Hepojoki, S., Niemimaa, J., Isoviita, V. M., Vaheri, A., Henttonen, H., & Vapalahti, O. (2014). Hantaviruses in Finnish soricomorphs: Evidence for two distinct hantaviruses carried by Sorex araneus suggesting ancient host-switch. *Infection, Genetics and Evolution, 27*, 51–61. https://doi.org/10.1016/j.meegid.2014.06.023

Ling, J., Smura, T., Tamarit, D., Huitu, O., Voutilainen, L., Henttonen, H., Vaheri, A., Vapalahti, O., & Sironen, T. (2018). Evolution and postglacial colonization of Seewis hantavirus with Sorex araneus in Finland. *Infection, Genetics and Evolution, 57*, 88–97. https://doi.org/10.1016/j.meegid.2017.11.010

Ling, J., Verner-Carlsson, J., Eriksson, P., Plyusnina, A., Lohmus, M., Jarhult, J. D., van de Goot, F., Plyusnin, A., Lundkvist, A., & Sironen, T. (2019). Genetic analyses of Seoul hantavirus genome recovered from rats (Rattus norvegicus) in the Netherlands unveils diverse routes of spread into Europe. *Journal of Medical Virology, 91*(5), 724–730. https://doi.org/10.1002/jmv.25390

Liu, R., Ma, H., Shu, J., Zhang, Q., Han, M., Liu, Z., Jin, X., Zhang, F., & Wu, X. (2019). Vaccines and therapeutics against Hantaviruses. *Frontiers in Microbiology, 10*, 2989. https://doi.org/10.3389/fmicb.2019.02989

Lober, C., Anheier, B., Lindow, S., Klenk, H. D., & Feldmann, H. (2001). The Hantaan virus glycoprotein precursor is cleaved at the conserved pentapeptide WAASA. *Virology, 289*(2), 224–229. https://doi.org/10.1006/viro.2001.1171

Lokugamage, K., Kariwa, H., Hayasaka, D., Cui, B. Z., Iwasaki, T., Lokugamage, N., Ivanov, L. I., Volkov, V. I., Demenev, V. A., Slonova, R., Kompanets, G., Kushnaryova, T., Kurata, T., Maeda, K., Araki, K., Mizutani, T., Yoshimatsu, K., Arikawa, J., & Takashima, I. (2002). Genetic characterization of hantaviruses transmitted by the Korean field mouse (Apodemus peninsulae), Far East Russia. *Emerging Infectious Diseases, 8*(8), 768–776. https://doi.org/10.3201/eid0808.010494

Lundkvist, A., & Niklasson, B. (1992). Bank vole monoclonal antibodies against Puumala virus envelope glycoproteins: Identification of epitopes involved in neutralization. *Archives of Virology, 126*(1–4), 93–105. https://doi.org/10.1007/BF01309687

Maes, P., Clement, J., & Van Ranst, M. (2009). Recent approaches in hantavirus vaccine development. *Expert Review of Vaccines, 8*(1), 67–76. https://doi.org/10.1586/14760584.8.1.67

Malinin, O. V., & Platonov, A. E. (2017). Insufficient efficacy and safety of intravenous ribavirin in treatment of haemorrhagic fever with renal syndrome caused by Puumala virus. *Infectious Diseases (London), 49*(7), 514–520. https://doi.org/10.1080/23744235.2017.1293841

Mayor, J., Engler, O., & Rothenberger, S. (2021). Antiviral efficacy of Ribavirin and Favipiravir against Hantaan Virus. *Microorganisms, 9*(6). https://doi.org/10.3390/microorganisms9061306

McClain, D. J., Summers, P. L., Harrison, S. A., Schmaljohn, A. L., & Schmaljohn, C. S. (2000). Clinical evaluation of a vaccinia-vectored Hantaan virus vaccine. *Journal of Medical Virology, 60*(1), 77–85. https://doi.org/10.1002/(sici)1096-9071(200001)60:1%3c77::aid-jmv13%3e3.0.co;2-s

McCormick, J. B., Sasso, D. R., Palmer, E. L., & Kiley, M. P. (1982). Morphological identification of the agent of Korean haemorrhagic fever (Hantaan virus)as a member of the Bunyaviridae. *Lancet, 1*(8275), 765–768. https://doi.org/10.1016/s0140-6736(82)91812-8

Meheretu, Y., Cizkova, D., Tesikova, J., Welegerima, K., Tomas, Z., Kidane, D., Girmay, K., Schmidt-Chanasit, J., Bryja, J., Gunther, S., Bryjova, A., Leirs, H., & Gouy de Bellocq, J. (2012). High diversity of RNA viruses in rodents, Ethiopia. *Emerging Infectious Diseases, 18*(12), 2047–2050. https://doi.org/10.3201/eid1812.120596

Meheretu, Y., Stanley, W. T., Craig, E. W., Gouy de Bellocq, J., Bryja, J., Leirs, H., Pahlmann, M., & Gunther, S. (2019). Tigray orthohantavirus infects two related rodent species adapted to different elevations in Ethiopia. *Vector Borne and Zoonotic Diseases, 19*(12), 950–953. https://doi.org/10.1089/vbz.2019.2452

Milholland, M. T., Castro-Arellano, I., Suzan, G., Garcia-Pena, G. E., Lee, T. E., Rohde, R. E., Alonso Aguirre, A., & Mills, J. N. (2018). Global Diversity and Distribution of Hantaviruses and Their Hosts. *Ecohealth, 15*(1), 163–208. https://doi.org/10.1007/s10393-017-1305-2

Mills, J. N. (2005). Regulation of rodent-borne viruses in the natural host: Implications for human disease. *Archives of Virology, 19*, 45–57. https://doi.org/10.1007/3-211-29981-5

Mir, M. A. (2010). Hantaviruses. *Clinics in Laboratory Medicine, 30*(1), 67–91. https://doi.org/10.1016/j.cll.2010.01.004

Mizumoto, K., Kagaya, K., & Chowell, G. (2020). Early epidemiological assessment of the transmission potential and virulence of coronavirus disease 2019 (COVID-19) in Wuhan City, China, January-February, 2020. *BMC Medicine, 18*(1), 217. https://doi.org/10.1186/s12916-020-01691-x

Muyangwa, M., Martynova, E. V., Khaiboullina, S. F., Morzunov, S. P., & Rizvanov, A. A. (2015). Hantaviral proteins: Structure, functions, and role in hantavirus infection. *Frontiers in Microbiology, 6*, 1326. https://doi.org/10.3389/fmicb.2015.01326

Myhrman, G. (1951). Nephropathia epidemica a new infectious disease in northern Scandinavia. *Acta Medica Scandinavica, 140*(1), 52–56. https://doi.org/10.1111/j.0954-6820.1951.tb10155.x

Noack, D., Goeijenbier, M., Reusken, C., Koopmans, M. P. G., & Rockx, B. H. G. (2020). Orthohantavirus pathogenesis and cell tropism. *Frontiers in Cellular and Infection Microbiology, 10*, 399. https://doi.org/10.3389/fcimb.2020.00399

Ohlopkova, O. V., Stolbunova, K. A., Popov, I. V., Popov, I. V., Kabwe, E., Davidyuk, Y. N., Stepanyuk, M. A., Moshkin, A. D., Kononova, Y. V., Lukbanova, E. A., Ermakov, A. M., Chikindas, M. L., Sobolev, I. A., Khaiboullina, S. F., & Shestopalov, A. M. (2024). Detection of Brno loanvirus (Loanvirus brunaense) in common noctule bats (Nyctalus noctula) in Southern Russia. *Brazilian Journal of Microbiology*. https://doi.org/10.1007/s42770-024-01587-5

Olsson, G. E., White, N., Ahlm, C., Elgh, F., Verlemyr, A. C., Juto, P., & Palo, R. T. (2002). Demographic factors associated with hantavirus infection in bank voles (Clethrionomys glareolus). *Emerging Infectious Diseases, 8*(9), 924–929. https://doi.org/10.3201/eid0809.020037

On the state of sanitary and epidemiological well-being of the population in the Russian Federation in 2022: State report. M.: Federal Service for Supervision of Consumer Rights Protection and Human Welfare, 2023. 368 p. https://rospotrebnadzor.ru/upload/iblock/b50/t4kqksh4b12a2iwjnha29922vu7naki5/GD-SEB.pdf.

Organization WH. COVID19 Strategy Update. 2020; 1–18. https://www.who.int/. COVID19 Strategy UpdaTE. Accessed 10 December 2020.

PAHO/WHO Hantavirus. Available online: https://www3.paho.org/hq/index.php?option=com_content&view=article&id=14911:hantavirus&Itemid=40721&lang=en#:~:text=Hantavirus%20(HV)%20is%20an%20emerging,of%20respiratory%20distress%20and%20hypotension (13 October 2022).

Pantophlet, R., & Burton, D. R. (2006). GP120: Target for neutralizing HIV-1 antibodies. *Annual Review of Immunology, 24*, 739–769. https://doi.org/10.1146/annurev.immunol.24.021605.090557

Park, K., Kim, C. S., & Moon, K. T. (2004). Protective effectiveness of hantavirus vaccine. *Emerging Infectious Diseases, 10*(12), 2218–2220. https://doi.org/10.3201/eid1012.040684

Park, S. M., & Kim, J. (2008). A soluble and heat-resistant form of hantavirus nucleocapsid protein for the serodiagnosis of HFRS. *Journal of Virological Methods, 147*(1), 1–9. https://doi.org/10.1016/j.jviromet.2007.08.001

Park, K., Kim, W. K., Lee, S. H., Kim, J., Lee, J., Cho, S., Lee, G. Y., No, J. S., Lee, K. H., & Song, J. W. (2021). A novel genotype of Hantaan orthohantavirus harbored by Apodemus agrarius chejuensis as a potential etiologic agent of hemorrhagic fever with renal syndrome in Republic of Korea. *PLoS Neglected Tropical Diseases, 15*(5), e0009400. https://doi.org/10.1371/journal.pntd.0009400

Pettersson, L., Thunberg, T., Rocklov, J., Klingstrom, J., Evander, M., & Ahlm, C. (2014). Viral load and humoral immune response in association with disease severity in Puumala hantavirus-infected patients—Implications for treatment. *Clinical Microbiology & Infection, 20*(3), 235–241. https://doi.org/10.1111/1469-0691.12259

Pljusnin, A., & Elliott, R. M. (2011). *Bunyaviridae: Molecular and cellular biology*. Caister Academic Press.

Plyusnin, A., & Morzunov, S. (2001). Virus evolution and genetic diversity of hantaviruses and their rodent hosts. *Hantaviruses*, 47–75.

Plyusnin, A., & Sironen, T. (2014). Evolution of hantaviruses: Co-speciation with reservoir hosts for more than 100 MYR. *Virus Research, 187*, 22–26.

Plyusnin, A., Vapalahti, O., Lundkvist, A., Henttonen, H., & Vaheri, A. (1996). Newly recognised hantavirus in Siberian lemmings. *Lancet, 347*(9018), 1835. https://doi.org/10.1016/s0140-6736(96)91655-4

Plyusnina, A., Ibrahim, I. N., & Plyusnin, A. (2009). A newly recognized hantavirus in the Asian house rat (Rattus tanezumi) in Indonesia. *Journal of General Virology, 90*(Pt 1), 205–209. https://doi.org/10.1099/vir.0.006155-0

Poor, A. *Cricetidae world rats and mice, voles, hamsters, and relatives*. Available online: https://animaldiversity.org/accounts/Cricetidae/.

Povalishina, T. (1965). On the influence of the human activity upon the existence and detection of natural foci of haemorrhagic fever with a renal syndrome. In B. Rasick & K. Heyberger (Ed.), *Theoretical questions of natural foci of diseases*. Czechoslovak Academy of Sciences.

Radosa, L., Schlegel, M., Gebauer, P., Ansorge, H., Heroldova, M., Janova, E., Stanko, M., Mosansky, L., Fricova, J., Pejcoch, M., Suchomel, J., Purchart, L., Groschup, M. H., Kruger, D. H., Ulrich, R. G., & Klempa, B. (2013). Detection of shrew-borne hantavirus in Eurasian pygmy shrew (Sorex minutus) in Central Europe. *Infection, Genetics and Evolution, 19*, 403–410. https://doi.org/10.1016/j.meegid.2013.04.008

Raharinosy, V., Olive, M. M., Andriamiarimanana, F. M., Andriamandimby, S. F., Ravalohery, J. P., Andriamamonjy, S., Filippone, C., Rakoto, D. A. D., Telfer, S., & Heraud, J. M. (2018).

Geographical distribution and relative risk of Anjozorobe virus (Thailand orthohantavirus) infection in black rats (Rattus rattus) in Madagascar. *Journal of Virology, 15*(1), 83. https://doi.org/10.1186/s12985-018-0992-9

Razzauti, M., Plyusnina, A., Henttonen, H., & Plyusnin, A. (2008). Accumulation of point mutations and reassortment of genomic RNA segments are involved in the microevolution of Puumala hantavirus in a bank vole (Myodes glareolus) population. *Journal of General Virology, 89*(Pt 7), 1649–1660. https://doi.org/10.1099/vir.0.2008/001248-0

Razzauti, M., Plyusnina, A., Henttonen, H., & Plyusnin, A. (2013). Microevolution of Puumala hantavirus during a complete population cycle of its host, the bank vole (Myodes glareolus). *PLoS ONE, 8*(5), e64447. https://doi.org/10.1371/journal.pone.0064447

Razzauti, M., Plyusnina, A., Niemimaa, J., Henttonen, H., & Plyusnin, A. (2012). Co-circulation of two Puumala hantavirus lineages in Latvia: A Russian lineage described previously and a novel Latvian lineage. *Journal of Medical Virology, 84*(2), 314–318. https://doi.org/10.1002/jmv.22263

Reusken, C., & Heyman, P. (2013). Factors driving hantavirus emergence in Europe. *Current Opinion in Virology, 3*(1), 92–99. https://doi.org/10.1016/j.coviro.2013.01.002

Rey, G.-C. A. (2021). The surface glycoproteins of hantaviruses. *Current Opinion in Virology, 50*, 87–94.

Reynes, J. M., Razafindralambo, N. K., Lacoste, V., Olive, M. M., Barivelo, T. A., Soarimalala, V., Heraud, J. M., & Lavergne, A. (2014). Anjozorobe hantavirus, a new genetic variant of Thailand virus detected in rodents from Madagascar. *Vector Borne and Zoonotic Diseases, 14*(3), 212–219. https://doi.org/10.1089/vbz.2013.1359

Rhen, T., & Cidlowski, J. A. (2005). Antiinflammatory action of glucocorticoids—New mechanisms for old drugs. *New England Journal of Medicine, 353*(16), 1711–1723. https://doi.org/10.1056/NEJMra050541

Rissanen, I., Krumm, S. A., Stass, R., Whitaker, A., Voss, J. E., Bruce, E. A., Rothenberger, S., Kunz, S., Burton, D. R., Huiskonen, J. T., Botten, J. W., Bowden, T. A., & Doores, K. J. (2021). Structural basis for a neutralizing antibody response elicited by a recombinant Hantaan Virus Gn Immunogen. *mBio, 12*(4), e0253120. https://doi.org/10.1128/mBio.02531-20

Rizvanov, A. A., Khaiboullina, S. F., & St Jeor, S. (2004). Development of reassortant viruses between pathogenic hantavirus strains. *Virology, 327*(2), 225–232. https://doi.org/10.1016/j.virol.2004.07.012

Rodriguez, L. L., Owens, J. H., Peters, C. J., & Nichol, S. T. (1998). Genetic reassortment among viruses causing hantavirus pulmonary syndrome. *Virology, 242*(1), 99–106.

Schlegel, M., Kindler, E., Essbauer, S. S., Wolf, R., Thiel, J., Groschup, M. H., Heckel, G., Oehme, R. M., & Ulrich, R. G. (2012). Tula virus infections in the Eurasian water vole in Central Europe. *Vector Borne and Zoonotic Diseases, 12*(6), 503–513. https://doi.org/10.1089/vbz.2011.0784

Schmaljohn, C. S. (2012). Vaccines for hantaviruses: Progress and issues. *Expert Review of Vaccines, 11*(5), 511–513. https://doi.org/10.1586/erv.12.15

Schmaljohn, C. S., Hasty, S. E., & Dalrymple, J. M. (1992). Preparation of candidate vaccinia-vectored vaccines for haemorrhagic fever with renal syndrome. *Vaccine, 10*(1), 10–13. https://doi.org/10.1016/0264-410x(92)90412-d

Schmaljohn, C. S., Hasty, S. E., Harrison, S. A., & Dalrymple, J. M. (1983). Characterization of Hantaan virions, the prototype virus of hemorrhagic fever with renal syndrome. *Journal of Infectious Diseases, 148*(6), 1005–1012. https://doi.org/10.1093/infdis/148.6.1005

Schmidt, J., Jandrig, B., Klempa, B., Yoshimatsu, K., Arikawa, J., Meisel, H., Niedrig, M., Pitra, C., Kruger, D. H., & Ulrich, R. (2005). Nucleocapsid protein of cell culture-adapted Seoul virus strain 80–39: Analysis of its encoding sequence, expression in yeast and immuno-reactivity. *Virus Genes, 30*(1), 37–48. https://doi.org/10.1007/s11262-004-4580-2

Sehgal, A., Mehta, S., Sahay, K., Martynova, E., Rizvanov, A., Baranwal, M., Chandy, S., Khaiboullina, S., Kabwe, E., & Davidyuk, Y. (2023). Hemorrhagic fever with renal syndrome in Asia: History, pathogenesis, diagnosis, treatment, and prevention. *Viruses, 15*(2). https://doi.org/10.3390/v15020561

Seitsonen, E., Hynninen, M., Kolho, E., Kallio-Kokko, H., & Pettila, V. (2006). Corticosteroids combined with continuous veno-venous hemodiafiltration for treatment of hantavirus pulmonary syndrome caused by Puumala virus infection. *European Journal of Clinical Microbiology and Infectious Diseases, 25*(4), 261–266. https://doi.org/10.1007/s10096-006-0117-z

Severson, W. E., Schmaljohn, C. S., Javadian, A., & Jonsson, C. B. (2003). Ribavirin causes error catastrophe during Hantaan virus replication. *Journal of Virology, 77*(1), 481–488. https://doi.org/10.1128/jvi.77.1.481-488.2003

Shastri, B., Kofman, A., Hennenfent, A., Klena, J. D., Nicol, S., Graziano, J. C., Morales-Betoulle, M., Cannon, D., Maradiaga, A., Tran, A., & Ramdeen, S. K. (2019). Domestically acquired Seoul virus causing hemophagocytic lymphohistiocytosis-Washington, DC, 2018. *Open Forum Infectious Diseases, 6*(10), ofz404. https://doi.org/10.1093/ofid/ofz404

Shen, J., Duan, H., Zhang, B., Wang, J., Ji, J. S., Wang, J., Pan, L., Wang, X., Zhao, K., Ying, B., Tang, S., Zhang, J., Liang, C., Sun, H., Lv, Y., Li, Y., Li, T., Li, L., Liu, H., Zhang, L., Wang, L., & Shi, X. (2020). Prevention and control of COVID-19 in public transportation: Experience from China. *Environmental Pollution, 266*(Pt 2), 115291. https://doi.org/10.1016/j.envpol.2020.115291

Shkair, L., Garanina, E. E., Martynova, E. V., Kolesnikova, A. I., Arkhipova, S. S., Titova, A. A., Rizvanov, A. A., & Khaiboullina, S. F. (2022). Immunogenic properties of MVs containing structural hantaviral proteins: An original study. *Pharmaceutics, 14*(1). https://doi.org/10.3390/pharmaceutics14010093

Sibold, C., Meisel, H., Kruger, D. H., Labuda, M., Lysy, J., Kozuch, O., Pejcoch, M., Vaheri, A., & Plyusnin, A. (1999). Recombination in Tula hantavirus evolution: Analysis of genetic lineages from Slovakia. *Journal of Virology, 73*(1), 667–675. https://doi.org/10.1128/JVI.73.1.667-675.1999

Singh, S., Numan, A., Sharma, D., Shukla, R., Alexander, A., Jain, G. K., Ahmad, F. J., & Kesharwani, P. (2022). Epidemiology, virology and clinical aspects of hantavirus infections: An overview. *International Journal of Environmental Health Research, 32*(8), 1815–1826. https://doi.org/10.1080/09603123.2021.1917527

Singhal, T. (2020). A review of Coronavirus disease-2019 (COVID-19). *Indian Journal of Pediatrics, 87*(4), 281–286. https://doi.org/10.1007/s12098-020-03263-6

Sironen, T., Vaheri, A., & Plyusnin, A. (2001). Molecular evolution of Puumala hantavirus. *Journal of Virology, 75*(23), 11803–11810. https://doi.org/10.1128/JVI.75.23.11803-11810.2001

Smadel, J. E. (1953). Epidemic hemorrhagic fever. *American Journal of Public Health and the Nations Health, 43*(10), 1327–1330.

Smorodintsev, A. A., Chudakov, V., & Churilov, A. (1959). Haemorrhagic Nephroso-Nephritis. *Haemorrhagic Nephroso-Nephritis.*

Sohn, Y. M., Rho, H. O., Park, M. S., Kim, J. S., & Summers, P. L. (2001). Primary humoral immune responses to formalin inactivated hemorrhagic fever with renal syndrome vaccine (Hantavax): Consideration of active immunization in South Korea. *Yonsei Medical Journal, 42*(3), 278–284. https://doi.org/10.3349/ymj.2001.42.3.278

Song, G. (1999). Epidemiological progresses of hemorrhagic fever with renal syndrome in China. *Chinese Medical Journal (England), 112*(5), 472–477. https://www.ncbi.nlm.nih.gov/pubmed/11593522

Song, J. W., Baek, L. J., Schmaljohn, C. S., & Yanagihara, R. (2007). Thottapalayam virus, a prototype shrewborne hantavirus. *Emerging Infectious Diseases, 13*(7), 980–985. https://doi.org/10.3201/eid1307.070031

Song, J. W., Kang, H. J., Song, K. J., Truong, T. T., Bennett, S. N., Arai, S., Truong, N. U., & Yanagihara, R. (2007). Newfound hantavirus in Chinese mole shrew, Vietnam. *Emerging Infectious Diseases, 13*(11), 1784–1787. https://doi.org/10.3201/eid1311.070492

Song, J. W., Song, K. J., Baek, L. J., Frost, B., Poncz, M., & Park, K. (2005). In vivo characterization of the integrin beta3 as a receptor for Hantaan virus cellular entry. *Experimental & Molecular Medicine, 37*(2), 121–127. https://doi.org/10.1038/emm.2005.16

Song, J. Y., Jeong, H. W., Yun, J. W., Lee, J., Woo, H. J., Bae, J. Y., Park, M. S., Choi, W. S., Park, D. W., Noh, J. Y., Cheong, H. J., & Kim, W. J. (2020). Immunogenicity and safety of a modified three-dose priming and booster schedule for the Hantaan virus vaccine (Hantavax): A multi-center phase III clinical trial in healthy adults. *Vaccine, 38*(50), 8016–8023. https://doi.org/10.1016/j.vaccine.2020.10.035

Song, J. Y., Woo, H. J., Cheong, H. J., Noh, J. Y., Baek, L. J., & Kim, W. J. (2016). Long-term immunogenicity and safety of inactivated Hantaan virus vaccine (Hantavax) in healthy adults. *Vaccine, 34*(10), 1289–1295. https://doi.org/10.1016/j.vaccine.2016.01.031

Souza, W. M., Bello, G., Amarilla, A. A., Alfonso, H. L., Aquino, V. H., & Figueiredo, L. T. (2014). Phylogeography and evolutionary history of rodent-borne hantaviruses. *Infection, Genetics and Evolution, 21*, 198–204. https://doi.org/10.1016/j.meegid.2013.11.015

Spiteri, G., Fielding, J., Diercke, M., Campese, C., Enouf, V., Gaymard, A., Bella, A., Sognamiglio, P., Sierra Moros, M. J., Riutort, A. N., Demina, Y. V., Mahieu, R., Broas, M., Bengner, M., Buda, S., Schilling, J., Filleul, L., Lepoutre, A., Saura, C., Mailles, A., Levy-Bruhl, D., Coignard, B., Bernard-Stoecklin, S., Behillil, S., van der Werf, S., Valette, M., Lina, B., Riccardo, F., Nicastri, E., Casas, I., Larrauri, A., Salom Castell, M., Pozo, F., Maksyutov, R. A., Martin, C., Van Ranst, M., Bossuyt, N., Siira, L., Sane, J., Tegmark-Wisell, K., Palmerus, M., Broberg, E. K., Beaute, J., Jorgensen, P., Bundle, N., Pereyaslov, D., Adlhoch, C., Pukkila, J., Pebody, R., Olsen, S., & Ciancio, B. C. (2020). First cases of coronavirus disease 2019 (COVID-19) in the WHO European Region, 24 January to 21 February 2020. *Eurosurveillance, 25*(9). https://doi.org/10.2807/1560-7917.ES.2020.25.9.2000178

Steer, A. (1955). Pathology of hemorrhagic fever: A comparison of the findings; 1951 and 1952. *The American Journal of Pathology, 31*(2), 201–221. https://www.ncbi.nlm.nih.gov/pubmed/14350062

Strakova, P., Dufkova, L., Sirmarova, J., Salat, J., Bartonicka, T., Klempa, B., Pfaff, F., Hoper, D., Hoffmann, B., Ulrich, R. G., & Ruzek, D. (2017). Novel hantavirus identified in European bat species Nyctalus noctula. *Infection, Genetics and Evolution, 48*, 127–130. https://doi.org/10.1016/j.meegid.2016.12.025

Sumibcay, L., Kadjo, B., Gu, S. H., Kang, H. J., Lim, B. K., Cook, J. A., Song, J. W., & Yanagihara, R. (2012). Divergent lineage of a novel hantavirus in the banana pipistrelle (Neoromicia nanus) in Cote d'Ivoire. *Journal of Virology, 9*, 34. https://doi.org/10.1186/1743-422X-9-34

Surveillance Atlas of Infectious Diseases. [online source]. http://atlas.ecdc.europa.eu/public/index.aspx

Taller, A. M., Xiao, S. Y., Godec, M. S., Gligic, A., Avsic-Zupanc, T., Goldfarb, L. G., Yanagihara, R., & Asher, D. M. (1993). Belgrade virus, a cause of hemorrhagic fever with renal syndrome in the Balkans, is closely related to Dobrava virus of field mice. *Journal of Infectious Diseases, 168*(3), 750–753. https://doi.org/10.1093/infdis/168.3.750

Taylor, S. L., Wahl-Jensen, V., Copeland, A. M., Jahrling, P. B., & Schmaljohn, C. S. (2013). Endothelial cell permeability during hantavirus infection involves factor XII-dependent increased activation of the kallikrein-kinin system. *PLoS Pathogens, 9*(7), e1003470. https://doi.org/10.1371/journal.ppat.1003470

Tian, H., & Stenseth, N. C. (2019). The ecological dynamics of hantavirus diseases: From environmental variability to disease prevention largely based on data from China. *PLoS Neglected Tropical Diseases, 13*(2), e0006901. https://doi.org/10.1371/journal.pntd.0006901

Tian, H., Yu, P., Bjornstad, O. N., Cazelles, B., Yang, J., Tan, H., Huang, S., Cui, Y., Dong, L., Ma, C., Ma, C., Zhou, S., Laine, M., Wu, X., Zhang, Y., Wang, J., Yang, R., Stenseth, N. C., & Xu, B. (2017). Anthropogenically driven environmental changes shift the ecological dynamics of hemorrhagic fever with renal syndrome. *PLoS Pathogens, 13*(1), e1006198. https://doi.org/10.1371/journal.ppat.1006198

Tkachenko, E. A., Dzagurova, T. K., & Tkachenko, P. E. (2014). Current status of Hantavirus vaccines development. In *Novel technologies for vaccine development* (pp. 113–151). Springer.

Tkachenko, E. A., Ishmukhametov, A. A., Dzagurova, T. K., Bernshtein, A. D., Morozov, V. G., Siniugina, A. A., Kurashova, S. S., Balkina, A. S., Tkachenko, P. E., Kruger, D. H., & Klempa, B.

(2019). Hemorrhagic fever with renal syndrome, Russia. *Emerging Infectious Diseases, 25*(12), 2325–2328. https://doi.org/10.3201/eid2512.181649

Ulrich, R., Koletzki, D., Lachmann, S., Lundkvist, A., Zankl, A., Kazaks, A., Kurth, A., Gelderblom, H. R., Borisova, G., Meisel, H., & Kruger, D. H. (1999). New chimaeric hepatitis B virus core particles carrying hantavirus (serotype Puumala) epitopes: Immunogenicity and protection against virus challenge. *Journal of Biotechnology, 73*(2–3), 141–153. https://doi.org/10.1016/s0168-1656(99)00117-0

Vaheri, A., Henttonen, H., Voutilainen, L., Mustonen, J., Sironen, T., & Vapalahti, O. (2013). Hantavirus infections in Europe and their impact on public health. *Reviews in Medical Virology, 23*(1), 35–49. https://doi.org/10.1002/rmv.1722

Vaheri, A., Vapalahti, O., & Plyusnin, A. (2008). How to diagnose hantavirus infections and detect them in rodents and insectivores. *Reviews in Medical Virology, 18*(4), 277–288. https://doi.org/10.1002/rmv.581

Van Epps, H. L., Schmaljohn, C. S., & Ennis, F. A. (1999). Human memory cytotoxic T-lymphocyte (CTL) responses to Hantaan virus infection: Identification of virus-specific and cross-reactive CD8(+) CTL epitopes on nucleocapsid protein. *Journal of Virology, 73*(7), 5301–5308. https://doi.org/10.1128/JVI.73.7.5301-5308.1999

Vial, P. A., Valdivieso, F., Calvo, M., Rioseco, M. L., Riquelme, R., Araneda, A., Tomicic, V., Graf, J., Paredes, L., Florenzano, M., Bidart, T., Cuiza, A., Marco, C., Hjelle, B., Ye, C., Hanfelt-Goade, D., Vial, C., Rivera, J. C., Delgado, I., Mertz, G. J., & Hantavirus Study Group in C. (2015). A non-randomized multicentre trial of human immune plasma for treatment of hantavirus cardiopulmonary syndrome caused by Andes virus. *Antiviral Therapy, 20*(4), 377–386. https://doi.org/10.3851/IMP2875

Vial, P. A., Valdivieso, F., Ferres, M., Riquelme, R., Rioseco, M. L., Calvo, M., Castillo, C., Diaz, R., Scholz, L., Cuiza, A., Belmar, E., Hernandez, C., Martinez, J., Lee, S. J., Mertz, G. J., & Hantavirus Study Group in C. (2013). High-dose intravenous methylprednisolone for hantavirus cardiopulmonary syndrome in Chile: A double-blind, randomized controlled clinical trial. *Clinical Infectious Diseases, 57*(7), 943–951. https://doi.org/10.1093/cid/cit394

Wagenknecht, H.-A. (2009). Book review. *Protein Science, 13*, 3331–3332. https://doi.org/10.1110/ps.041082704

Wang, C. Q., Gao, J. H., Li, M., Guo, W. P., Lu, M. Q., Wang, W., Hu, M. X., Li, M. H., Yang, J., Liang, H. J., Tian, X. F., Holmes, E. C., & Zhang, Y. Z. (2014). Co-circulation of Hantaan, Kenkeme, and Khabarovsk Hantaviruses in Bolshoy Ussuriysky Island, China. *Virus Research, 191*, 51–58. https://doi.org/10.1016/j.virusres.2014.07.021

Wang, D., Hu, B., Hu, C., Zhu, F., Liu, X., Zhang, J., Wang, B., Xiang, H., Cheng, Z., Xiong, Y., Zhao, Y., Li, Y., Wang, X., & Peng, Z. (2020). Clinical characteristics of 138 hospitalized patients with 2019 novel Coronavirus-Infected Pneumonia in Wuhan, China. *JAMA, 323*(11), 1061–1069. https://doi.org/10.1001/jama.2020.1585

Wang, H., Yoshimatsu, K., Ebihara, H., Ogino, M., Araki, K., Kariwa, H., Wang, Z., Luo, Z., Li, D., Hang, C., & Arikawa, J. (2000). Genetic diversity of hantaviruses isolated in china and characterization of novel hantaviruses isolated from Niviventer confucianus and Rattus rattus. *Virology, 278*(2), 332–345. https://doi.org/10.1006/viro.2000.0630

Wang, H., Yoshimatsu, K., Ebihara, H., Ogino, M., Araki, K., Kariwa, H., ... & Arikawa, J. (2000). Genetic diversity of hantaviruses isolated in China and characterization of novel hantaviruses isolated from Niviventer confucianus and Rattus rattus. *Virology, 278*(2), 332–345.

Wang, J. J., Wei, Z. Z., Wei, J., Ma, C. A., Dong, J. H., Lu, X. L., Zheng, Y., Yu, P. B., Qu, J. H., & Dong, L. F. (2012). Long term epidemiological effects of vaccination on hemorrhagical fever with renal syndrome (HFRS) in Shaanxi provincial HFRS epidemic areas. *Zhonghua Liu Xing Bing Xue Za Zhi, 33*(3), 309–312. https://www.ncbi.nlm.nih.gov/pubmed/22613385

Wang, M., Wang, J., Wang, T., Li, J., Hui, L., & Ha, X. (2013). Thrombocytopenia as a predictor of severe acute kidney injury in patients with Hantaan virus infections. *PLoS ONE, 8*(1), e53236. https://doi.org/10.1371/journal.pone.0053236

Wang, M., Zhu, Y., Wang, J., Lv, T., & Jin, B. (2011). Identification of three novel CTL epitopes within nucleocapsid protein of Hantaan virus. *Viral Immunology, 24*(6), 449–454. https://doi.org/10.1089/vim.2011.0026

Watson, D. C., Sargianou, M., Papa, A., Chra, P., Starakis, I., & Panos, G. (2014). Epidemiology of Hantavirus infections in humans: A comprehensive, global overview. *Critical Reviews in Microbiology, 40*(3), 261–272. https://doi.org/10.3109/1040841X.2013.783555

Weiss, S., Sudi, L. E., Dux, A., Mangu, C. D., Ntinginya, N. E., Shirima, G. M., Kondgen, S., Schubert, G., Witkowski, P. T., Muyembe, J. J., Ahuka, S., Klempa, B., Leendertz, F. H., & Kruger, D. H. (2022). Kiwira virus, a newfound Hantavirus discovered in free-tailed Bats (Molossidae) in East and Central Africa. *Viruses, 14*(11). https://doi.org/10.3390/v14112368

Weiss, S., Witkowski, P. T., Auste, B., Nowak, K., Weber, N., Fahr, J., Mombouli, J. V., Wolfe, N. D., Drexler, J. F., Drosten, C., Klempa, B., Leendertz, F. H., & Kruger, D. H. (2012). Hantavirus in bat, Sierra Leone. *Emerging Infectious Diseases, 18*(1), 159–161. https://doi.org/10.3201/eid1801.111026

Witkowski, P. T., Drexler, J. F., Kallies, R., Lickova, M., Bokorova, S., Maganga, G. D., Szemes, T., Leroy, E. M., Kruger, D. H., Drosten, C., & Klempa, B. (2016). Phylogenetic analysis of a newfound bat-borne hantavirus supports a laurasiatherian host association for ancestral mammalian hantaviruses. *Infection, Genetics and Evolution, 41*, 113–119. https://doi.org/10.1016/j.meegid.2016.03.036

Wu, D., Lu, J., Cao, L., Ma, X., Liu, Q., Liu, Y., & Zhang, Z. (2020). Positive effects of COVID-19 control measures on pneumonia prevention. *International Journal of Infectious Diseases, 96*, 548–549. https://doi.org/10.1016/j.ijid.2020.05.069

Wu, D., Lu, J., Liu, Y., Zhang, Z., & Luo, L. (2020). Positive effects of COVID-19 control measures on influenza prevention. *International Journal of Infectious Diseases, 95*, 345–346. https://doi.org/10.1016/j.ijid.2020.04.009

Wu, J. T., Leung, K., & Leung, G. M. (2020). Nowcasting and forecasting the potential domestic and international spread of the 2019-nCoV outbreak originating in Wuhan, China: A modelling study. *Lancet, 395*(10225), 689–697. https://doi.org/10.1016/S0140-6736(20)30260-9

Xiao, Y., Li, Y., Li, Y., Yu, C., Bai, Y., Wang, L., & Wang, Y. (2021). Estimating the long-term epidemiological trends and seasonality of hemorrhagic fever with renal syndrome in China. *Infection and Drug Resistance, 14*, 3849–3862. https://doi.org/10.2147/IDR.S325787

Xu, L., Wu, J., He, B., Qin, S., Xia, L., Qin, M., Li, N., & Tu, C. (2015). Novel hantavirus identified in black-bearded tomb bats, China. *Infection, Genetics and Evolution, 31*, 158–160. https://doi.org/10.1016/j.meegid.2015.01.018

Xu, R., Yang, X. Y., Yang, D. F., Zou, C. Y., Gong, P. L., & Zeng, F. D. (2009). Phase I evaluation of the safety and pharmacokinetics of a single-dose intravenous injection of a murine monoclonal antibody against Hantaan virus in healthy volunteers. *Antimicrobial Agents and Chemotherapy, 53*(12), 5055–5059. https://doi.org/10.1128/AAC.00728-09

Xu, Z., Wei, L., Wang, L., Wang, H., & Jiang, S. (2002). The in vitro and in vivo protective activity of monoclonal antibodies directed against Hantaan virus: Potential application for immunotherapy and passive immunization. *Biochemical and Biophysical Research Communications, 298*(4), 552–558. https://doi.org/10.1016/s0006-291x(02)02491-9

Yamanishi, K., Tanishita, O., Tamura, M., Asada, H., Kondo, K., Takagi, M., Yoshida, I., Konobe, T., & Fukai, K. (1988). Development of inactivated vaccine against virus causing haemorrhagic fever with renal syndrome. *Vaccine, 6*(3), 278–282. https://doi.org/10.1016/0264-410x(88)90224-1

Yanagihara, R., Gu, S. H., Arai, S., Kang, H. J., & Song, J. W. (2014). Hantaviruses: Rediscovery and new beginnings. *Virus Research, 187*, 6–14. https://doi.org/10.1016/j.virusres.2013.12.038

Yashina, L. N., Abramov, S. A., Zhigalin, A. V., Smetannikova, N. A., Dupal, T. A., Krivopalov, A. V., Kikuchi, F., Senoo, K., Arai, S., Mizutani, T., Suzuki, M., Cook, J. A., & Yanagihara, R. (2021). Geographic distribution and phylogeny of soricine shrew-borne Seewis virus and Altai virus in Russia. *Viruses, 13*(7). https://doi.org/10.3390/v13071286

Yashina, L. N., Panov, V. V., Abramov, S. A., Smetannikova, N. A., Luchnikova, E. M., Dupal, T. A., Krivopalov, A. V., Arai, S., & Yanagihara, R. (2022). Academ virus, a novel Hantavirus in the Siberian Mole (Talpa altaica) from Russia. *Viruses, 14*(2). https://doi.org/10.3390/v14020309

Yi, Y., Park, H., & Jung, J. (2018). Effectiveness of inactivated hantavirus vaccine on the disease severity of hemorrhagic fever with renal syndrome. *Kidney Research and Clinical Practice, 37*(4), 366–372. https://doi.org/10.23876/j.krcp.18.0044

Ying, X., Lai, X., Jin, X., Cai, L., & Li, X. (2020). Continuous renal replacement therapy rescues severe haemorrhagic fever with renal syndrome in pregnancy: A case report. *BMC Infectious Diseases, 20*(1), 920. https://doi.org/10.1186/s12879-020-05638-8

Zana, B., Kemenesi, G., Buzas, D., Csorba, G., Gorfol, T., Khan, F. A. A., Tahir, N., Zeghbib, S., Madai, M., Papp, H., Foldes, F., Urban, P., Herczeg, R., Toth, G. E., & Jakab, F. (2019). Molecular identification of a novel hantavirus in Malaysian bronze tube-nosed bats (Murina aenea). *Viruses, 11*(10). https://doi.org/10.3390/v11100887

Zeller, H. G., Karabatsos, N., Calisher, C. H., Digoutte, J. P., Cropp, C. B., Murphy, F. A., & Shope, R. E. (1989). Electron microscopic and antigenic studies of uncharacterized viruses. II. Evidence suggesting the placement of viruses in the family Bunyaviridae. *Archives of Virology, 108*(3–4), 211–227. https://doi.org/10.1007/BF01310935

Zhang, X. K., Takashima, I., & Hashimoto, N. (1989). Characteristics of passive immunity against hantavirus infection in rats. *Archives of Virology, 105*(3–4), 235–246. https://doi.org/10.1007/BF01311360

Zhang, Y., Yuan, J., Yang, X., Zhou, J., Yang, W., Peng, C., Zhang, H. L., & Shi, Z. (2011). A novel hantavirus detected in Yunnan red-backed vole (Eothenomys miletus) in China. *Journal of General Virology, 92*(Pt 6), 1454–1457. https://doi.org/10.1099/vir.0.030122-0

Zhang, Y. Z. (2014). Discovery of hantaviruses in bats and insectivores and the evolution of the genus Hantavirus. *Virus Research, 187*, 15–21. https://doi.org/10.1016/j.virusres.2013.12.035

Zhang, Y. Z., Xiao, D. L., Wang, Y., Wang, H. X., Sun, L., Tao, X. X., & Qu, Y. G. (2004). The epidemic characteristics and preventive measures of hemorrhagic fever with syndromes in China. *Zhonghua Liu Xing Bing Xue Za Zhi, 25*(6), 466–469. https://www.ncbi.nlm.nih.gov/pubmed/15231118

Zhang, Y. Z., Zou, Y., Fu, Z. F., & Plyusnin, A. (2010). Hantavirus infections in humans and animals, China. *Emerging Infectious Diseases, 16*(8), 1195–1203. https://doi.org/10.3201/eid1608.090470

Zheng, Y., Zhou, B. Y., Wei, J., Xu, Y., Dong, J. H., Guan, L. Y., Ma, P., Yu, P. B., & Wang, J. J. (2018). Persistence of immune responses to vaccine against haemorrhagic fever with renal syndrome in healthy adults aged 16–60 years: Results from an open-label 2-year follow-up study. *Infectious Diseases (London), 50*(1), 21–26. https://doi.org/10.1080/23744235.2017.1353704

Zou, L. X., & Sun, L. (2020). Analysis of hemorrhagic fever with renal syndrome using wavelet tools in Mainland China, 2004–2019. *Frontiers in Public Health, 8*, 571984. https://doi.org/10.3389/fpubh.2020.571984

Zou, Y., Wang, J. B., Gaowa, H. S., Yao, L. S., Hu, G. W., Li, M. H., Chen, H. X., Plyusnin, A., Shao, R., & Zhang, Y. Z. (2008). Isolation and genetic characterization of hantaviruses carried by Microtus voles in China. *Journal of Medical Virology, 80*(4), 680–688. https://doi.org/10.1002/jmv.21119

Chapter 3

Action against cholera | UNICEF Malawi [Internet]. 2023 [cited 2023 May 2]. Available from: https://www.unicef.org/malawi/reports/action-against-cholera

Africa CDC. ommuniqué from Africa CDC on the Southern Africa Development Community (SADC) Extra Ordinary Virtual Summit of Heads of State and Government on the Cholera situation in the region [Internet]. 2024 February. Available from: https://africacdc.org/news-item/communique-from-africa-cdc-on-the-southern-africa-development-community-sadc-extra-ordinary-virtual-summit-of-heads-of-state-and-government-on-the-cholera-situation-in-the-region/

Ali, M., Nelson, A. R., Lopez, A. L., Sack, D. A. (2015, June 4). Updated global burden of cholera in endemic countries. Remais JV, editor. *PLOS Neglected Tropical Diseases, 9*(6), e0003832.

Bangert, M., Molyneux, D. H., Lindsay, S. W., Fitzpatrick, C., & Engels, D. (2017, April 4). The cross-cutting contribution of the end of neglected tropical diseases to the sustainable development goals. *Infectious Diseases of Poverty, 6*(1), 73.

Bompangue Nkoko, D., Giraudoux, P., Plisnier, P. D., Tinda, A. M., Piarroux, M., Sudre, B., et al. (2011, November) Dynamics of cholera outbreaks in Great Lakes region of Africa, 1978-2008. *Emerging Infectious Diseases, 17*(11), 2026–2034.

Cholera - Malawi [Internet]. [cited 2023 May 2]. Available from: https://www.who.int/emergencies/disease-outbreak-news/item/2022-DON435

Christaki, E., Dimitriou, P., Pantavou, K., & Nikolopoulos, G. K. (2020). The impact of climate change on cholera: A review on the global status and future challenges. *Atmosphere, 11*(5), 449.

Clemens, J. D. (2011, May 24). Vaccines in the time of cholera. *Proceedings of the National Academy of Sciences of the United States of America, 108*(21), 8529–8530.

Cocquyt, C., & Vyverman, W. (2005). Phytoplankton in Lake Tanganyika: A comparison of community composition and biomass off Kigoma with previous studies 27 years ago. *Journal of Great Lakes Research., 31*(4), 535–546.

Colwell, R. R., & Huq, A. (1994, December 15). Environmental reservoir of Vibrio cholerae. The causative agent of cholera. *Annals of the New York Academy of Sciences, 740*, 44–54.

Deployments from the oral cholera vaccine stockpile, 2013–2017. *The Weekly Epidemiological Record,* 2017 August 11, *92*(32), 437–442.

Dudley, J. P., Hoberg, E. P., Jenkins, E. J., Parkinson, A. J. (2015, December). Climate change in the North American Arctic: A one health perspective. *Ecohealth, 12*(4), 713–725.

Gaffga, N. H., Tauxe, R. V., & Mintz, E. D. (2007). Cholera: A new homeland in Africa? *American Journal of Tropical Medicine and Hygiene, 77*(4), 705.

Harris, E. (2023, April 25). WHO warns "very high" global risk as cholera cases spread. *JAMA, 329*(16), 1340.

Hecky, R., Bugenyi, F., Ochumba, P., Talling, J., Mugidde, R., Gophen, M., et al. (1994). Deoxygenation of the deep water of Lake Victoria, East Africa. *Limnology and Oceanography, 39*(6), 1476–1481.

Hsiao, A., Ahmed, A. S., Subramanian, S., Griffin, N. W., Drewry, L. L., Petri, W. A., et al. (2014). Members of the human gut microbiota involved in recovery from Vibrio cholerae infection. *Nature, 515*(7527), 423–426.

Hunter, P. R. (2003). Climate change and waterborne and vector-borne disease. *Journal of Applied Microbiology, 94*(Suppl), 37S–46S.

Ilboudo, P. G., Mengel, M. A., Gessner, B. D., Ngwira, B., Cavailler, P., Le Gargasson, J. B. (2021, March 10). Cost-effectiveness of a reactive oral cholera immunization campaign using Shanchol^{TM} in Malawi. *Cost Effectiveness and Resource Allocation, 19*, 17.

Kaponda, P., Muthukrishnan, S., Barber, R., & Holm, R. H. (2019). Drinking water quality and human dimensions of cholera patients to inform evidence-based prevention investment in Karonga District, Malawi. *Water Supply, 19*(7), 2079–2087.

Kaseya, J., & Dereje, N., Tajudeen, R., Ngongo, A. N., Ndembi, N., & Fallah, M. P. (2024, March 7). Climate change and malaria, dengue and cholera outbreaks in Africa: a call for concerted actions. *BMJ Global Health, 9*(3).

Khonje, A., Metcalf, C. A., Diggle, E., Mlozowa, D., Jere, C., Akesson, A. et al. (2012, June) Cholera outbreak in districts around Lake Chilwa, Malawi: Lessons learned. *Malawi Medical Journal, 24*(2), 29–33.

Khoury, P. (2023, January 19). Cholera is back but the world is looking away. *BMJ, 380*, 141.

Legros, D. D. Ending cholera: a global roadmap to 2030.

Luchen, C. C., Mwaba, J., Ng'ombe, H., Alabi, P. I. O., Simuyandi, M., Chilyabanyama, O. N., et al. (2021). Effect of HIV status and retinol on immunogenicity to oral cholera vaccine in adult population living in an endemic area of Lukanga Swamps, Zambia. *PLoS One, 16*(12), e0260552.

Malawi Cholera Flash Appeal 2023. (2023, February–June) - Malawi | ReliefWeb [Internet]. 2023 [cited 2023 May 2]. Available from: https://reliefweb.int/report/malawi/malawi-cholera-flash-appeal-2023-february-june-2023

Malawi's Cholera Outbreak Could Spill Over into Neighboring Countries | Think Global Health [Internet]. Council on Foreign Relations. [cited 2023 May 3]. Available from: https://www.thinkglobalhealth.org/article/malawis-cholera-outbreak-could-spill-over-neighboring-countries

Malawi's worst cholera epidemic in decades sparks massive demand for vaccines | Gavi, the Vaccine Alliance [Internet]. [cited 2023 May 2]. Available from: https://www.gavi.org/vaccineswork/malawis-worst-cholera-epidemic-decades-sparks-massive-demand-vaccines-stocks-run

Mehandru, S., Poles, M. A., Tenner-Racz, K., Horowitz, A., Hurley, A., Hogan, C., et al. (2004, September 20). Primary HIV-1 infection is associated with preferential depletion of CD4+ T lymphocytes from effector sites in the gastrointestinal tract. *Journal of Experimental Medicine, 200*(6), 761–770.

Mendelsohn, J., & Dawson, T. (2008, March). Climate and cholera in KwaZulu-Natal, South Africa: The role of environmental factors and implications for epidemic preparedness. *International Journal of Hygiene and Environmental Health, 211*(1–2), 156–162.

Mengel, M. A., Delrieu, I., Heyerdahl, L., & Gessner, B. D. (2014). Cholera outbreaks in Africa. In G. B. Nair & Y. Takeda (Eds.), *Cholera outbreaks [Internet]*. Springer Berlin Heidelberg [cited 2023 May 2]. pp. 117–144. (Current Topics in Microbiology and Immunology; Vol. 379). Available from: https://doi.org/10.1007/82_2014_369

Morton, S., Pencheon, D., & Squires, N. (2017, October). Sustainable Development Goals (SDGs), and their implementation. *British Medical Bulletin., 24*, 1–10.

Multi-country outbreak of cholera, External situation report #1 - 28 March 2023 [Internet]. [cited 2023 May 2]. Available from: https://www.who.int/publications/m/item/multi-country-outbreak-of-cholera--external-situation-report--1---28-march-2023

Ng'ombe, H., Simuyandi, M., Mwaba, J., Luchen, C. C., & Alabi, P., Chilyabanyama, O. N., et al. (2022, January 5). Immunogenicity and waning immunity from the oral cholera vaccine (Shanchol™) in adults residing in Lukanga Swamps of Zambia. Borrow R, editor. *PLoS ONE, 17*(1), e0262239.

Nkoane, M. A., & Adefolalu, A. O. (2024). Rapid-onset diarrhoea in HIV patient: The importance of suspecting cholera in non-endemic areas. *Southern African Journal of Infectious Diseases, 39*(1), 619.

O'Reilly, C. M., Alin, S. R., Plisnier, P. D., Cohen, A. S., & McKee, B. A. (2003). Climate change decreases aquatic ecosystem productivity of Lake Tanganyika, Africa. *Nature, 424*(6950), 766–768.

OCHA. Malawi Cholera Flash Appeal 2023 (February–June 2023) [Internet]. 2023 Jun [cited 2025 March 5]. Available from: https://www.unocha.org/publications/report/malawi/malawi-cholera-flash-appeal-2023-february-june-2023

Oxfam/ile. Southern African countries struggling with cholera outbreak [Internet]. 2024 Dec [cited 2025 March 3]. Available from: https://www.rural21.com/english/news/detail/article/southern-african-countries-struggling-with-cholera-outbreak.html

Perez-Saez, J., Lessler, J., Lee, E. C., Luquero, F. J., Malembaka, E. B., Finger, F., et al. (2022, June). The seasonality of cholera in sub-Saharan Africa: A statistical modelling study. *The Lancet Global Health, 10*(6), e831–839.

Rasam, A., Ghazali, R., Noor, A., Mohd, W., & Hamid, J., Bazlan, M., et al. (2014). Spatial epidemiological techniques in cholera mapping and analysis towards a local scale predictive modelling. In IOP Publishing (p. 012095).

Responding to the Cholera outbreak in Malawi | UNICEF Malawi [Internet]. [cited 2023 May 2]. Available from: https://www.unicef.org/malawi/responding-cholera-outbreak-malawi

Roadmap 2030 – Global Task Force on Cholera Control [Internet]. [cited 2023 May 2]. Available from: https://www.gtfcc.org/about-cholera/roadmap-2030/

Schwartz, K., Hammerl, J. A., Göllner, C., Strauch, E. (2019, April 12). Environmental and clinical strains of Vibrio cholerae Non-O1, Non-O139 from Germany possess similar virulence gene profiles. *Frontiers in Microbiology, 10*, 733.

Sévère, K., Anglade, S. B., Bertil, C., Duncan, A., Joseph, P., Deroncenay, A., et al. (2016, November 2). Clinical features of human immunodeficiency virus-infected patients presenting with Cholera in Port-au-Prince, Haiti. *American Journal of Tropical Medicine and Hygiene, 95*(5), 999–1003.

Shaikh, H., Lynch, J., Kim, J., & Excler, J. L. (2020, February 29). Current and future cholera vaccines. *Vaccine, 38*, A118–126.

Shariff, S., Kantawala, B., Siddiq, A., Oseili, T., Nazir, A., & Uwishema, O. (2024). Cholera outbreak in Malawi: Empirical assessment and lessons learnt. *IJS Global Health, 7*(3), e0262.

Sinyange, N., Brunkard, J. M., Kapata, N., Mazaba, M. L., Musonda, K. G., Hamoonga, R., et al. (2018, May 18). Cholera epidemic—Lusaka, Zambia, October 2017-May 2018. *MMWR Morbidity and Mortality Weekly Report, 67*(19), 556–559.

Smith, A. M., Sekwadi, P., Erasmus, L. K., Lee, C. C., Stroika, S. G., Ndzabandzaba, S., et al. (2023, August). Imported Cholera cases, South Africa, 2023. *Emerging Infectious Diseases, 29*(8), 1687–1690.

Social capital, collective action and access to water in rural Kenya - PubMed [Internet]. [cited 2023 April 26]. Available from: https://pubmed.ncbi.nlm.nih.gov/25181474/

Song, K. R., Lim, J. K., Park, S. E., Saluja, T., Cho, S. I., Wartel, T. A., et al. (2021, December 15). Oral Cholera vaccine efficacy and effectiveness. *Vaccines (Basel), 9*(12), 1482.

UNAIDS. Eastern and Southern Africa-Regional Profile [Internet]. 2024 [cited 2025 March 5]. Available from: https://www.unaids.org/sites/default/files/media_asset/2024-unaids-global-aids-update-eastern-southern-africa_en.pdf

UNICEF. As cholera cases continue to rise in parts of Southern Africa, UNICEF calls for increased focus on children in the cholera response [Internet]. 2024 Jan [cited 2025 March 3]. Available from: https://www.unicef.org/press-releases/cholera-cases-continue-rise-parts-southern-africa-unicef-calls-increased-focus

Utsalo, S. J., Eko, F. O., Umoh, F., & Asindi, A. A. (1999, April). Faecal excretion of Vibrio cholerae during convalescence of cholera patients in Calabar, Nigeria. *European Journal of Epidemiology, 15*(4), 379–381.

Vollmer, M. K., Bootsma, H. A., Hecky, R. E., Patterson, G., Halfman, J. D., Edmond, J. M., et al. (2005). Deep-water warming trend in Lake Malawi, East Africa. *Limnology and Oceanography, 50*(2), 727–732.

von Seidlein, L., Wang, X. Y., Macuamule, A., Mondlane, C., Puri, M., Hendriksen, I., et al. (2008, May). Is HIV infection associated with an increased risk for cholera? Findings from a case-control study in Mozambique. *Tropical Medicine & International Health, 13*(5), 683–688.

Wendel, J. (2015). Climate change predicted to worsen spread of cholera. *Eos, Transactions American Geophysical Union.*

WHO. Cholera Africa [Internet]. 2023 April [cited 2024 March 5]. Available from: https://www.arcgis.com/apps/dashboards/8a0bb70fc8ae41d285d47797465b817a

WHO. Global strategic preparedness, readiness and response plan for cholera [Internet]. 2023 [cited 2025 March 6]. Available from: https://cdn.who.int/media/docs/default-source/documents/emergencies/global-cholera-sprrp-v7-2023-05-19_cleared.pdf?sfvrsn=7b5f7ced_1&download=true

WHO/Africa. Understanding the link between Climate Change and Cholera in Africa. [Internet]. 2024 [cited 2025 March 5]. Available from: https://files.aho.afro.who.int/afahobckpcontainer/production/files/Analytical_Brief_on_Climate_Change_and_Cholera_in_the_African_Region.pdf

Wierzba, T. F. (2019, June 3). Oral cholera vaccines and their impact on the global burden of disease. *Human Vaccines & Immunotherapeutics, 15*(6), 1294–1301.

Wise, J. (2023, February 9). Cholera: Malawi is in grip of its deadliest outbreak. *BMJ, 380*, 328.

Chapter 4

Abesig, J., Chen, Y., Wang, H., et al. (2020). Prevalence of viral hepatitis B in Ghana between 2015 and 2019: A systematic review and meta-analysis. *PLoS ONE, 15*, e0234348.

Afum, T., Asare, P., Asante-Poku, A., et al. (2021). Diagnosis of tuberculosis among COVID-19 suspected cases in Ghana. *PLoS ONE, 16*(12), e0261849. https://doi.org/10.1371/journal.pone.0261849

Agyapong, O. P., Fobil, J. N., & Badu, E. K. (2021). Challenges in malaria control in Ghana: Perspectives from healthcare providers. *Malaria Journal, 20*(1), 79.

Alene, K. A., Wangdi, K., & Clements, A. C. A. (2020). Impact of the COVID-19 pandemic on tuberculosis control: An overview. *Tropical Medicine & Infectious Disease, 5*(3), 123. https://doi.org/10.3390/tropicalmed5030123

Alhassan, R. K., Nutor, J. J., & Arhinful, D. K. (2020). Reducing health inequities in tuberculosis control: The role of community-based interventions in Ghana. *BMC Public Health, 20*(1), 110. https://doi.org/10.1186/s1288902009110w

Amekudzi, L. K., Adukpo, D. C., & Agyapong, E. (2018). Environmental factors affecting malaria transmission in Ghana: A review. *Ghana Journal of Science, 58*(2), 61–75.

Amponsah-Dacosta, E., & Hepburn, A. J. (2021). The epidemiology of hepatitis B in sub-Saharan Africa. *Journal of Hepatology, 75*(4), 1041–1054.

Anarfi, J. K., & Owusu, A. Y. (2020). HIV/AIDS in Ghana: A socio-cultural perspective. *African Journal of AIDS Research, 19*(3), 175–185.

Asamoah, C. K., Asamoah, B. O., & Agardh, A. (2017). A generation at risk: A cross-sectional study on HIV/AIDS knowledge and stigmatizing behaviors among young women in Ghana. *Global Health Action, 10*(1), 1331538. https://doi.org/10.1080/16549716.2017.1331538

Asante, F. A., & Asenso-Okyere, W. K. (2003). Economic burden of malaria in Ghana. *Tropical Medicine & International Health, 8*(1), 49–57. https://doi.org/10.1046/j.1365-3156.2003.00956.x

Asante, K. P., Owusu-Agyei, S., & Cairns, M. (2018). Malaria prevention and control in Ghana: Progress and challenges. *Journal of Tropical Medicine, 2018*, 1–8. https://doi.org/10.1155/2018/8454732

Attipoe, L., Nyarko, S. H., & Badoe, E. A. (2019). HIV and hepatitis B co-infection: Challenges and opportunities in Ghana. *BMC Infectious Diseases, 19*(1), 89.

Ayeh-Kumi, P. F., Addo, M. M., & Obeng, P. (2021). Advances in HIV prevention and treatment: The Ghanaian context. *AIDS Research and Therapy, 18*(1), 53.

Badoe, E. A., & Essuman, R. (2019). Liver cancer in Ghana: A growing epidemic. *Ghana Medical Journal, 53*(3), 125–131.

Boah, M., Yeboah, D., Kpordoxah, M. R., & Adokiya, M. N. (2023). Temporal trend analysis of the HIV/AIDS burden before and after ART implementation in Ghana. *BMC Public Health, 23*, 1399. https://doi.org/10.1186/s12889023163213

Chanda-Kapata, P., Ntoumi, F., Kapata, N., et al. (2022). Tuberculosis, HIV/AIDS, and malaria health services in sub-Saharan Africa: A situation analysis of the disruptions and impact of the COVID-19 pandemic. *International Journal of Infectious Diseases, 124*(Suppl 1), S41-46.

Croxford, S., Kitching, A., Desai, S., et al. (2017). Mortality and causes of death in people with HIV in the ART era. *The Lancet Public Health, 2*(1), e35–e46. https://doi.org/10.1016/S24682667(16)300202

Dapaah, J. M., Senah, K. A., & Akuffo, C. O. (2017). Integrating HIV services into maternal and child healthcare: Perspectives from healthcare providers in Ghana. *Reproductive Health, 14*(1), 115.

Friedland, G., Churchyard, G., & Nardell, E. (2020a). Tuberculosis and HIV co-infection: Current state of knowledge and research priorities. *The Lancet Infectious Diseases, 20*(1), e22–e31. https://doi.org/10.1016/S14733099(19)304773

Fobil, J. N., Levey, R., & Agyeman-Duah, R. (2020). Stigma and discrimination: Barriers to HIV testing and treatment in Ghana. *PLoS ONE, 15*(7), e0235337.

Friedland, G., Churchyard, G., & Nardell, E. (2020b). Tuberculosis and HIV coinfection: Current state of knowledge and research priorities. *The Lancet Infectious Diseases, 20*(1), e22–e31. https://doi.org/10.1016/S14733099(19)304773

Ghana AIDS Commission. (2020). National HIV and AIDS Strategic Plan 2021–2025. Accra, Ghana.

Ghana Health Service. (2020). Annual malaria report. Accra, Ghana.

Ghana Health Service (GHS). (2022a). National Tuberculosis Control Programme Annual Report. Accra, Ghana.

Ghana Health Service (GHS). (2022b). National Malaria Control Programme Annual Report. Accra, Ghana.

Ghana Health Service. (2023). *National HIV/AIDS response*. Ghana Health Service.

Ghana Malaria Indicator Survey (GMIS). (2022). *Ghana Malaria Indicator Survey Report*. Ghana Statistical Service.

Heuschen, A. K., Abdul-Mumin, A., Abubakari, A., et al. (2023). Effects of the COVID-19 pandemic on general health and malaria control in Ghana: A qualitative study with mothers and healthcare professionals. *Malaria Journal, 22*, 78. https://doi.org/10.1186/s12936-023-04513-6

Lartey, M., Adjei, A. A., & Yawson, A. E. (2015). Addressing hepatitis B in Ghana: Current strategies and future directions. *African Journal of Health Sciences, 25*(3), 219–226.

Loembé, M. M., & Nkengasong, J. N. (2021). COVID-19 vaccine access in Africa: Global distribution, vaccine platforms, and challenges ahead. *Immunity, 54*(7), 1353–1362. https://doi.org/10.1016/j.immuni.2021.06.017

Martinson, F. E., Weigle, K. A., Mushahwar, I. K., Weber, D. J., Royce, R., & Lemon, S. M. (1996). Seroepidemiological survey of hepatitis B in Ghanaian children. *Journal of Medical Virology, 48*, 278–283.

Mills, E. J., Bakanda, C., Birungi, J., et al. (2011). Life expectancy of persons receiving combination ART in low-income countries. *Annals of Internal Medicine, 155*(4), 209–216. https://doi.org/10.7326/000348191554201108160003 58

National Malaria Control Programme (NMCP). (2022). *Annual malaria report*. Ghana Health Service.

National Tuberculosis Control Programme (NTCP). (2022). Annual Report on TB in Ghana. Accra, Ghana.

Nketiah-Amponsah, E., Afful-Mensah, G., & Ampaw, S. (2020). HIV-related stigma and access to healthcare in Ghana. *AIDS Research and Therapy, 17*(1), 1–10. https://doi.org/10.1186/s12981020002901

Nonvignon, J., Aikins, M., & Chinbuah, M. A. (2016). Economic burden of malaria on households and the healthcare system in Ghana. *Tropical Medicine & International Health, 21*(3), 392–400.

Obeng, A. F., Attipoe, L., & Asare, D. (2022). The state of HIV care in Ghana: Achievements and future prospects. *Global Health Action, 15*(1), 199–211.

Obuobi, D., Nimo, J., & Kyei, K. (2021). Mother-to-child transmission of hepatitis B: A public health concern in Ghana. *International Journal of Maternal and Child Health, 9*(1), 45–54.

Ofori-Asenso, R., & Agyeman, A. A. (2016). Hepatitis B in Ghana: A systematic review and meta-analysis. *BMC Infectious Diseases, 16*, 130. https://doi.org/10.1186/s1287901614665

Owusu-Dabo, E., Adjei, G., Meyer, C. G., & Browne, E. (2018). Tuberculosis epidemiology and control in Ghana. *Infectious Diseases, 50*(8), 601–610. https://doi.org/10.1080/23744235.2018.1486855

Owusu-Sekyere, E., & Opoku, A. (2015). Economic impact of malaria in Ghana: A household-level analysis. *Journal of African Economies, 24*(3), 295–319.

Schweitzer, A., Horn, J., Mikolajczyk, R. T., Krause, G., & Ott, J. J. (2015). Estimations of worldwide prevalence of chronic hepatitis B virus infection: A systematic review of data published between 1965 and 2013. *The Lancet, 386*(10003), 1546–1555.

Udoakang, A. J., Djomkam Zune, A. L., Tapela, K., Nganyewo, N. N., Olisaka, F. N., Anyigba, C. A., Tawiah-Eshun, S., Owusu, I. A., Paemka, L., Awandare, G. A., & Quashie, P. K. (2023).

The COVID-19, tuberculosis, and HIV/AIDS: Ménage à trois. *Frontiers in Immunology, 14*, 1104828. https://doi.org/10.3389/fimmu.2023.1104828
UNAIDS. (2023a). *Country factsheets: Ghana.* Retrieved from https://aidsinfo.unaids.org
UNAIDS. (2023b). *Ghana country fact sheet: HIV and AIDS statistics.* Retrieved from https://www.unaids.org/en/regionscountries/countries/ghana
UNAIDS. (2023c). *Global AIDS monitoring report.* UNAIDS.
Watson, O. J., Barnsley, G., Toor, J., Hogan, A. B., Winskill, P., & Ghani, A. C. (2022). Global impact of the first year of COVID-19 vaccination: A mathematical modeling study. *The Lancet Infectious Diseases, 22*(9), 1293–1302. https://doi.org/10.1016/S1473-3099(22)00320-6
World Bank. (2016). *Tuberculosis in Ghana: A situation analysis.* World Bank.
World Health Organization (WHO). (2020). *Global tuberculosis report 2020.* WHO.
World Health Organization (WHO). (2023a). *Global tuberculosis report 2023.* WHO.
World Health Organization. (2023b). *World malaria report.* WHO.
Yeboah-Manu, D., Asante-Poku, A., & Owusu, A. (2016). Multi-drug resistant tuberculosis in Ghana: Burden and strategies for control. *International Journal of Infectious Diseases, 46*, 5–10.
Zaidi, J., Grapsa, E., Tanser, F., et al. (2013). Dramatic increase in HIV prevalence after ART scale-up. *AIDS, 27*(14), 2301–2305. https://doi.org/10.1097/QAD.0b013e328362e832
Zumla, A., Raviglione, M., Hafner, R., & von Reyn, C. F. (2013). Tuberculosis. *The New England Journal of Medicine, 368*(8), 745–755. https://doi.org/10.1056/NEJMra1200894

Chapter 5

Abdul-Mumin, A., Abubakari, A., Agbozo, F., Abdul-Karim, A., Nuertey, B. D., Mumuni, K., Anna-Katharina, H., Lisa, H., Claudia, M. D., Olaf, M., & Albrecht, J. (2021). Field evaluation of specificity and sensitivity of a standard SARS-CoV-2 antigen rapid diagnostic test: A prospective study at a teaching hospital in Northern Ghana. *PLOS Global Public Health, 1*(12), e0000040. https://doi.org/10.1371/journal.pgph.0000040
Aboagye, F. T., Annison, L., Hackman, H. K., Acquah, M. E., Ashong, Y., Owusu-Frimpong, I., Egyam, B. C., Annison, S., Osei-Adjei, G., & Antwi-Baffour, S. (2024). Comparative evaluation of RT-PCR and antigen-based rapid diagnostic tests (Ag-RDTs) for SARS-CoV-2 detection: Performance, variant specificity, and clinical implications. *Microbiology Spectrum Virology, 12*(6). https://doi.org/10.1128/spectrum.00073-24
Abu-Faraj, Zia (2020). Freitas, A. R. R., Beckedorff, O. A., Cavalcanti, L. P. G., Siqueira, A. M., Castro, D. B., Costa, C. F. D., Lemos, D. R. Q., & Barros, E. N. C. (2021). The emergence of novel SARS-CoV-2 variant P.1 in Amazonas (Brazil) was temporally associated with a change in the age and sex profile of COVID-19 mortality: A population based ecological study. *Lancet Regional Health. Americas, 1*, 100021. https://doi.org/10.1016/j.lana.2021.100021
Adjaottor, E. S., Addo, F.-M., Ahorsu, F. A., Chen, H.-P., & Ahorsu, D. K. (2022). Predictors of COVID-19 stress and COVID-19 vaccination acceptance among adolescents in Ghana. *International Journal of Environmental Research and Public Health, 19*, 7871. https://doi.org/10.3390/ijerph19137871
Adu, P., Popoola, T., Iqbal, N., et al. (2024). Cross-country assessment of the unique contributions of psychological factors to vaccination: Perspectives on the COVID-19 pandemic. *Journal of Health Psychology, 30* (9):2385–2399. https://doi.org/10.1177/13591053241266592
Afrifa-Anane, G. F., Larbi, R. T., Addo, B., Agyekum, M. W., Kyei-Arthur, F., Appiah, M., et al. (2022). Facilitators and barriers to COVID-19 vaccine uptake among women in two regions of Ghana: A qualitative study. *PLoS ONE, 17*(8), e0272876. https://doi.org/10.1371/journal.pone.0272876
Asante, I. A., Lwanga, C. N., Takyi, C., Sekyi-Yorke, A. N., Quarcoo, J. A., Odikro, M. A., Kploanyi, E. E., Donkor, I. O., Addo-Lartey, A., Duah, N. A., Odumang, D. A., Lomotey, E. S., Boatemaa,

L., Kwasah, L., Nyarko, S. O., Affram, Y., Asiedu-Bekoe, F., & Kenu, E. (2024). Detection of SARS-CoV-2 variants imported through land borders at the height of the COVID-19 pandemic in Ghana, 2022. *Cureus, 16*(8), e68220. https://doi.org/10.7759/cureus.68220

Assan, A., Hussein, H., & Agyeman-Duah, D. N. (2022). COVID-19 lockdown implementation in Ghana: Lessons learned and hurdles to overcome. *Journal of Public Health Policy, 43*, 129–139. https://doi.org/10.1057/s41271-021-00330-w

Bani, S., Amakye, E. K., Akomea, S., Nyarko, E. N., Dodoo, D., Aidoo, C., Fynn-Buadu, M., Adom, M., Bani, F., & Christian, O. C. (2024). An evaluation of the sensitivity and specificity of three COVID-19 rapid immunochromatographic test kits compared to real-time reverse transcriptase-polymerase chain reaction (rRT-PCR) among clinical samples. *Cureus, 16*(6), e63294. https://doi.org/10.7759/cureus.63294

Chtioui, M. J., Grati, H., Harzallah, N., Christine, M., Jebali, O., Trabelsi, A., Ahmed, M. B., Thabet, L., Mhalla, S., Moussa, M. B., Messaoud, T., Romdhane, H. B., Toumi, A., & Hamouda, C. (2020). Rapid diagnostic tests: Pros, cons and potential use in the COVID-19 management in Tunisia. *La Tunisie Medicale, 98*(8–9), 639–642.

COVID-19 Updates | Ghana; https://ghs.gov.gh/covid19/. Accessed 7 April 2004.

Dadzie, A., Kuffour, A. S., Turkson, A., et al. (2024). COVID-19 in patients presenting with malaria-like symptoms at a primary healthcare facility in Accra, Ghana. *Plos ONE, 19*(2), e0298088. https://doi.org/10.1371/journal.pone.0298088

Ghana Health Service. (2024a). Dashboard. Accessed 19 December 2024.

Ghana Health Service. (2024b). Dashboard. Accessed 19 December 2023.

Harapan, H., Itoh, N., Yufika, A., Winardi, W., Keam, S., Te, H., ... Mudatsir, M. (2020). Corona virus disease 2019 (COVID-19): A literature review. *Journal of Infection and Public Health, 13*(5), 667–673. https://doi.org/10.1016/j.pulmoe.2020.10.013

Ismaila, H., Asamani, J. A., Lokossou, V. K., Oduro-Mensah, E., Nabyonga-Orem, J., & Akoriyea, S. K. (2021). The cost of clinical management of SARS-COV-2 (COVID-19) infection by level of disease severity in Ghana: A protocol-based cost of illness analysis. *BMC Health Services Research, 21*(1), 1–10.

Lee, Y. K., & Song, H. S. (2024). Recent advances in electrochemical and Nanophotonic biosensors for SARS-Cov-2 detection. *BioChip Journal, 18*, 171–185. https://doi.org/10.1007/s13206-024-00138-2

Liu, Y. C., Kuo, R. L., & Shih, S. R. (2020). COVID-19: The first documented Corona virus pandemic in history. *Biomedical Journal, 43*(4), 328–333.

Mallari, E. U., Keller, S., Febre, J. F., Timbol, J., Powers, R., Peregrino, R. R., Slyzkii, A., Mulder, C., Magno, M. V., & Spruijt, I. (2023). Feasibility and acceptability of COVID-19 self-testing in the Philippines. *PHA, 13*(4), 119–122. e-ISSN 2220-8372.

MOH, 2020 (Covid-19 Guidelines for Ghana).

Morang'a, C. M., Ngoi, J. M., Gyamfi, J., Amuzu, D. S. Y., Nuertey, B., Soglo, P., Appiah, V., Asante, I. A., Owusu-Oduro, P., Armoo, S., Adu-Gyasi, D., Amoako, N., Oliver-Commey, J., Owusu, M., Sylverken, A., Fenteng, E. D., M'cormack, V. V., ei-Maya, F. T., Quansah, E. B., Ayivor-Djanie, R., Amoako, E. K., Ogbe, I. T., Yemi, B. K., Osei-Wusu, I., Mettle, D. N. A., Saiid, S., Tapela, K., Dzabeng, F., Magnussen, V., Quaye, J., Opurum, P. C., Carr, R. A., Ababio, P. T., Abass, A.-K., Akoriyea, S. K., Amoako, E., Kumi-Ansah, F., Boakye, O. D., Mibut, D. K., Odoom, T., Ofori-Boadu, L., Allegye-Cudjoe, E., Dassah, S., Asoala, V., Asante, K. P., Phillips, R. O., Osei-Atweneboana, M. Y., Gyapong, J. O., Kuma-Aboagye, P., Ampofo, W. K., Duedu, K. O., Ndam, N. T., Bediako, Y., Quashie, P. K., Amenga-Etego, L. N., & Awandare, G. A. (2022). *Genetic diversity of SARS-CoV-2 infections in Ghana from 2020–2021.* 13, 2494 | https://doi.org/10.1038/s41467-022-30219-5 | www.nature.com/naturecommunications

Ngoi, J. M., Quashie, P. K., Morang'a, C. M., Bonney, J. H., Amuzu, D. S., Kumordjie, S., Asante, I. A., Bonney, E. Y., Eshun, M., Boatemaa, L., Magnusen, V., Kotey, E. N., Ndam, N. T., Tei-Maya, F., Arjarquah, A. K., Obodai, E., Otchere, I. D., Bediako, Y., Mutungi, J. K., Amenga-Etego, L. N., Odoom, J. K., Anang, A. K., Kyei, G. B., Adu, B., Ampofo, W. K., Awandare, G.A. (2021). Genomic analysis of SARS-CoV-2 reveals local viral evolution in Ghana. *Exp Biol Med*

(Maywood), 246 (8): 960–970. https://doi.org/10.1177/1535370220975351. Epub 2020 Dec 16. PMID: 33325750; PMCID: PMC7746953.

Nyazika, T. K., Kaela, R., Mugoni, M., Musomekwa, K., Kyei-Baafour, E., Chiwanda, S., Mapondera, P. T., Makawa, T. S., Sithole, E. M., Mavunganidze, G., Manasa, J., Jambo, K. C., & Musarurwa, C. (2020). Implementation of antibody rapid diagnostic testing versus real-time reverse transcription-PCR sample pooling in the screening of COVID-19: A case of different testing strategies in Africa. *mSphere, 5*, e00524-20. https://doi.org/10.1128/mSphere.00524-20.

Ofori-Adjei, D., Lartey, M., & Koram, K. A. (2020). Ghana and the COVID-19 pandemic. *Ghana Medical Journal, 54*(4 supplement), 1–2. https://doi.org/10.4314/gmj.v54i4s.1

Torres-Castro, R., Vasconcello-Castilloa, L., Alsina-Restoy, X., Solis-Navarroa, L., Burgos, F., Puppo, H., & Vilaró, J. (2021). Respiratory function in patients post-infection by COVID-19: A systematic review and meta-analysis. *Pulmonology, 27*, 328–337.

Villar, J., Ariff, S., Gunier, R. B., Thiruvengadam, R., Rauch, S., Kholin, A., Roggero, P., Prefumo, F., Silva do Vale, M., Arturo Cardona-Perez, J., Maiz, N., Cetin, I., Savasi, V., Deruelle, P., Easter, S. R., Sichitiu, J., Conti, C. P. S., Ernawati, E., Mhatre, M., Teji, J. S., Liu, B., Capelli, C., Oberto, M., Salazar, L., Gravett, M. G., Cavoretto, P. I., Nachinab, V. B., Galadanci, H., Oros, D., Ayede, A. I., Sentilhes, L., Bako, B., Savorani, M., Cena, H., Garcia-May, P. K., Etuk, S., Casale, R., Abd-Elsalam, S., Ikenoue, S., Aminu, M. B., Vecciarelli, C., Duro, E. A., Usman, M. A., John-Akinola, Y., Nieto, R., Ferrazzi, E., Bhutta, Z. A., Langer, A., Kennedy, S. H., & Papageorghiou, A. T. (2021). Maternal and neonatal morbidity and mortality among pregnant women with and without COVID-19 infection. *JAMA Pediatrics, 175*(8).

Wang, C., et al. (2020) A Novel Coronavirus Outbreak of Global Health Concern. *The Lancet, 395*, 470–473. https://doi.org/10.1016/S0140-6736(20)30185-9

WHO dashboard. Accessed 28 February 2025.

Winter, A. K., & Hegde, S. T. (2020). The important role of serology for COVID-19 control. *The Lancet Infectious Diseases, 20*, 758–759. https://doi.org/10.1016/S1473-3099(20)30322-4

Chapter 6

Areri, H., Marshall, A., & Harvey, G. (2020). Factors influencing self-management of adults living with HIV on antiretroviral therapy in Northwest Ethiopia: A cross-sectional study. *BMC Infectious Diseases, 20*, 879. https://doi.org/10.1186/s12879-020-05618-y

Armitage, R., & Nellums, L. B. (2020). COVID-19 and the consequences of isolating the elderly. *The Lancet Public Health, 5*(5), e256.

BHIVA, DAIG, EACS, GESIDA & Polish Scientific AIDS Society. (2021). *Statement on risk of COVID-19 for people living with HIV (PLWH)*. https://www.bhiva.org/joint-statement-on-risk-of-COVID-19-for-PLWH-and-SARS-CoV-2-vaccine-advice. Accessed on 1 December 2024.

Bouabida, K., Chaves, B. G., & Anane, E. (2023). Challenges and barriers to HIV care engagement and care cascade. *Frontiers in Reproductive Health, 5*, 1201087.

Brandt, C., Zvolensky, M. J., Woods, S. P., Gonzalez, A., Safren, S. A., & O'Cleirigh, C. M. (2017). Anxiety symptoms and disorders among adults living with HIV and AIDS: A critical review and integrative synthesis of the empirical literature. *Clinical Psychology Review, 51*, 164–184.

Brazier, E., Tymejczyk, O., Wools-Kaloustian, K., Jiamsakul, A., Torres, M. T. L., Lee, J. S., et al. (2024). Long-term HIV care outcomes under universal HIV treatment guidelines: A retrospective cohort study in 25 countries. *PLoS Medicine, 21*(3), e1004367. https://doi.org/10.1371/journal.pmed.1004367

Brown, M. J., & Weissman, S. B. (2020). The impact of COVID-19 on older adults living with HIV: HIV care and psychosocial effects. *Journal of Gerontological Social Work, 63*(6–7), 602–606.

Burke, R. M., Sabet, N., Ellis, J., Rangaraj, A., Lawrence, D. S., Jarvis, J. N., Falconer, J., Tugume, L., Bidwell, G., Berhanu, R. H., & MacPherson, P. (2025). Causes of hospitalisation among people living with HIV worldwide, 2014–23: A systematic review and meta-analysis. *The Lancet HIV*.

Chenneville, T., Gabbidon, K., Hanson, P., & Holyfield, C. (2020). The impact of COVID-19 on HIV treatment and research: A call to action. *International Journal of Environmental Research and Public Health, 17*(12), 4548.

Collins, C., Isbell, M. T., Karim, Q. A., Sohn, A. H., Beyrer, C., & Maleche, A. (2023). Leveraging the HIV response to strengthen pandemic preparedness. *PLOS Global Public Health, 3*(1), e0001511.

Cooley, S. A., Nelson, B., Doyle, J., Rosenow, A., & Ances, B. M. (2021). Collateral damage: Impact of SARS-CoV-2 pandemic in people living with HIV. *Journal of Neurovirology, 27*, 168–170.

International AIDS Society. (2020). COVID-19 *DSD resources community responses and perspectives*. http://www.differentiatedcare.org/Resources/Resource-Library/COVID-19-DSD-Resources-Community-responses. Accessed 27 February 2024.

Dadi, T. L., Tegene, Y., Vollebregt, N., Medhin, G., & Spigt, M. (2024). The importance of self-management for better treatment outcomes for HIV patients in a low-income setting: Perspectives of HIV experts and service providers. *AIDS Research and Therapy, 21*, 28. https://doi.org/10.1186/s12981-024-00612-9

Dandachi, D., Dang, B. N., Lucari, B., Teti, M., & Giordano, T. P. (2020). Exploring the attitude of patients with HIV about using telehealth for HIV care. *AIDS Patient Care and STDs, 34*(4), 166–172.

Finmark Trust. (2020). *Livelihood impacts of COVID-19 in Kenya, Nigeria and South Africa*. Tech Central. https://techcentral.co.za/livelihood-impacts-of-covid-19-in-kenya-nigeria-and-south-africa/175855/. Accessed 25 February 2024.

Friedland, B. A., Gottert, A., Hows, J., Baral, S. D., Sprague, L., Nyblade, L., McClair, T. L., Anam, F., Geibel, S., Kentutsi, S., & Tamoufe, U. (2020). The people living with HIV stigma Index 2.0: Generating critical evidence for change worldwide. *AIDS, 34*, S5–S18.

Gandhi, R. T., Bedimo, R., Hoy, J. F., Landovitz, R. J., Smith, D. M., Eaton, E. F., Lehmann, C., Springer, S. A., Sax, P. E., Thompson, M. A., & Benson, C. A. (2023). Antiretroviral drugs for treatment and prevention of HIV infection in adults: 2022 recommendations of the International Antiviral Society–USA panel. *JAMA, 329*(1), 63–84.

Gangcuangco, L. M. A., & Eustaquio, P. C. (2023). The state of the HIV Epidemic in the Philippines: Progress and challenges in 2023. *Tropical Medicine and Infectious Disease, 8*(5), 258.

Global Fund. (2021). *COVID-19 situation report #35*. https://www.theglobalfund.org/en/COVID-19/news. Accessed 27 February 2024.

Gwadz, M., Campos, S., Freeman, R., Cleland, C. M., Wilton, L., Sherpa, D., ... & Leonard, N. R. (2021). Black and Latino persons living with HIV evidence risk and resilience in the context of COVID-19: A mixed-methods study of the early phase of the pandemic. *AIDS and Behavior, 25*, 1340–1360.

Ho, C. S., Chee, C. Y., & Ho, R. C. (2020). Mental health strategies to combat the psychological impact of COVID-19 beyond paranoia and panic. *Annals of the Academy of Medicine, Singapore, 49*(1), 1–3.

Hoffmann, C., Casado, J. L., Härter, G., Vizcarra, P., Moreno, A., Cattaneo, D., Meraviglia, P., Spinner, C. D., Schabaz, F., Grunwald, S., & Gervasoni, C. (2021). Immune deficiency is a risk factor for severe COVID-19 in people living with HIV. *HIV Medicine, 22*(5), 372–378.

Hogan, A. B., Jewell, B. L., Sherrard-Smith, E., Vesga, J. F., Watson, O. J., Whittaker, C., ... & Hallett, T. B. (2020). Potential impact of the COVID-19 pandemic on HIV, tuberculosis, and malaria in low-income and middle-income countries: A modelling study. *The Lancet Global Health, 8*(9), e1132–e1141.

Hosken, G. (2020, May 17). Coronavirus fears keep HIV, TB patients from medication. *Sunday Times, Johannesburg*. https://www.timeslive.co.za/sunday-times/news/2020-05-17-coronavirus-fears-keep-hiv-tb-patients-from-medication/. Accessed 25 February 2024.

Ijumba, P. (2002). 'Voices' of primary health care facility workers: Human resources. *South African Health Review, 2002*(1), 181–200.

Jewell, B. L., Mudimu, E., Stover, J., Ten Brink, D., Phillips, A. N., Smith, J. A., ... & Kelly, S. L. (2020). Potential effects of disruption to HIV programmes in sub-Saharan Africa caused by COVID-19: Results from multiple mathematical models. *The Lancet HIV*, *7*(9), e629–e640.

Jewell, B. L., Smith, J. A., & Hallett, T. B. (2020). Understanding the impact of interruptions to HIV services during the COVID-19 pandemic: A modelling study. *EClinicalMedicine, 26.*

John, M.E. and Chipwaza, B. (2022). HIV status disclosure among adults attending care and treatment clinic in Kilombero district, South-Eastern Tanzania. *International Journal of Africa Nursing Sciences, 17*, 100434. https://doi.org/10.1016/j.ijans.2022.100434

Jones, D. L., Ballivian, J., Rodriguez, V. J., Uribe, C., Cecchini, D., Salazar, A. S., ... & Alcaide, M. L. (2021). Mental health, coping, and social support among people living with HIV in the Americas: a comparative study between Argentina and the USA during the SARS-CoV-2 pandemic. *AIDS and Behavior, 25*, 2391–2399.

Kemp, C. G., Lipira, L., Huh, D., Nevin, P. E., Turan, J. M., Simoni, J. M., Cohn, S. E., Bahk, M., Berzins, B., Andrasik, M., & Mugavero, M. J. (2019). HIV stigma and viral load among African-American women receiving treatment for HIV. *AIDS, 33*(9), 1511–1519.

Kowalska, J. D., Skrzat-Klapaczyńska, A., Bursa, D., Balayan, T., Begovac, J., Chkhartishvili, N., … & ECEE Network Group, 2020 Kowalska, J. D., Skrzat-Klapaczyńska, A., Bursa, D., Balayan, T., Begovac, J., Chkhartishvili, N., ... & ECEE Network Group. (2020). HIV care in times of the COVID-19 crisis—Where are we now in Central and Eastern Europe? *International Journal of Infectious Diseases, 96*, 311–314.

Laurence, J. (2020). Why aren't people living with HIV at higher risk for developing severe coronavirus disease 2019 (COVID-19)? *AIDS Patient Care and STDs, 34*(6), 247–248.

Lazarus, J. V., Wohl, D. A., Cascio, M., Guaraldi, G., Rockstroh, J., Hodson, M., Richman, B., Brown, G., Anderson, J., & Fuster-RuizdeApodaca, M. J. (2023). Long-term success for people living with HIV: A framework to guide practice. *HIV Medicine, 24*, 8–19.

Lee, K. W., Yap, S. F., Ngeow, Y. F., & Lye, M. S. (2021). COVID-19 in people living with HIV: A systematic review and meta-analysis. *International Journal of Environmental Research and Public Health, 18*(7), 3554.

Liu, Y., Gayle, A. A., Wilder-Smith, A., & Rocklöv, J. (2020). The reproductive number of COVID-19 is higher compared to SARS coronavirus. *Journal of Travel Medicine.*

Lo Hog Tian, J. M., Watson, J. R., Ibáñez-Carrasco, F., Tran, B., Parsons, J. A., Maunder, R. G., Card, K. G., Baral, S., Hui, C., Boni, A. R., & Ajiboye, M. (2021). Impact of experienced HIV stigma on health is mediated by internalized stigma and depression: Results from the people living with HIV stigma index in Ontario. *BMC Public Health, 21*, 1–10.

Madzima, B., Makoni, T., Mugurungi, O., Mudariki, G., Mpofu, A., Dube, F., ... & Taramusi, I. (2022). The impact of the COVID-19 pandemic on people living with HIV in Zimbabwe. *African Journal of AIDS Research, 21*(2), 194–200.

Marbaniang, I., Sangle, S., Nimkar, S., Zarekar, K., Salvi, S., Chavan, A., ... & Mave, V. (2020). The burden of anxiety during the COVID-19 pandemic among people living with HIV (PLHIV) in Pune, India. *Research Square*, rs-3.

McCluskey, S. M., Pepperrell, T., Hill, A., Venter, W. D., Gupta, R. K., & Siedner, M. J. (2021). Adherence, resistance, and viral suppression on dolutegravir in sub-Saharan Africa: Implications for the TLD era. *AIDS, 35*(Supplement 2), S127–S135.

Moranguinho, I., Taveira, N., & Bártolo, I. (2023). Antiretroviral treatment of HIV-2 infection: Available drugs, resistance pathways, and promising new compounds. *International Journal of Molecular Sciences, 24*(6), 5905.

Payagala, S., & Pozniak, A. (2024). The global burden of HIV. *Clinics in Dermatology, 42*(2), 119–127.

Pham, M. D., Nguyen, H. V., Anderson, D., Crowe, S., & Luchters, S. (2022). Viral load monitoring for people living with HIV in the era of test and treat: Progress made and challenges ahead–a systematic review. *BMC Public Health, 22*(1), 1203.

Poteat, T. C., Reisner, S. L., Miller, M., & Wirtz, A. L. (2020). COVID-19 vulnerability of transgender women with and without HIV infection in the Eastern and Southern US. *medRxiv.*

Paramesha, A. E., & Chacko, L. K. (2019). Predictors of adherence to antiretroviral therapy among PLHIV. *Indian Journal of Public Health, 63*(4), 367–376.

Salinas-Escudero, G., Toledano-Toledano, F., García-Peña, C., Parra-Rodríguez, L., Granados-García, V., & Carrillo-Vega, M. F. (2021). Disability-adjusted life years for the COVID-19 pandemic in the Mexican population. *Frontiers in Public Health, 9*, 686700.

Sanchez, T. H., Zlotorzynska, M., Rai, M., & Baral, S. D. (2020). Characterizing the impact of COVID-19 on men who have sex with men across the United States in April 2020. *AIDS and Behavior, 24*(7), 2024–2032.

Santos, G. M., Ackerman, B., Rao, A., Wallach, S., Ayala, G., Lamontage, E., ... & Howell, S. (2021). Economic, mental health, HIV prevention and HIV treatment impacts of COVID-19 and the COVID-19 response on a global sample of cisgender gay men and other men who have sex with men. *AIDS and Behavior, 25*, 311–321.

Schramm, B., Temfack, E., Descamps, D., Nicholas, S., Peytavin, G., Bitilinyu-Bangoh, J. E., Storto, A., Lê, M. P., Abdi, B., Ousley, J., & Kalua, T. (2022). Viral suppression and HIV-1 drug resistance 1 year after pragmatic transitioning to dolutegravir first-line therapy in Malawi: A prospective cohort study. *The Lancet HIV, 9*(8), e544–e553.

Shaw, J., & Matin, N. (2022). Opportunistic infections in HIV. *Medicine, 50*(5), 294–297.

Simon, M., Derrick, S., Kosanam, S., & Pasupula, R. (2024). Pill Burden: A Major Barrier to HAART adherence and Fixed Dose Combinations (FDCS) as its Solution-A mini-review. *Current HIV Research, 22*(3), 143–152.

Stangl, A. L., Lloyd, J. K., Brady, L. M., Holland, C. E., & Baral, S. (2013). A systematic review of interventions to reduce HIV-related stigma and discrimination from 2002 to 2013: How far have we come? *Journal of the International AIDS Society, 16*, 18734.

Stelzle, D., Rangaraj, A., Jarvis, J. N., Razakasoa, N. H., Perrin, G., Low-Beer, D., Doherty, M., Ford, N., & Dalal, S. (2025). Prevalen ce of advanced HIV disease in sub-Saharan Africa: A multi-country analysis of nationally representative household surveys. *The Lancet Global Health, 13*(3).

Sukmaningrum, E., Levy, J., Negara, M. D., Devika, D., Wardhani, B. D. K., Wulandari, L. P. L., & Januraga, P. P. (2024). Lived experience, social support, and challenges to health service use during the COVID-19 pandemic among HIV key populations in Indonesia. *BMC Health Services Research, 24*(1), 774.

Tasnim, S., Hossain, M. M., & Mazumder, H. (2020). Impact of rumors and misinformation on COVID-19 in social media. *Journal of Preventive Medicine and Public Health, 53*(3), 171–174.

UNAIDS (Joint United Nations Programme on HIV/AIDS). (2024). *The urgency of now: AIDS at a crossroads*. Geneva. Licence: CC BY-NC-SA 3.0 IGO [Online]. Available: https://www.unaids.org/sites/default/files/media_asset/2024-unaids-global-aids-update_en.pdf (10 November 2024).

Walker, P. G., Whittaker, C., Watson, O. J., Baguelin, M., Winskill, P., Hamlet, A., ... & Ghani, A. C. (2020). The impact of COVID-19 and strategies for mitigation and suppression in low-and middle-income countries. *Science, 369*(6502), 413–422.

Woldegeorgis, B. Z., Zekarias, Z., Adem, B. G., Obsa, M. S., & Kerbo, A. A. (2023). Prevalence and determinants of opportunistic infections among HIV-infected adults receiving antiretroviral therapy in Ethiopia: A systematic review and meta-analysis. *Frontiers in Medicine, 10*, 1087086.

World Health Organization (WHO). (2020a). *Mental health and psychosocial considerations during the COVID-19 outbreak*. Available online: https://www.who.int/docs/default-source/coronaviruse/mental-health-considerations. Accessed on 26 April 2024.

World Health Organization (WHO). (2020b). *Maintaining essential health services: Operational guidance for the COVID-19 context interim guidance*. https://www.who.int/emergencies/diseases/novel-coronavirus-2019/technical-guidance/maintaining-essential-health-services-and-systems. Accessed 19 March 2023.

World Health Organization (WHO). (2024). *HIV statistics, globally and by WHO region, 2024. Global HIV programme*. https://www.who.int/teams/global-hiv-hepatitis-and-stis-programmes/hiv/strategic-information/hiv-data-and-statistics Accessed 20 December 2024

Yuvaraj, A., Mahendra, V. S., Chakrapani, V., Yunihastuti, E., Santella, A. J., Ranauta, A., & Doughty, J. (2020). HIV and stigma in the healthcare setting. *Oral Diseases, 26*, 103–111.

Chapter 7

Aboobakur, M., Latheef, A., Mohamed, A. J., Moosa, S., Pandey, R. M., Krishnan, A., & Prabhakaran, D. (2010). Surveillance for non-communicable disease risk factors in Maldives: Results from the first STEPS survey in male. *International Journal of Public Health, 55*(5), 489–496. https://doi.org/10.1007/s00038-009-0114-y

Alicea-Planas, J., Trudeau, J. M., & Vásquez Mazariegos, W. F. (2021). COVID-19 risk perceptions and social distancing practice in Latin America. *Hispanic Health Care International, 19*(4), 254–259. https://doi.org/10.1177/1540415320985141

Bardosh, K., Jean, L., Desir, L., Yoss, S., Poovey, B., Beau de Rochars, M. V., & Noland, G. S. (2023). Was lockdown worth it? Community perspectives and experiences of the Covid-19 pandemic in remote southwestern Haiti. *Social Science & Medicine, 331*, 116076. https://doi.org/10.1016/J.SOCSCIMED.2023.116076

Baroux, N., Magnat, É., Cauchy, M., Cantin, J.-F., Cohen, R., & Domingue-Mena, P. (2024). Prévalence de la maladie rénale chronique stades 3–5 en Nouvelle-Calédonie. *Néphrologie & Thérapeutique, 20*(3), 1–9. https://doi.org/10.1684/ndt.2024.77

Bell, L., van Gemert, C., Merilles, O. E., Cash, H. L., Stoové, M., & Hellard, M. (2022). The impact of COVID-19 on public health systems in the Pacific Island countries and territories. *The Lancet Regional Health—Western Pacific, 25*, 100498. https://doi.org/10.1016/j.lanwpc.2022.100498

Blanc, J., Louis, E. F., Joseph, J., Castor, C., & Jean-Louis, G. (2020). What the world could learn from the Haitian resilience while managing COVID-19. *Psychological Trauma: Theory, Research, Practice, and Policy, 12*(6), 569–571. https://doi.org/10.1037/tra0000903

Bovet, P., Viswanathan, B., Shamlaye, C., Romain, S., & Gedeon, J. (2010). Addressing non-communicable diseases in the Seychelles: towards a comprehensive plan of action. *Global Health Promotion, 17*(2_suppl), 37–40. https://doi.org/10.1177/1757975910363930

Caribbean Public Health Agency-CARPHA. (2017). Promoting healthy diets, food security, and sustainable development in the Caribbean through joint policy action caricom technical brief. *Report*, (High Level Meeting to Develop a Roadmap on Multi-Sectoral Action in Countries to Prevent Childhood Obesity through Improved Food and Nutrition Security Barbados, 9–10 February 2017), 1.

Chand, S. S., Chand, A. A., & Chand, K. K. (2021). The use of careFiji app for contact tracing during the COVID-19 pandemic: Digital gap and challenges faced in Fiji. *International Journal of Surgery, 92*, 106023. https://doi.org/10.1016/j.ijsu.2021.106023

Dookeeram, D., Hariharan, S., Hambleton, I., Ali, K., Teelucksingh, S., Ramsewak, S., … Maharaj, S. B. (2023). Experiences with SARS-CoV-2 (Covid-19) in Trinidad and Tobago, a small island developing state: Realities and opportunities. *The Lancet Regional Health—Americas, 26*, 100589. https://doi.org/10.1016/j.lana.2023.100589

Foster, N., Thow, A. M., Unwin, N., Alvarado, M., & Samuels, T. A. (2018). Regulatory measures to fight obesity in Small Island Developing States of the Caribbean and Pacific, 2015–2017. *Revista Panamericana de Salud Pública, 42*, 1–7. https://doi.org/10.26633/RPSP.2018.191

Fujita, Y., & Sabogal, A. (2021). *Perspective of localization of aid during COVID-19 reflecting on the tensions between the top-down and bottom-up responses to the health emergency in Haiti.* Retrieved from www.iss.nl/en/library

Haidar, F., Issa, N., Gourinat, A. C., Savalle, M., Elodie, C., & Wyburn, K. (2022). The "New Caledonia COVID-19 Paradox": Dramatic indirect impact of the pandemic on organ donation and transplantation in a non-prevalence country. *Néphrologie & Thérapeutique, 18*(5), 472. https://doi.org/10.1016/j.nephro.2022.07.034

Hale, T., Phillips, T., Petherick, A., Kira, B., Angrist, N., Aymar, K., & Webster, S. (2020). *Lockdown rollback checklist: Do countries meet WHO recommendations for rolling back lockdown?*

Hennis, A. J. M., Fraser, H. S., Jonnalagadda, R., Fuller, J., & Chaturvedi, N. (2004). Explanations for the high risk of diabetes-related amputation in a Caribbean population of Black African descent and potential for prevention. *Diabetes Care, 27*(11), 2636–2641. https://doi.org/10.2337/diacare.27.11.2636

Hunte, S.-A., Pierre, K., St. Rose, R., & Simeon, D. T. (2020). Health systems' resilience: COVID-19 response in Trinidad and Tobago. *The American Journal of Tropical Medicine and Hygiene, 103*(2), 590–592. https://doi.org/10.4269/ajtmh.20-0561

International Diabetes Federation (IDF). (2025). *IDF Diabetes Atlas 2025*. Retrieved from https://diabetesatlas.org/resources/idf-diabetes-atlas-2025/

Kerbaj, J., Cazorla, C., De Greslan, T., Serie, M., Gourinat, A.-C., & Marot, B. (2020). COVID-19: The New Caledonia experience. *Clinical Infectious Diseases, 71*(16), 2279–2281. https://doi.org/10.1093/cid/ciaa600

Kianersi, S., Jules, R., Zhang, Y., Luetke, M., & Rosenberg, M. (2021). Associations between hurricane exposure, food insecurity, and microfinance; A cross-sectional study in Haiti. *World Development, 145*, 105530. https://doi.org/10.1016/J.WORLDDEV.2021.105530

Kousi, T., Vivacqua, D., Dalal, J., James, A., Câmara, D. C. P., Botero Mesa, S., … Hofer, C. B. (2022). COVID-19 pandemic in Africa's island nations during the first 9 months: A descriptive study of variation in patterns of infection, severe disease, and response measures. *BMJ Global Health, 7*(3), e006821. https://doi.org/10.1136/bmjgh-2021-006821

Kyu, H. H., Abate, D., Abate, K. H., Abay, S. M., Abbafati, C., Abbasi, N., … Murray, C. J. L. (2018). Global, regional, and national disability-adjusted life-years (DALYs) for 359 diseases and injuries and healthy life expectancy (HALE) for 195 countries and territories, 1990–2017: A systematic analysis for the Global Burden of Disease Study 2017. *The Lancet, 392*(10159), 1859–1922. https://doi.org/10.1016/S0140-6736(18)32335-3

Madewell, Z. J., Yang, Y., Longini, I. M., Halloran, M. E., & Dean, N. E. (2021). Factors associated with household transmission of SARS-CoV-2. *JAMA Network Open, 4*(8), e2122240. https://doi.org/10.1001/jamanetworkopen.2021.22240

Maharaj, S. B., Ramsewak, S. S., Dookeram, D., & Franco, D. (2021). Did vaccine inequity lead to the second wave of COVID-19 infections in Trinidad and Tobago? *BMJ Global Health, 6*(8), e007096. https://doi.org/10.1136/bmjgh-2021-007096

Mayr, V., Nußbaumer-Streit, B., & Gartlehner, G. (2020). Quarantine alone or in combination with other public health measures to control COVID-19: A rapid review (review). *Gesundheitswesen (Bundesverband der Arzte des Offentlichen Gesundheitsdienstes (Germany)), 82*(6), 501–506. https://doi.org/10.1055/a-1164-6611

Mcclure, H. (2021). *Surviving the pandemic: COVID-19 in the Pacific and health security*. Retrieved from https://pacificsecurity.net/resource/development-bulletin-82/

Moury, P.-H., Gourinat, A.-C., Riou, O., Laumond, S., Dupont-Rouzeyrol, M., Cazorla, C., & Mangeas, M. (2021). Successful COVID-19 elimination after an alpha variant outbreak in a "safe travel zone." *Travel Medicine and Infectious Disease, 44*, 102202. https://doi.org/10.1016/j.tmaid.2021.102202

Murphy, M. M., Jeyaseelan, S. M., Howitt, C., Greaves, N., Harewood, H., Quimby, K. R., … Hambleton, I. R. (2020). COVID-19 containment in the Caribbean: The experience of small island developing states. *Research in Globalization, 2*, 100019. https://doi.org/10.1016/j.resglo.2020.100019

Musango, L., Veerapa-Mangroo, L., Joomaye, Z., Ghurbhurrun, A., Vythelingam, V., & Paul, E. (2021). Key success factors of Mauritius in the fight against COVID-19. *BMJ Global Health, 6*(3), e005372. https://doi.org/10.1136/bmjgh-2021-005372

Nair, D., Thekkur, P., Fernando, M., Kumar, A. M. V., Satyanarayana, S., Chandraratne, N., … Harries, A. D. (2023). Outcomes and challenges in noncommunicable disease care provision in health facilities supported by primary health care system strengthening project in Sri Lanka: A mixed-methods study. *Healthcare, 11*(2), 202. https://doi.org/10.3390/healthcare11020202

Ochida, N., Dupont-Rouzeyrol, M., Moury, P.-H., Demaneuf, T., Gourinat, A.-C., Mabon, S., … Mangeas, M. (2023). Evaluating the strategies to control SARS-CoV-2 Delta variant spread in New Caledonia, a zero-COVID country until September 2021. *IJID Regions, 8*, 64–70. https://doi.org/10.1016/j.ijregi.2023.06.004

OECD. (2021). *COVID-19 pandemic Towards a blue recovery in small island developing states.*

Ordunez, P., Prieto-Lara, E., Pinheiro Gawryszewski, V., Hennis, A. J. M., & Cooper, R. S. (2015). Premature mortality from cardiovascular disease in the Americas—Will the goal of a decline of "25% by 2025" be met? *PLOS ONE, 10*(10), e0141685. https://doi.org/10.1371/journal.pone.0141685

Ramphul, K. (2022). The fight against COVID-19 in the small island of Mauritius. *Acta Bio-Medica: Atenei Parmensis, 92*(6), e2021452. https://doi.org/10.23750/abm.v92i6.12199

Razzaghi, H., Martin, D. N., Quesnel-Crooks, S., Hong, Y., Gregg, E., Andall-Brereton, G., … Saraiya, M. (2019). 10-year trends in noncommunicable disease mortality in the Caribbean region. *Revista Panamericana de Salud Pública*, 1–11. https://doi.org/10.26633/RPSP.2019.37

Reading, P. C., & Strugnell, R. A. (2021). COVID-19 in Fiji. *Microbiology Australia, 42*(4), 192–195. https://doi.org/10.1071/MA21053

Resiere, D., Mehdaoui, H., Dyer, H., Chabartier, C., Cabié, A., Inamo, J., … Kallel, H. (2021). Covid-19 in the Caribbean: Lessons learned from the ongoing international medical and scientific cooperation. *Globalization and Health, 17*(1), 55. https://doi.org/10.1186/s12992-021-00706-3

Rivera-Andrade, A., & Luna, M. A. (2014). Trends and heterogeneity of cardiovascular disease and risk factors across Latin American and Caribbean countries. *Progress in Cardiovascular Diseases, 57*(3), 276–285. https://doi.org/10.1016/j.pcad.2014.09.004

Sahadeo, N. S. D., Nicholls, S., Moreira, F. R. R., O'Toole, Á., Ramkissoon, V., Whittaker, C., … Carrington, C. V. F. (2023). Implementation of genomic surveillance of SARS-CoV-2 in the Caribbean: Lessons learned for sustainability in resource-limited settings. *PLOS Global Public Health, 3*(2), e0001455. https://doi.org/10.1371/journal.pgph.0001455

Schwalb, A., Armyra, E., Méndez-Aranda, M., & Ugarte-Gil, C. (2022). COVID-19 in Latin America and the Caribbean: Two years of the pandemic. *Journal of Internal Medicine, 292*(3), 409–427. https://doi.org/10.1111/joim.13499

Sharma, N., Balak, D., Prakash, S., & Maguire, J. (2022). Descriptive analysis of deaths associated with COVID-19 in Fiji, 15 April to 14 November 2021. *Western Pacific Surveillance and Response Journal, 13*(4), 64–71. https://doi.org/10.5365/wpsar.2022.13.4.964

Singh, S., & Goel, D. (n.d.). *On the countries of Indian Ocean region.*

Taylor, R., Badcock, J., King, H., Pargeter, K., Zimmet, P., Fred, T., … Wang, R. L. (1992). Dietary intake, exercise, obesity and noncommunicable disease in rural and urban populations of three Pacific Island countries. *Journal of the American College of Nutrition, 11*(3), 283–293. https://doi.org/10.1080/07315724.1992.10718229

Umakanthan, S., Bukelo, M. M., & Gajula, S. S. (2022). The commonwealth Caribbean COVID-19: Regions resilient pathway during pandemic. *Frontiers in Public Health, 10*. https://doi.org/10.3389/fpubh.2022.844333

Vos, T., Lim, S. S., Abbafati, C., Abbas, K. M., Abbasi, M., Abbasifard, M., … Murray, C. J. L. (2020). Global burden of 369 diseases and injuries in 204 countries and territories, 1990–2019: A systematic analysis for the Global Burden of Disease Study 2019. *The Lancet, 396*(10258), 1204–1222. https://doi.org/10.1016/S0140-6736(20)30925-9

WHO-Mauritius Country Office. (2020). *Best practices and experience of Mauritius' preparedness and response to COVID-19 pandemic.* Retrieved from https://www.afro.who.int/sites/default/files/2021-01/MauritiusInter-ActionReview1COVID-19 Report.pdf

WHO. (2023). *Country disease outlook, Seychelles.* Retrieved from https://www.afro.who.int/sites/default/files/2023-08/Seychelles.pdf

Wickramasinghe, D., & Fernando, V. K. (2022). Sri Lanka's fight against COVID-19: A brief overview. In *Pandemic risk, response, and resilience* (pp. 129–142). https://doi.org/10.1016/B978-0-323-99277-0.00031-0

World Health Organization. (2020). Older people, and people with pre-existing conditions (such as heart diseases, diabetes, respiratory conditions) appear to be more susceptible to becoming severely ill with the virus. Retrieved May 26, 2025, from https://www.who.int/publications-detail/clinical-management-of-severeacute-respiratory-. Acesso em: 12 Maio 2022. website: https://www.who.int/publications-detail/clinical-management-of-severe-acute-respiratory-

Yisahak, S. F., Beagley, J., Hambleton, I. R., & Narayan, K. M. V. (2014). Diabetes in North America and the Caribbean: An update. *Diabetes Research and Clinical Practice, 103*(2), 223–230. https://doi.org/10.1016/j.diabres.2013.11.009

- World Health Organization (WHO) COVID-19 Dashboard.
- United Nations Development Programme (UNDP) Island Vulnerability Reports.
- Ministry of Health – Fiji, New Zealand, Maldives, etc.
- Academic Journals on Public Health and Island Economies.

https://www.worldbank.org/en/country/caribbean/brief/the-economic-impact-of-non-communicable-diseases-in-the-caribbean

https://data.worldbank.org/indicator/SP.POP.TOTL

https://www.worldbank.org/en/region/lac/publication/noncommunicable-diseases-care-in-the-eastern-caribbean

https://caribbean.eclac.org/information-resources/website/caribbean-public-health-agency-carpha-coronavirus-disease-2019-covid

https://paho-covid19-response-who.hub.arcgis.com/

https://www.camcouncils.org/

https://doi.org/10.1787/532b0e2d-en

Chapter 8

Aboobakur, M., Latheef, A., Mohamed, A. J., Moosa, S., Pandey, R. M., Krishnan, A., & Prabhakaran, D. (2010). Surveillance for non-communicable disease risk factors in Maldives: Results from the first STEPS survey in male. *International Journal of Public Health, 55*(5), 489–496. https://doi.org/10.1007/s00038-009-0114-y

Alicea-Planas, J., Trudeau, J. M., & Vásquez Mazariegos, W. F. (2021). COVID-19 risk perceptions and social distancing practice in Latin America. *Hispanic Health Care International, 19*(4), 254–259. https://doi.org/10.1177/1540415320985141

Bardosh, K., Jean, L., Desir, L., Yoss, S., Poovey, B., Beau de Rochars, M. V., & Noland, G. S. (2023). Was lockdown worth it? Community perspectives and experiences of the Covid-19 pandemic in remote southwestern Haiti. *Social Science & Medicine, 331*, 116076. https://doi.org/10.1016/J.SOCSCIMED.2023.116076

Baroux, N., Magnat, É., Cauchy, M., Cantin, J.-F., Cohen, R., & Domingue-Mena, P. (2024). Prévalence de la maladie rénale chronique stades 3–5 en Nouvelle-Calédonie. *Néphrologie & Thérapeutique, 20*(3), 1–9. https://doi.org/10.1684/ndt.2024.77

Bell, L., van Gemert, C., Merilles, O. E., Cash, H. L., Stoové, M., & Hellard, M. (2022). The impact of COVID-19 on public health systems in the Pacific Island countries and territories. *The Lancet Regional Health—Western Pacific, 25*, 100498. https://doi.org/10.1016/j.lanwpc.2022.100498

Blanc, J., Louis, E. F., Joseph, J., Castor, C., & Jean-Louis, G. (2020). What the world could learn from the Haitian resilience while managing COVID-19. *Psychological Trauma: Theory, Research, Practice, and Policy, 12*(6), 569–571. https://doi.org/10.1037/tra0000903

Bovet, P., Viswanathan, B., Shamlaye, C., Romain, S., & Gedeon, J. (2010). Addressing non-communicable diseases in the Seychelles: Towards a comprehensive plan of action. *Global Health Promotion, 17*(2_suppl), 37–40. https://doi.org/10.1177/1757975910363930

Caribbean Public Health Agency-CARPHA. (2017). Promoting healthy diets, food security, and sustainable development in the Caribbean through joint policy action caricom technical brief. *Report*, (High Level Meeting to Develop a Roadmap on Multi-Sectoral Action in Countries to Prevent Childhood Obesity through Improved Food and Nutrition Security Barbados, 9–10 February 2017), 1.

Chand, S. S., Chand, A. A., & Chand, K. K. (2021). The use of careFiji app for contact tracing during the COVID-19 pandemic: Digital gap and challenges faced in Fiji. *International Journal of Surgery, 92*, 106023. https://doi.org/10.1016/j.ijsu.2021.106023

Dookeeram, D., Hariharan, S., Hambleton, I., Ali, K., Teelucksingh, S., Ramsewak, S., … Maharaj, S. B. (2023). Experiences with SARS-CoV-2 (Covid-19) in Trinidad and Tobago, a small island developing state: Realities and opportunities. *The Lancet Regional Health—Americas, 26*, 100589. https://doi.org/10.1016/j.lana.2023.100589

Foster, N., Thow, A. M., Unwin, N., Alvarado, M., & Samuels, T. A. (2018). Regulatory measures to fight obesity in Small Island Developing States of the Caribbean and Pacific, 2015–2017. *Revista Panamericana de Salud Pública, 42*, 1–7. https://doi.org/10.26633/RPSP.2018.191

Fujita, Y., & Sabogal, A. (2021). *Perspective of localization of aid during COVID-19 Reflecting on the tensions between the top-down and bottom-up responses to the health emergency in Haiti.* Retrieved from www.iss.nl/en/library

Haidar, F., Issa, N., Gourinat, A. C., Savalle, M., Elodie, C., & Wyburn, K. (2022). The "New Caledonia COVID-19 Paradox": Dramatic indirect impact of the pandemic on organ donation and transplantation in a non-prevalence country. *Néphrologie & Thérapeutique, 18*(5), 472. https://doi.org/10.1016/j.nephro.2022.07.034

Hale, T., Phillips, T., Petherick, A., Kira, B., Angrist, N., Aymar, K., & Webster, S. (2020). *Lockdown rollback checklist: Do countries meet WHO recommendations for rolling back lockdown?*

Hennis, A. J. M., Fraser, H. S., Jonnalagadda, R., Fuller, J., & Chaturvedi, N. (2004). Explanations for the high risk of diabetes-related amputation in a caribbean population of Black African descent and potential for prevention. *Diabetes Care, 27*(11), 2636–2641. https://doi.org/10.2337/diacare.27.11.2636

Hunte, S.-A., Pierre, K., St. Rose, R., & Simeon, D. T. (2020). Health systems' resilience: COVID-19 response in Trinidad and Tobago. *The American Journal of Tropical Medicine and Hygiene, 103*(2), 590–592. https://doi.org/10.4269/ajtmh.20-0561

International Diabetes Federation (IDF). (2025). *IDF Diabetes Atlas 2025.* Retrieved from https://diabetesatlas.org/resources/idf-diabetes-atlas-2025/

Kerbaj, J., Cazorla, C., De Greslan, T., Serie, M., Gourinat, A.-C., & Marot, B. (2020). COVID-19: The new Caledonia experience. *Clinical Infectious Diseases, 71*(16), 2279–2281. https://doi.org/10.1093/cid/ciaa600

Kianersi, S., Jules, R., Zhang, Y., Luetke, M., & Rosenberg, M. (2021). Associations between hurricane exposure, food insecurity, and microfinance; A cross-sectional study in Haiti. *World Development, 145*, 105530. https://doi.org/10.1016/J.WORLDDEV.2021.105530

Kousi, T., Vivacqua, D., Dalal, J., James, A., Câmara, D. C. P., Botero Mesa, S., … Hofer, C. B. (2022). COVID-19 pandemic in Africa's island nations during the first 9 months: A descriptive study of variation in patterns of infection, severe disease, and response measures. *BMJ Global Health, 7*(3), e006821. https://doi.org/10.1136/bmjgh-2021-006821

Kyu, H. H., Abate, D., Abate, K. H., Abay, S. M., Abbafati, C., Abbasi, N., … Murray, C. J. L. (2018). Global, regional, and national disability-adjusted life-years (DALYs) for 359 diseases and injuries and healthy life expectancy (HALE) for 195 countries and territories, 1990–2017: A systematic analysis for the Global Burden of Disease Study 2017. *The Lancet, 392*(10159), 1859–1922. https://doi.org/10.1016/S0140-6736(18)32335-3

Madewell, Z. J., Yang, Y., Longini, I. M., Halloran, M. E., & Dean, N. E. (2021). Factors associated with household transmission of SARS-CoV-2. *JAMA Network Open, 4*(8), e2122240. https://doi.org/10.1001/jamanetworkopen.2021.22240

Maharaj, S. B., Ramsewak, S. S., Dookeram, D., & Franco, D. (2021). Did vaccine inequity lead to the second wave of COVID-19 infections in Trinidad and Tobago? *BMJ Global Health, 6*(8), e007096. https://doi.org/10.1136/bmjgh-2021-007096

Mayr, V., Nußbaumer-Streit, B., & Gartlehner, G. (2020). Quarantine alone or in combination with other public health measures to control COVID-19: A rapid review (review). *Gesundheitswesen*

(*Bundesverband der Arzte des Offentlichen Gesundheitsdienstes (Germany)*), *82*(6), 501–506. https://doi.org/10.1055/a-1164-6611

Mcclure, H. (2021). *Surviving the pandemic: COVID-19 in the Pacific and health security*. Retrieved from https://pacificsecurity.net/resource/development-bulletin-82/

Moury, P.-H., Gourinat, A.-C., Riou, O., Laumond, S., Dupont-Rouzeyrol, M., Cazorla, C., & Mangeas, M. (2021). Successful COVID-19 elimination after an alpha variant outbreak in a "safe travel zone." *Travel Medicine and Infectious Disease, 44*, 102202. https://doi.org/10.1016/j.tmaid.2021.102202

Murphy, M. M., Jeyaseelan, S. M., Howitt, C., Greaves, N., Harewood, H., Quimby, K. R., … Hambleton, I. R. (2020). COVID-19 containment in the Caribbean: The experience of small island developing states. *Research in Globalization, 2*, 100019. https://doi.org/10.1016/j.resglo.2020.100019

Musango, L., Veerapa-Mangroo, L., Joomaye, Z., Ghurbhurrun, A., Vythelingam, V., & Paul, E. (2021). Key success factors of Mauritius in the fight against COVID-19. *BMJ Global Health, 6*(3), e005372. https://doi.org/10.1136/bmjgh-2021-005372

Nair, D., Thekkur, P., Fernando, M., Kumar, A. M. V., Satyanarayana, S., Chandraratne, N., … Harries, A. D. (2023). Outcomes and challenges in noncommunicable disease care provision in health facilities supported by primary health care system strengthening project in Sri Lanka: A mixed-methods study. *Healthcare, 11*(2), 202. https://doi.org/10.3390/healthcare11020202

Ochida, N., Dupont-Rouzeyrol, M., Moury, P.-H., Demaneuf, T., Gourinat, A.-C., Mabon, S., … Mangeas, M. (2023). Evaluating the strategies to control SARS-CoV-2 Delta variant spread in New Caledonia, a zero-COVID country until September 2021. *IJID Regions, 8*, 64–70. https://doi.org/10.1016/j.ijregi.2023.06.004

OECD. (2021). *COVID-19 pandemic towards a blue recovery in small island developing states*.

Ordunez, P., Prieto-Lara, E., Pinheiro Gawryszewski, V., Hennis, A. J. M., & Cooper, R. S. (2015). Premature mortality from cardiovascular disease in the Americas—Will the goal of a decline of "25% by 2025" be met? *PLOS ONE, 10*(10), e0141685. https://doi.org/10.1371/journal.pone.0141685

Ramphul, K. (2022). The fight against COVID-19 in the small island of Mauritius. *Acta Bio-Medica: Atenei Parmensis, 92*(6), e2021452. https://doi.org/10.23750/abm.v92i6.12199

Razzaghi, H., Martin, D. N., Quesnel-Crooks, S., Hong, Y., Gregg, E., Andall-Brereton, G., … Saraiya, M. (2019). 10-year trends in noncommunicable disease mortality in the Caribbean region. *Revista Panamericana de Salud Pública*, 1–11. https://doi.org/10.26633/RPSP.2019.37

Reading, P. C., & Strugnell, R. A. (2021). COVID-19 in Fiji. *Microbiology Australia, 42*(4), 192–195. https://doi.org/10.1071/MA21053

Resiere, D., Mehdaoui, H., Dyer, H., Chabartier, C., Cabié, A., Inamo, J., … Kallel, H. (2021). Covid-19 in the Caribbean: Lessons learned from the ongoing international medical and scientific cooperation. *Globalization and Health, 17*(1), 55. https://doi.org/10.1186/s12992-021-00706-3

Rivera-Andrade, A., & Luna, M. A. (2014). Trends and heterogeneity of cardiovascular disease and risk factors across Latin American and Caribbean countries. *Progress in Cardiovascular Diseases, 57*(3), 276–285. https://doi.org/10.1016/j.pcad.2014.09.004

Sahadeo, N. S. D., Nicholls, S., Moreira, F. R. R., O'Toole, Á., Ramkissoon, V., Whittaker, C., … Carrington, C. V. F. (2023). Implementation of genomic surveillance of SARS-CoV-2 in the Caribbean: Lessons learned for sustainability in resource-limited settings. *PLOS Global Public Health, 3*(2), e0001455. https://doi.org/10.1371/journal.pgph.0001455

Schwalb, A., Armyra, E., Méndez-Aranda, M., & Ugarte-Gil, C. (2022). COVID-19 in Latin America and the Caribbean: Two years of the pandemic. *Journal of Internal Medicine, 292*(3), 409–427. https://doi.org/10.1111/joim.13499

Sharma, N., Balak, D., Prakash, S., & Maguire, J. (2022). Descriptive analysis of deaths associated with COVID-19 in Fiji, 15 April to 14 November 2021. *Western Pacific Surveillance and Response Journal, 13*(4), 64–71. https://doi.org/10.5365/wpsar.2022.13.4.964

Singh, S., & Goel, D. (n.d.). *On the countries of Indian Ocean region*.

Taylor, R., Badcock, J., King, H., Pargeter, K., Zimmet, P., Fred, T., … Wang, R. L. (1992). Dietary intake, exercise, obesity and noncommunicable disease in rural and urban populations of three Pacific Island countries. *Journal of the American College of Nutrition, 11*(3), 283–293. https://doi.org/10.1080/07315724.1992.10718229

Umakanthan, S., Bukelo, M. M., & Gajula, S. S. (2022). The commonwealth Caribbean COVID-19: Regions resilient pathway during pandemic. *Frontiers in Public Health, 10.* https://doi.org/10.3389/fpubh.2022.844333

Vos, T., Lim, S. S., Abbafati, C., Abbas, K. M., Abbasi, M., Abbasifard, M., … Murray, C. J. L. (2020). Global burden of 369 diseases and injuries in 204 countries and territories, 1990–2019: A systematic analysis for the Global Burden of Disease Study 2019. *The Lancet, 396*(10258), 1204–1222. https://doi.org/10.1016/S0140-6736(20)30925-9

WHO-Mauritius Country Office. (2020). *Best practices and experience of Mauritius' preparedness and response to COVID-19 pandemic.* Retrieved from https://www.afro.who.int/sites/default/files/2021-01/MauritiusInter-ActionReview1COVID-19Report.pdf

WHO. (2023). *Country disease outlook, Seychelles.* Retrieved from https://www.afro.who.int/sites/default/files/2023-08/Seychelles.pdf

Wickramasinghe, D., & Fernando, V. K. (2022). Sri Lanka's fight against COVID-19: A brief overview. In *Pandemic risk, response, and resilience* (pp. 129–142). https://doi.org/10.1016/B978-0-323-99277-0.00031-0

World Health Organization. (2020). Older people, and people with pre-existing conditions (such as heart diseases, diabetes, respiratory conditions) appear to be more susceptible to becoming severely ill with the virus. Retrieved May 26, 2025, from https://www.who.int/publications-detail/clinical-management-of-severeacute-respiratory-. Acesso em: 12 Maio 2022. website: https://www.who.int/publications-detail/clinical-management-of-severe-acute-respiratory-

Yisahak, S. F., Beagley, J., Hambleton, I. R., & Narayan, K. M. V. (2014). Diabetes in North America and the Caribbean: An update. *Diabetes Research and Clinical Practice, 103*(2), 223–230. https://doi.org/10.1016/j.diabres.2013.11.009

- World Health Organization (WHO) COVID-19 Dashboard.
- United Nations Development Programme (UNDP) Island Vulnerability Reports.
- Ministry of Health – Fiji, New Zealand, Maldives, etc.
- Academic Journals on Public Health and Island Economies.

https://www.worldbank.org/en/country/caribbean/brief/the-economic-impact-of-non-communicable-diseases-in-the-caribbean

https://data.worldbank.org/indicator/SP.POP.TOTL

https://www.worldbank.org/en/region/lac/publication/noncommunicable-diseases-care-in-the-eastern-caribbean

https://caribbean.eclac.org/information-resources/website/caribbean-public-health-agency-carpha-coronavirus-disease-2019-covid

https://paho-covid19-response-who.hub.arcgis.com/

https://www.camcouncils.org/

https://doi.org/10.1787/532b0e2d-en

Chapter 9

Albarino, C. G., Shoemaker, T., Khristova, M. L., et al. (2013). Genomic analysis of filoviruses associated with four viral hemorrhagic fever outbreaks in Uganda and the Democratic Republic of the Congo in 2012. *Virology, 442*(2), 97–100.

Baron, R. C., McCormick, J. B., & Zubeir, O. A. (1983). Ebola virus disease in southern Sudan: Hospital dissemination and intrafamilial spread. *Bulletin of the World Health Organization, 61*(6), 997–1003.

Bompangue Nkoko, D., Giraudoux, P., Plisnier, P. D., Tinda, A. M., Piarroux, M., & Sudre B., et al. (2011, November). Dynamics of cholera outbreaks in Great Lakes region of Africa, 1978–2008. *Emerging Infectious Diseases, 17*(11), 2026–2034.

Brown et al. (2016). *Tropical Medicine and Infectious Disease 1*(1), 8; https://doi.org/10.3390/tropicalmed1010008 (Table 2).

CDC, Africa, African union, technical facts sheet, 2024.

Centers for disease control and prevention. https://www.cdc.gov/ebola/outbreaks/index.html#cdc_listing_res2-references

Chirisa, I., Nyamadzawo, L., Bandauko, E., et al. (2015). The 2008/2009 cholera outbreak in Harare, Zimbabwe: Case of failure in urban environmental health and planning. *Reviews on Environmental Health, 30*, 117–124.

Declaration de son Excellence Monsieur le Ministre de la Santé Publique annonçant la fin de l'épidémie de FHV à virus Ebola dans les zones de santé de Mweka, Luebo et Bulape dans la Province du Kasai Occidental [PDF- 579KB]. Mardi, le 20 novembre 2007. Dr Victor Makwenge Kaput, Ministre de la Santé Publique.

Djuicy, D. D., Sadeuh-Mba, S. A., Bilounga, C. N., Yonga, M. G., Tchatchueng-Mbougua, J. B., Essima, G. D. et al. (2024). Early release—Concurrent Clade I and Clade II Monkeypox Virus Circulation, Cameroon, 1979–2022. *Emerging Infectious Diseases Journal—CDC, 30*(3). https://wwwnc.cdc.gov/eid/article/30/3/23-0861_article

Emond, R. T., Evans, B., Bowen, E. T., et al. (1977). A case of Ebola virus infection. *British Medical Journal, 2*(6086), 541–544.

Eozenou, P. (1980). Enquête rétrospective sur un cas de monkeypox en République Unie Du Cameroun. *Bull OCEAC, 2*(3), 23–26.

European Centre for Disease Prevention and Control (ECDC)—Risk assessment: Monkeypox multi-country outbreak.

Fine P. E. M., Jezek, Z., Grab, B., & Dixon, H. (1988, September). The transmission potential of monkeypox virus in human populations. *International Journal of Epidemiology, 17*(3), 643–650. https://doi.org/10.1093/ije/17.3.643

Formenty, P., Libama, F., Epelboin, A., et al. (2003). Outbreak of Ebola hemorrhagic fever in the Republic of Congo, 2003: A new strategy? *Médecine Tropicale (Marseille), 63*(3), 291–295.

Georges, A. J., Leroy, E. M., Renaud, A. A., et al. (1999). Ebola hemorrhagic fever outbreaks in Gabon, 1994–1997: Epidemiologic and health control issues. *Journal of Infectious Diseases, 179*, S65-75.

Gessain, A., Nakoune, E., & Yazdanpanah, Y. (2022). Monkeypox. *New England Journal of Medicine, 387*, 1783–1793.

Hassan, O. B., & Nellums, L. B. (2021). Cholera during COVID-19: The forgotten threat for forcibly displaced populations. *EclinicalMedicine, 32*, 100753. https://doi.org/10.1016/j.eclinm.2021.100753

Hayes, C. G., Burans, J. P., Ksiazek, T. G., et al. (1992). Outbreak of fatal illness among captive macaques in the Philippines caused by an Ebola-related filovirus. *American Journal of Tropical Medicine and Hygiene, 46*(6), 664–671.

Laurenson-Schafer, H., Sklenovská, N., Hoxha, A., Kerr, S. M., Ndumbi, P., Fitzner, J., Almiron, M., de Sousa, L. A, Briand, S., Cenciarelli, O., Colombe, S., Doherty, M., Fall, I. S., García-Calavaro, C., Haussig, J. M., Kato, M., Mahamud, A. R., Morgan, O. W., Nabeth, P., Naiene, J. D., Navegantes, W. A., Ogundiran, O., Okot, C., Pebody, R., Matsui, T., López-Gatell Ramírez, H., Smallwood, C., Tasigchana, R. F. P., Vaughan, A. M., Williams, G. S., WHO Mpox Surveillance and Analytics team†, Mala, P. O., Lewis, R. F., Pavlin, B. I., Olivier le Polain de Waroux. (2023). Description of the first global outbreak of Mpox: An analysis of global surveillance data. *Lancet Global Health, 11*, e1012–1023.

Heymann, D. (1980). Rapport initial d'une enquête Ebola-Monkeypox à Moloundou (Cameroun, février 1980). *Bull OCEAC, 7*, 58–60.

Heymann, D. L., Weisfeld, J. S., Webb, P. A., et al. (1980). Ebola hemorrhagic fever: Tandala, Zaire, 1977–1978. *Journal of Infectious Diseases., 142*(3), 372–376.

https://www.afro.who.int/health-topics/ebola-disease

Izudi, J., & Bajunirwe, F. (2024). Case fatality rate for Ebola disease, 1976–2022: A meta-analysis of global data. *Journal of Infection and Public Health, 17*(1), 25–34. https://doi.org/10.1016/j.jiph.2023.10.020

Jadhav, V., Paul, A., Trivedi, V., Bhatnagar, R., Bhalsinge, R., & Jadhav, S. V. (2025, March 7). Global epidemiology, viral evolution, and public health responses: A systematic review on Mpox (1958-2024). *Journal of Global Health, 15*, 04061. https://doi.org/10.7189/jogh.15.04061. PMID: 40048320; PMCID: PMC11893143.

Jahrling, P. B., Geisbert, T. W., Dalgard, D. W., et al. (1990). Preliminary report: Isolation of Ebola virus from monkeys imported to USA. *Lancet, 335*(8688), 502–505.

Jezek, Z., & Fenner, F. (1988). Epidemiology of human monkeypox. In J. L. Melnick (Ed.), *Human monkeypox* (pp. 81–110). S Karger AG.

Khan, A. S., Tshioko, F. K., Heymann, D. L., et al. (1999). The reemergence of Ebola Hemorrhagic fever, Democratic Republic of the Congo, 1995. *Journal of Infectious Diseases, 179*, S76–S86.

Kirsch, T. D., Moseson, H., Massaquoi, M., Nyenswah, T. G., Goodermote, R., Rodriguez-Barraquer, I., Lessler, J., Cumings, D. A. T., & Peters, D. H. (2017). Impact of interventions and the incidence of ebola virus disease in Liberia—Implications for future epidemics. *Health Policy and Planning, 32*(2), 205–214. https://doi.org/10.1093/heapol/czw113

Le Guenno, B., Formenty, P., Wyers, M., et al. (1995). Isolation and partial characterisation of a new strain of Ebola virus. *Lancet, 345*, 1271–1274.

MacNeil, A., Farnon, E. C., Morgan, O. W., et al. (2011). Filovirus outbreak detection and surveillance: Lessons from Bundibugyo. *Journal of Infectious Diseases., 204*, S761–S767.

Maganga, G. D., Kapetshi, J., Berthet, N., et al. (2014). Ebola virus disease in the Democratic Republic of Congo [PDF—1.91MB]. *New England Journal of Medicine, 371*, 2083–2091.

Makuntima, N. T., Bompangue, D., Moore, S., de Richemond, N. M., Vandevelde, T., Mwamba, D., Colwell, R., & Muyembe, J. J. (2023, December 4). Cholera resurgence potentially induced by the consequences of climate in the El Niño phenomenon: An urgent call for strengthened cholera elimination in Africa. *The Pan African Medical Journal, 4*(46), 96. https://doi.org/10.11604/pamj.2023.46.96.42258.PMID:38405090;PMCID:PMC10891368

Mandal, S., Mandal, M. D., & Pal, N. K. (2011). Cholera: A great global concern. *Asian Pacific Journal of Tropical Medicine, 4*(7), 573–580. https://doi.org/10.1016/S1995-7645(11)60149-1

Milleliri, J. M., Tévi-Benissan, C., Baize, S., et al. (2004). Les épidémies de fièvre hémorragique due au virus Ebola au Gabon (1994–2002): Aspects épidémiologiques et réflexions sur les mesures de contrôle. *Bulletin De La Societe De Pathologie Exotique, 97*(3), 199–205.

Miranda, M. E., White, M. E., Dayrit, M. M., Hayes, C. G., Ksiazek, T. G., & Burans, J. P. (1991). Seroepidemiological study of filovirus related to Ebola in the Philippines. *Lancet, 337*, 425–426.

Musa, S. S., Ezie, K. N., Scott, G. Y., et al. (2022, July 16). The challenges of addressing the cholera outbreak in Cameroon. *Public Health in Practice (Oxford), 4*, 100295. Published 2022. https://doi.org/10.1016/j.puhip.2022.100295

Nigerian CDC National Monkeypox Public Health Response Guidelines. https://ncdc.gov.ng/themes/common/docs/protocols/96_1577798337

Okware, S. I., Omaswa, F. G., Zaramba, S., et al. (2002). An outbreak of Ebola in Uganda. *Tropical Medicine and International Health, 7*(12), 1068–1075.

Olawade, D. B., Wada, O. Z., Fidelis, S. C., Oluwole, O. S., & Alisi, C. S., & Orimabuyaku, N.F., Clement David-Olawade, A. (2024, October 28). Strengthening Africa's response to Mpox (monkeypox): Insights from historical outbreaks and the present global spread. *Science in One Health, 3*, 100085. https://doi.org/10.1016/j.soh.2024.100085. PMID: 39583938; PMCID: PMC11582772.

Olu, O. O., Usman, A., Ameda, I. M., Ejiofor, N., Mantchombe, F., Chamla, D., & Nabyonga-Orem, J. (2023, November 14). The Chronic Cholera situation in Africa: Why are African countries unable to tame the well-known lion? *Health Services Insights, 16*, 11786329231211964. https://doi.org/10.1177/11786329231211964. PMID: 38028119; PMCID: PMC10647958.

Parker, S., & Buller, R. M. (2013). A review of experimental and natural infections of animals with monkeypox virus between 1958 and 2012. *Future Virology, 8*, 129–157.

Roess, A. A., Monroe, B. P., Kinzoni, E. A., Gallagher, S., Ibata, S. R., Badinga, N., Molouania, T. M., Mabola, F. S., Mombouli, J. V., Carroll, D. S., Macneil, A., Benzekri, N. A., Moses, C., Damon, I. K., & Reynolds, M. G. (2011). Assessing the effectiveness of a community intervention for Monkeypox Prevention in the Congo Basin. *PLoS Neglected Tropical Diseases, 5*(10), e1356. https://doi.org/10.1371/journal.pntd.0001356

Rollin, P. E., Williams, J., Bressler, D., et al. (1999). Isolated cases of Ebola (subtype Reston) virus among quarantined non-human primates recently imported from the Philippines to the United States. *Journal of Infectious Diseases, 179*(suppl 1), S108–S114.

Shoemaker, T., MacNeil, A., Balinandi, S., et al. (2012). Reemerging Sudan Ebola Virus disease in Uganda, 2011. *Emerging Infectious Diseases, 18*(9), 1480–1483.

Tchokoteu, P. F., Kago, I., Tetanye, E., Ndoumbe, P., Pignon, D., & Mbede J. (1991). Variola or a severe case of varicella? A case of human variola due to monkeypox virus in a child from the Cameroon. *Annales de la Société Belge de Médecine Tropicale [Internet], 71*(2), 123–128. http://www.ncbi.nlm.nih.gov/pubmed/1656900

Ugwu, C. L. J, Bragazzi, N. L., Wu, J., Kong, J. D., Asgary, A., Orbinski, J., & Woldegerima, W. A. (2025, February 3). Risk factors associated with human Mpox infection: A systematic review and meta-analysis. *BMJ Global Health, 10*(2), e016937. https://doi.org/10.1136/bmjgh-2024-016937. PMID: 39900427; PMCID: PMC11795413.

US CDC—2022 Monkeypox Outbreak Global Map | Monkeypox | Poxvirus | CDC.

von Magnus, P., Andersen, E. K., Petersen, K. B., & Birch-Andersen, A. (1959). A pox-like disease in cynomolgus monkeys. *Acta Pathologica Et Microbiologica Scandinavica, 46*, 156–176.

WHO—Director-General's statement on the report of the meeting of the IHR 2005 emergency committee regarding the multi-country monkeypox outbreak.

WHO—Laboratory testing for the monkeypox virus: Interim guidance.

WHO—Meeting of the international health regulations (2005) emergency committee regarding the multi-country monkeypox outbreak.

WHO—Monkeypox factsheet.

WHO—multi-country monkeypox outbreak in non-endemic countries.

WHO. (2022a, May 29). *Multi-country monkeypox outbreak in non-endemic countries: Update.* https://www.who.int/emergencies/disease-outbreak-news/item/2022-DON388. Accessed February 20, 2025.

WHO. (2022b, July 23). *WHO Director-General's statement at the press conference following IHR Emergency Committee regarding the multi-country outbreak of monkeypox—23 July 2022.* https://www.who.int/director-general/speeches/detail/who-director-general-sstatement-on-the-press-conference-following-IHR-emergencycommittee-regarding-the-multi--country-outbreak-of-monkeypox--23-july-2022. Accessed February 16, 2025.

World Health organization. Ebolavirus Disease: Vaccines. https://www.who.int/news-room/questions-and-answers/item/ebola-vaccines

World Health Organization. (1978a). Ebola haemorrhagic fever in Sudan, 1976. Report of a WHO/International Study Team. *Bulletin of the World Health Organization, 56*(2), 247–270.

World Health Organization. (1978b). Ebola haemorrhagic fever in Zaire, 1976. Report of an International Commission. *Bulletin of the World Health Organization, 56*(2), 271–293.

World Health Organization. (1992). Viral haemorrhagic fever in imported monkeys. *Weekly Epidemiological Record, 67*(24), 183.

World Health Organization. (1996). Ebola haemorrhagic fever—South Africa. *Weekly Epidemiological Record., 71*(47), 359.

World Health Organization. (2003). Outbreak(s) of Ebola haemorrhagic fever, Congo and Gabon, October 2001–July 2002. *Weekly Epidemiological Report, 78*(26), 223–225.

World Health Organization. (2004, January 6) Ebola haemorrhagic fever in the Republic of the Congo—Update 6.

World Health Organization. (2005). Outbreak of Ebola haemorrhagic fever in Yambio, South Sudan, April–June 2004. *Weekly Epidemiological Record, 80*(43), 370–375.
World Health Organization. (2007). Ebola virus haemorrhagic fever, Democratic Republic of the Congo—Update. *Weekly Epidemiological Record, 82*(40), 345–346.
World Health Organization. (2009a, February 17). End of the Ebola outbreak in the Democratic Republic of the Congo. *Global Alert and Response.*
World Health Organization. (2009b). Ebola Reston in pigs and humans, Philippines. *Weekly Epidemiological Record, 84*(7), 49–50.
Word Health Organization. (2014a, October 9). Ebola Virus Disease—Spain.
World Health Organization. (2014b, December 2). *WHO congratulates Spain on ending Ebola Transmission.*
World Health Organization. (2014c, December 30). *Ebola Virus Disease—United Kingdom.* Disease Outbreak News.
World Health Organization. (2015, May 15). *Ebola Virus Disease—Italy.* Disease Outbreak News.
World Health Organization. (2023a). *Call for urgent and collective action to fight Cholera.* World Health Organization.
World Health Organization. (2023b). Cholera—Global situation. Geneva.
World Health Organization. Regional Office for Africa. (2024). *Monthly Regional Cholera Bulletin: December 2024.* World Health Organization. Regional Office for Africa. https://iris.who.int/handle/10665/380302

Chapter 10

Ascuntar, M. (2020). Community first: The key to stopping the Ebola epidemic—Humanitarian Practice Network. *Humanitarian Practice Network.* Retrieved from https://odihpn.org/publication/community-first-the-key-to-stopping-the-ebola-epidemic/
Bausch, D. G., & Schwarz, L. (2014). Outbreak of Ebola Virus disease in Guinea: Where ecology meets economy. *PLOS Neglected Tropical Diseases, 8*(7), e3056. https://doi.org/10.1371/JOURNAL.PNTD.0003056
Bedson, J., Jalloh, M. F., Pedi, D., Bah, S., Owen, K., Oniba, A., … Hébert-Dufresne, L. (2020). Community engagement in outbreak response: Lessons from the 2014–2016 Ebola outbreak in Sierra Leone. *BMJ Global Health, 5*(8). https://doi.org/10.1136/BMJGH-2019-002145
Breman, J. G., Heymann, D. L., Lloyd, G., McCormick, J. B., Miatudila, M., Murphy, F. A., … Johnson, K. M. (2016). Discovery and description of Ebola Zaire Virus in 1976 and relevance to the West African epidemic during 2013–2016. *The Journal of Infectious Diseases, 214*(Suppl 3), S93. https://doi.org/10.1093/INFDIS/JIW207
Diane Djiomba Njankou, S., & Nyabadza, F. (2023). Modeling the potential influence of economic migration on Ebola virus disease transmission dynamics. *Frontiers in Applied Mathematics and Statistics, 9.* https://doi.org/10.3389/fams.2023.1024571
Duah, J. K., Dotun-Olujinmi, O., Johnson, J. A., & Greenhill, R. G. (2023). Points of entry dynamics: Understanding the cross-border threats for Ebola virus disease and COVID-19 in Ghana using a logic model approach. *Journal of Public Health in Africa, 14*(4), 7. https://doi.org/10.4081/jphia.2023.2264
Gonsalves, G., & Staley, P. (2014). Panic, paranoia, and public health—The AIDS epidemic's lessons for Ebola. *New England Journal of Medicine, 371*(25), 2348–2349. https://doi.org/10.1056/NEJMP1413425/SUPPL_FILE/NEJMP1413425_DISCLOSURES.PDF
Gonzalez, A., Nikparvar, B., Matson, M. J., Seifert, S. N., Ross, H. D., Munster, V., & Bharti, N. (2023). Human movement and transmission dynamics early in Ebola outbreaks. *MedRxiv,* 2023.12.18.23300175. https://doi.org/10.1101/2023.12.18.23300175
Houlihan, C. F., McGowan, C. R., Dicks, S., Baguelin, M., Moore, D. A. J., Mabey, D., … Glynn, J. R. (2017). Ebola exposure, illness experience, and Ebola antibody prevalence in international

responders to the West African Ebola epidemic 2014–2016: A cross-sectional study. *PLOS Medicine, 14*(5), e1002300. https://doi.org/10.1371/JOURNAL.PMED.1002300

Huber, C., Watts, A., Thomas-Bachli, A., McIntyre, E., Tuite, A., Khan, K., … Merrill, R. D. (2022). Using spatial and population mobility models to inform outbreak response approaches in the Ebola affected area, Democratic Republic of the Congo, 2018–2020. *Spatial and Spatio-Temporal Epidemiology, 44*, 100558. https://doi.org/10.1016/J.SSTE.2022.100558

Jacobsen, K. H., Aguirre, A. A., Bailey, C. L., Baranova, A. V., Crooks, A. T., Croitoru, A., … Agouris, P. (2016). Lessons from the Ebola outbreak: Action items for emerging infectious disease preparedness and response. *EcoHealth, 13*(1), 200–212. https://doi.org/10.1007/s10393-016-1100-5

Kaawa-Mafigiri, D., Kato, F., & Schmidt-Sane, M. (n.d.). *TDDA briefing key considerations for epidemic response and preparedness in Uganda tackling deadly diseases in Africa: Key considerations for epidemic response and preparedness in Uganda.*

Kabami, Z., Ario, A. R., Harris, J. R., Ninsiima, M., Ahirirwe, S. R., Ocero, J. R. A., … Nabadda, S. (2024). Ebola disease outbreak caused by the Sudan virus in Uganda, 2022: A descriptive epidemiological study. *The Lancet Global Health, 12*(10), e1684–e1692. https://doi.org/10.1016/S2214-109X(24)00260-2

Kamorudeen, R. T., Adedokun, K. A., & Olarinmoye, A. O. (2020). Ebola outbreak in West Africa, 2014–2016: Epidemic timeline, differential diagnoses, determining factors, and lessons for future response. *Journal of Infection and Public Health, 13*(7), 956–962. https://doi.org/10.1016/j.jiph.2020.03.014

Kemp, E. (2020). *Humanitarian exchange special feature responding to Ebola in the Democratic Republic of Congo 02 | Responding to Ebola in the Democratic Republic of Congo.* Retrieved from www.elrha.org/r2hc.

Kinsman, J. (2012). "A time of fear": Local, national, and international responses to a large Ebola outbreak in Uganda. *Globalization and Health, 8*(1), 1–12. https://doi.org/10.1186/1744-8603-8-15/FIG.S/2

Konyndyk, J. (2019). *Struggling with scale: Ebola's lessons for the next pandemic CGD BRIEF.* Retrieved from https://www.unicef.org/esa/sanitation-and-hygiene

McPake, B., Witter, S., Ssali, S., Wurie, H., Namakula, J., & Ssengooba, F. (2015). Ebola in the context of conflict affected states and health systems: Case studies of Northern Uganda and Sierra Leone. *Conflict and Health, 9*(1), 1–9. https://doi.org/10.1186/S13031-015-0052-7/TABLES/1

Mugamba, S., Nanyondo, J., & Millard, M. (2020). *Community engagement: The key to successful Ebola research.* Retrieved from https://odihpn.org/publication/community-engagement-the-key-to-successful-ebola-research/

Ninsiima, L. R., Mor, S. M., Romano, J. S., Namakula, L. N., Kankya, C., Kungu, J., … Nyakarahuka, L. (2024). Perceived drivers of the Ebola virus disease outbreak in Mubende and Kassanda districts, Uganda: A qualitative study. *BMJ Public Health, 2*(2), e001267. https://doi.org/10.1136/BMJPH-2024-001267

Rajapakse, N., & Dixit, D. (2020). Human and novel coronavirus infections in children: A review. *Paediatrics and International Child Health*, 1–20. https://doi.org/10.1080/20469047.2020.1781356

Richards, F. O., Klein, R. E., de León, O., Mendizábal-Cabrera, R., Morales, A. L., Cama, V., … Rizzo, N. (2016). A knowledge, attitudes and practices survey conducted three years after halting ivermectin mass treatment for onchocerciasis in Guatemala. *PLoS Neglected Tropical Diseases.* https://doi.org/10.1371/journal.pntd.0004777

Richards, P. (2020). Ebola and COVID-19 in Sierra Leone: Comparative lessons of epidemics for society. *Journal of Global History, 15*(3), 493–507. https://doi.org/10.1017/S1740022820000303

Rwagasore, E., Nsekuye, O., El-Khatib, Z., Kabeja, A., Mucunguzi, V. H., Nizeyimana, P., … Muvunyi, C. M. (2023). Lessons learned from Sudan Ebola Virus Disease (SUDV) preparedness in Rwanda: A comprehensive review and way forward. *Journal of Epidemiology and Global Health, 13*(3), 528–538. https://doi.org/10.1007/S44197-023-00133-0/FIG.S/6

Ryan, C. S., Belizaire, M. R. D., Nanyunja, M., Olu, O. O., Ahmed, Y. A., Latt, A., … Talisuna, A. O. (2022). Sustainable strategies for Ebola virus disease outbreak preparedness in Africa: A case study on lessons learnt in countries neighbouring the Democratic Republic of the Congo. *Infectious Diseases of Poverty, 11*(1). https://doi.org/10.1186/S40249-022-01040-5,

Saurabh, S., & Prateek, S. (2017). Role of contact tracing in containing the 2014 Ebola outbreak: A review. *African Health Sciences, 17*(1), 225–236. https://doi.org/10.4314/ahs.v17i1.28

Shin, Y. A., & Yeo, J. (2020). Response to Ebola virus outbreak in a refugee camp. In *Cultural competency for emergency and crisis management* (pp. 197–209). https://doi.org/10.4324/978 0367321888-14

Spengler, J. R., Estrada-Peña, A., Garrison, A. R., Schmaljohn, C., Spiropoulou, C. F., Bergeron, É., & Bente, D. A. (2016). A chronological review of experimental infection studies of the role of wild animals and livestock in the maintenance and transmission of Crimean-Congo hemorrhagic fever virus. *Antiviral Research, 135*, 31–47. https://doi.org/10.1016/j.antiviral.2016.09.013

Towner, J. S., Rollin, P. E., Bausch, D. G., Sanchez, A., Crary, S. M., Vincent, M., … Nichol, S. T. (2004). Rapid diagnosis of Ebola hemorrhagic fever by reverse transcription-PCR in an outbreak setting and assessment of patient viral load as a predictor of outcome. *Journal of Virology, 78*(8), 4330–4341. https://doi.org/10.1128/JVI.78.8.4330-4341.2004.

UNICEF. (2021). UNICEF Eastern and Southern Africa. In *Sanitation and hygiene* (p. 11). Retrieved from https://www.unicef.org/esa/reports/ebola-virus-disease

Wilkinson, A., & Leach, M. (2015). Briefing: Ebola–myths, realities, and structural violence. *African Affairs, 114*(454), 136–148. https://doi.org/10.1093/AFRAF/ADU080

MIX
Papier aus verantwortungsvollen Quellen
Paper from responsible sources
FSC® C105338

If you have any concerns about our products,
you can contact us on
ProductSafety@springernature.com

In case Publisher is established outside the EU,
the EU authorized representative is:
Springer Nature Customer Service Center GmbH
Europaplatz 3, 69115 Heidelberg, Germany

Printed by Libri Plureos GmbH
in Hamburg, Germany